The **Business** of

Bridal Beauty

Online Services

Milady Online
To access a wide variety of Milady products and services on the World Wide Web,
point your browser to:

http://www.milady.com

Delmar Online
To access a wide variety of Delmar products and services on the World Wide Web,
point your browser to:

http://www.delmar.com
or email: info@delmar.com

thomson.com
To access International Thomson Publishing's
home site for information on more than 34 publishers
and 20,000 products, point your browser to:

http://www.thomson.com
or email: findit@kiosk.thomson.com

A service of **I(T)P**®

The **Business** of
Bridal Beauty

by Gretchen Maurer

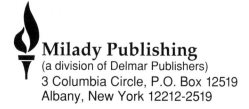

Milady Publishing
(a division of Delmar Publishers)
3 Columbia Circle, P.O. Box 12519
Albany, New York 12212-2519

NOTICE TO THE READER

Cover Design: Spiral Design Studio

Milady Staff
Publisher: Gordon Miller
Acquisitions Editor: Joseph Miranda
Project/Developmental Editor: NancyJean Downey
Production Manager: Brian Yacur
Production and Art/Design Coordinator: Suzanne Nelson

COPYRIGHT © 1998
Milady Publishing
(a division of Delmar Publishers)
an International Thomson Publishing company **I(T)P**®

Printed in the United States of America
Printed and distributed simultaneously in Canada

For more information, contact:
Milady/SalonOvations Publishing
3 Columbia Circle , Box 12519
Albany, New York 12212-2519

1 2 3 4 5 6 7 8 9 10 XXX 03 02 01 00 99 98

Library of Congress Cataloging-in-Publication Data

Maurer, Gretchen.
    The business of bridal beauty / by Gretchen Maurer.
       p. cm.
    Includes bibliographical references.
    ISBN: 1-56253-338-X
    1. Beauty shops—Management. 2. Bridal shops—Management. 3. Weddings—Planning. I. Title.
TT965.M39 1998
646.7'2'0688—dc21

97-38364
CIP

Table of Contents

Chapter *8*

Chapter *9*

PREFACE

Modern Bride magazine graciously sent me the results of their "Health and Beauty Survey 1996." The results should make the salon industry take their bridal client very seriously.

❧ 93% of brides-to-be will make a personal care change during their engagement

❧ 78% will hire a professional to do their wedding-day hair

Many will be looking to you and your salon for help. Are you ready?

The Business of Bridal Beauty addresses every area of beauty having to do with servicing brides and their wedding parties. *The Business of Bridal Beauty* covers the business end of setting up and marketing a bridal department, to the training of a bridal team. It is packed with information and ideas and tips that work.

The Business of Bridal Beauty is an informative yet enjoyable book to read. It is full of quotes as well as humorous personal experiences from notable professionals in our industry. As a member of the Association of Bridal Consultants, I have access to the top professionals in the bridal industry as well. Their insight and wisdom provide vital information to those who wish to embark on this specialized service.

Here are further results of the Health and Beauty survey conducted by *Modern Bride* magazine. Brides consider the following subjects in the bridal magazines "extremely" or "very" interesting:

❧ Wedding-day hairstyles (88%)

❧ Tips for keeping your hairstyle looking great all day (88%)

❧ Choosing the right hairstyle for your headpiece (84%)

❧ How to keep makeup fresh all day (82%)[1]

These statistics alone should send chills up the spine of every salon professional who has yet to market the bride. Hopefully, since you have this book in your hand, you are looking to learn how to get your piece of this multibillion-dollar industry.

The bride is unique. This is her most special day. To fully understand the bridal client, you must understand her personality and her image. By successfully putting together a total look for the bride on her big day you will ensure a salon client for life.

I don't have to tell you servicing brides can be stressful. As Denise Pereau of Salon Pereau in Cherry Hill, New Jersey, says, "Servicing brides is a necessary evil. Most salons die with the aging of their clients. Brides keep youth coming through the doors."

The problems that arise in servicing this client come up because there has not been any specific information developed or systems created for the salon and stylist to follow. That is until now.

The benefit of *The Business of Bridal Beauty* is that you will learn to capitalize on a client who is already coming to your salon. It will also show you how to obtain more brides and keep them coming back.

The Business of Bridal Beauty will become a reference book that you will go back to again and again. It is so packed with information that it is impossible to take it all in with one reading. Brides will love the choices of hairstyles available. The step-by-step instruction and my years of teaching experience will make your practice sessions enjoyable. This is an area of the beauty industry that can excite your entire salon and from which you and your salon can profit.

The Business of Bridal Beauty has been a pleasure to put together. Everything I have written about I have experienced. I am behind the chair just like you.

—GRETCHEN MAURER

DEDICATION

This book is dedicated to my teachers, Miss Nancy, Miss Nicky, and Miss Candy, of the Valley Academy School of Hairdressing in Ansonia, Connecticut, which has closed.

Thank you for being strong leaders in the field of cosmetology. Thank you for teaching me the basics and foundations of dressing hair. Thank you for making me do a head of pincurls, finger waves, and an updo *every day*! Thank you for being old fashioned, for the basics are never basic—they are the foundation on which we build our career.

The publisher would like to thank the following professionals who reviewed this book: Charlotte Drake, Newport Beach, California; Candi Ekstrom, Altamont Springs, Florida; Julia Hobday, Arlington, Virginia; and Jamie Rines Jones, Blairsville, Georgia.

PART 1

INTRODUCTION

WHY BRIDES?

In 1996 the oldest baby boomer turned fifty. Just who are these baby boomers we have been hearing about? They are known as the Post-War generation. They are the children of the troops who returned from World War II and the Korean War. They are the generation who lived in peace between these wars and the Vietnam War. And they got busy making babies!

The salon industry has capitalized on this age group for the last ten years with the concept and creation of day spas and related services. These women and men need youth-enhancing services and stress-relieving services and they have the money to spend. Hence, day spas, skin care products, and the like.

I have watched the advertisements in the fashion magazines in the last fifteen to twenty years go from mostly makeup ads to increasing numbers of skin care ads. Now there are as many skin care ads sharing the pages with the makeup ads. But what does all of this have to do with brides? Plenty! These Post-War babies are making a new generation of brides and grooms. Their adult children are the next wave of clients. Here comes the bride!

Many fifty-year olds have children approaching marriage. The baby boomers' "babies" stand to provide brides to the salon industry for the next twenty years!

Barbara Landon, head of *Modern Bride* magazine Research Department, told me weddings have been flat for the last three to four years. She said statistics provided by the Department of Health and Human Resources have shown a 1% rise in marriages in 1995 from 1994. We can only expect that figure to continue to rise.

> **H**ere comes the bride!

Seven in ten engaged women will spend more than usual on skin care, hair care, and makeup for their wedding day and or honeymoon, and 7% of these brides already purchase their hair care products at the salon. Once engaged, that number rises to 50%.[1] Brides are willing to spend more on hair care products and are willing to come to the salon to do it. What else are you offering the bride?

The Business of Bridal Beauty covers everything you need to know to properly service the bride and her party. From the headpiece to the toe polish. From that first phone call to the wedding day. Everything you need know at the right time is right here.

You have the information in your hands. You have the talent and desire. Now make the time!

Cynthia Zahn, who answers questions on salon services for *Modern Salon* magazine readers, had this to say to a budding colorist who wrote in: "Feed your talent with practice."[2] I wish I had said that. I am proud to quote it. If there is one thing I wish to stress is that practice makes perfect. Is anyone perfect? NO! So never stop practicing!

Take the time necessary to read, study, and practice the styles in this book. Read it from start to finish, beginning to end—and read it again! Practice, practice, and practice some more.

The wedding bells are ringing, the brides are coming. So get ready. Let *The Business of Bridal Beauty* make a perfect marriage between you, your future bridal clients, and the bridal beauty industry.

Seven in ten engaged women will spend more than usual on skin care, hair care, and makeup for their wedding day and/or honeymoon.

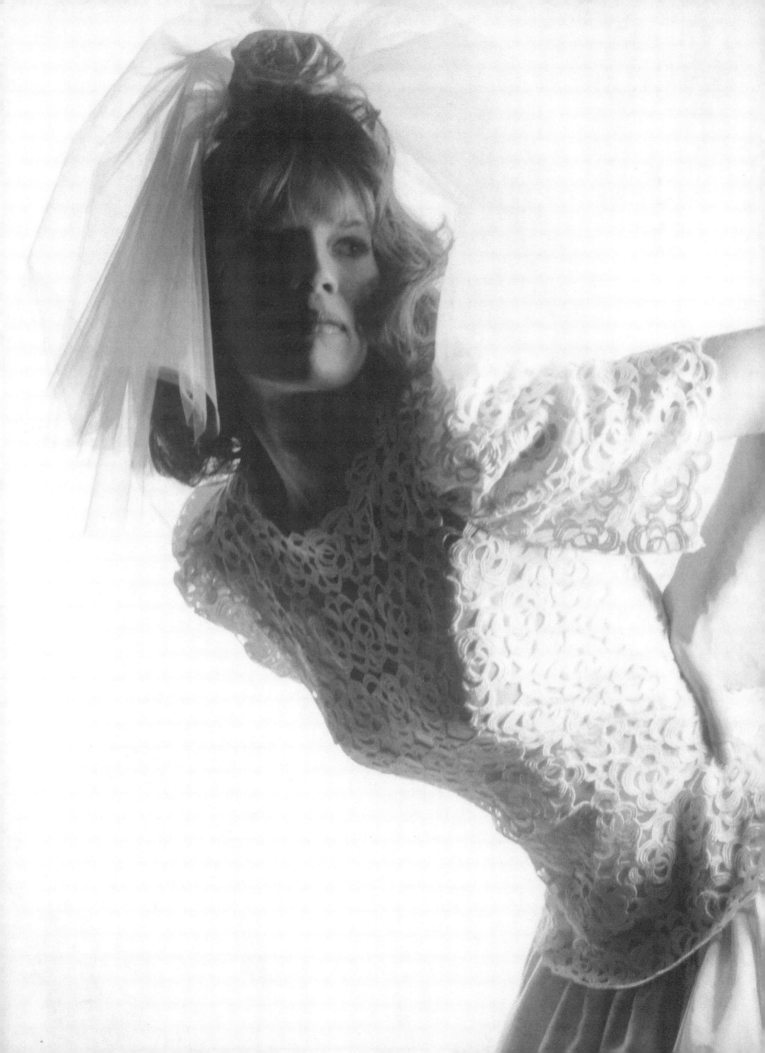

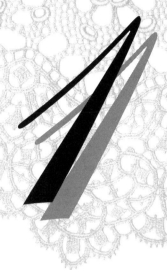

CHAPTER 1

Your Bridal Image

*W*hat is *image?*

Webster's *New World Dictionary* says (as it's fourth definition):

> *Image: 4. a: a mental picture of something; conception; idea; impression; b: the concept of a person, product, institution, etc., held by the general public, often one deliberately created by publicity, advertising, propaganda, etc.*[1]

Conception? Impression? Propaganda? Deliberately created and held by the general public? Look how much control we have. We hold the power to affect people's idea and impression of us and our salon. But some of us are too impressed with ourselves to notice we are not impressing those who count—our paying clients. Having a poor attitude or a big ego will eventually hurt your client base. On the other hand, being average and stuck in a creative void will hurt just as much if not more. I had a stylist ask me how can she get more style-oriented clients into her chair. My response was, "What is the salon's image? Are you attractive to a more progressive client? Are you wearing the new cuts and colors yourself?" Image counts. Image sells.

THE IMPORTANCE OF IMAGE

Politicians understand the importance of image. All you need do is watch a candidate prepare for a political debate and you will see how much of the image is premeditated. The candidates are taped, coached, and molded into what they think we want to see. What color tie they wear and the color of their suit is considered, plus what side of the TV screen they are standing on. It is all calculated and defined with a purpose.

Groups of voters are studied and separated. Commercials are run during different times of the day to reach certain groups. Each commercial is designed to target and emotionally move the group who the advertisers think are most likely to be watching. Some of the "groups" are the elderly, minorities, single mothers, working families, etc.

Advertisers bank on image. Artists embody their image. Fashion designers define it, and we interpret it. Yet, as hairdressers, we tend to throw this term around too loosely. We spend far more time on classes improving our technical skills, too much money on our wardrobes, and far too little time developing ourselves.

In defense I must add that there are not as many classes offered to improve our interpersonal skills and image as there are malls to shop in. One task is fun and the other is not so fun. Yet, clothes are temporary until the styles change and image enhancing is life changing—and speaking of change, presenting a positive image with strong interpersonal skills will deposit more change in the bank in the long run. Image enhancing by way of the mall depletes your account.

*A*dvertisers bank on image. Artists embody their image. Fashion designers define it, and we interpret it.

It's up to you. Are you going to make a withdrawal or a deposit on your personal image account?

THE SALON'S IMAGE

Image may mean the difference between a client walking in your door or right past it. Image is how your ad looks in the yellow pages, but is blown out of the water when the receptionist poorly handles a client over the phone. Image is how your new client is handled the first time compared to the fiftieth time. As a consumer we are always making a choice, as a person we will always have an opinion.

An image check of one's salon should be ongoing. The importance of image is just that, important! Your image and your salon's image is created and controllable by you and your employees. The salon location and economic climate of the area all have a bearing on the image of the salon, but don't fall into the trap of blaming economics. To see if you're playing the blame game, check out your local players. Is there a high-end salon in your town doing well? What are they doing that you are not? Are you that salon? Make sure you stay on top, and don't get too comfortable.

Excellent work and service should be a given. Cleanliness, pleasant phone manners, and organization need to be continually checked. Consider what Paul Hawken wrote in his book, *Growing a Business.*

We always hear that the customer comes first, the customer is always right, stay close to the customer. These credos are fine but a credo is not a business. The service provided by a company will not be guided by a sign posted on the wall. It will be guided by the views and ethics of the founders, owners, managers, and every last employee. The motto on the wall will have meaning only if it is truly the conviction of the person in charge."[2]

Image, motto, mission statement. Whatever you call it, it means nothing, if it's meaningless to those who must execute it.

Your image as perceived by a prospective bride is key to whether she will trust you for the most important beauty day of her life.

Vincent Farricielli, of V.Farricielli of New Haven, Connecticut, says this about image:

Today's bride wants only the best, and if your salon has a high image for being an expert in your field, especially a high image in the community, as well as a trained staff to address the needs of the bride, then your salon will be the only place she will want to have her hair done on her wedding day."[3]

The salon's image will set the tone for the bridal client the salon will attract. Read that again, please. Brides come in all shapes and sizes, with a variety of budgets. This book is your tool, your road map for financial success with the bridal client.

CONDUCT A SURVEY

Who are your brides? Conduct a survey!

To learn who your current bridal clients are, ask clients who have been married within the last three years if

> "Today's bride wants only the best…[so] your salon [should] be the only place she will want to have her hair done on her wedding day."

Who are
your brides?
Conduct a survey!

they are willing to be part of a survey. Explain that the questions are designed to help your salon learn more about brides and what is important to them concerning their wedding.

Here are some tips in conducting the survey:

❧ Make sure the entire staff knows about the survey before it is started.

❧ Let the staff be involved in the developing of the survey.

❧ Take the survey over a six-month period.

❧ Include the past brides as well as any brides-to-be.

❧ Post signs regarding the survey around the salon. You will be sure to have volunteers.

❧ Have the survey neatly arranged and professionally printed on one side of paper.

❧ Keep copies of the survey handy.

❧ Place the copies on a clipboard with a pen attached.

❧ Have a few or more clipboards set up as needed.

❧ Have a box or basket in which the clients can place their completed survey.

❧ Thank them for participating.

Make good use of the information you receive. After you have your results you will have a better idea and knowledge about brides as well as the complications involving weddings. You will also know which bridal shops to approach and network with. Most important, you and your staff will know how to better service your future bridal clients. If you or any of your staff, especially the male stylists, have never been married, you will all benefit greatly from the results of this survey. It will provide a window into this important day from the bride's point of view.

Questions to Ask

Here are a few questions to get you started on compiling your survey. Add any other information that you feel will be important to your salon. Set up the questions in a survey format like the one shown. Leave plenty of room for the answers. Someone with word processing knowledge can easily do this. Ask around—your clients are a rich source of help. Or you may wish to contact a photocopy shop which offers this service.

CLIENT SURVEY

Where did you purchase your wedding gown? _____

Were you happy with the service you received from the bridal gown salon?
Yes_____ No_____

Explain_____

Did you have a predetermined price you wanted to spend on your dress?
Yes_____ No_____

Did you stick to it? Yes_____ No_____

Did you pay more or less? _____
Why?_____

Did you have a budget set up for the entire wedding?
Yes_____ No_____

Did you stick to it? Yes_____ No_____

Please explain_____

_____

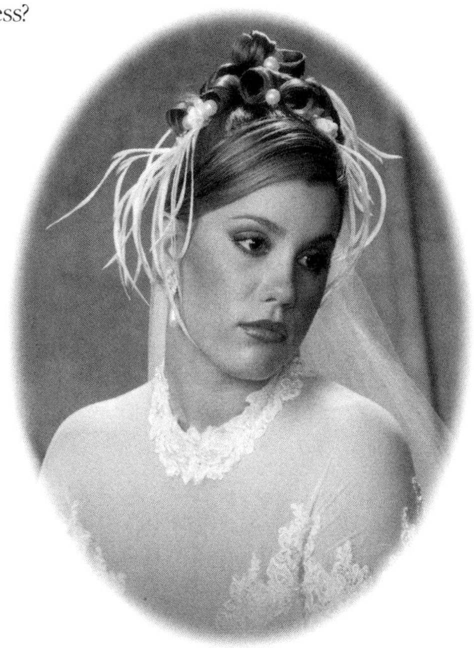

Did you figure salon services into your budget?
Yes_____ No_____

Did you have a salon do your hair on your wedding day?
Yes_____ No_____

Were you happy with the experience? Yes_____ No_____

Please explain _____

Did you try other salon services around the time of your wedding that you
normally do not receive? (such as waxing, skin care, massage, etc.)
Yes_____ No_____
Which ones?_____

What was important to you regarding other businesses that you used for your
wedding? Price?_____Service?_____ Both?_____

What did you like most about your wedding experience?

_____

_____

What did you like least?

_____

_____

What, if anything, would you do differently if you had to do it all again?

_____

_____

If you want to believe you are a team, then each player should feel of equal worth.

With the results you will be able to see if your bridal clients were motivated by price or if they were willing to pay more for excellent service. The answers to the following questions will clarify these issues:

🖎 What experience impressed them most?

🖎 Did some go over their budget?

🖎 What was it that they went over on?

🖎 Was it worth it to them?

🖎 What made it worth it?

Besides having concrete information to build from, there will be the buzz of wedding talk in the air for six months. This will provide insight for those staff members who have no idea how important a wedding day is to the bride. I see this scenario over and over when a bride chooses a single friend to be her maid of honor. I hear stories of how the maid of honor is not doing her share. The problem stems from a lack of communication on the bride's part. How can anyone know what to do if not specifically told what is expected? Never assume people know what to do. This extends from owners to managers, managers to staff, and in all relationships.

Therefore, in getting the salon prepared to take on more and more wedding parties, make sure your staff is involved and in the know from the beginning. Having everyone on the same page in its development is key. If you want to believe you are a team, then each player should feel of equal worth.

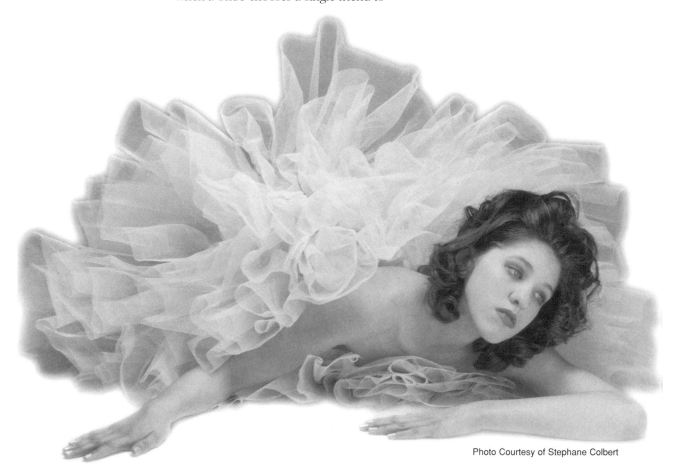

Photo Courtesy of Stephane Colbert

Image Reminders

❧ Getting the salon's image defined is first.

❧ Instilling its importance to your staff, their paycheck, and the salon's longevity is crucial.

❧ Learning what is important to the bride is your information for building a successful bridal department.

❧ Follow through.

❧ Commitment from the owner is the glue that holds it all together.

Make your salon experience worth it to the bride! You are mining an untapped resources that have been right under your nose.

I had one bride recently who came to us because we presented a well-established, organized wedding department. She had received our wedding department brochure through the mail and came in for her complimentary consultation armed with information. Shortly before the wedding day she typed up a detailed list of who was coming into the salon the morning of the wedding. The list was headed by the names of the wedding party, under which she added a computer graphic of a champagne bottle popping open. After each attendant's name was a description of how long or short her hair was. Then she listed what each person was having done, whether it was to be an updo or blow-out, etc., and each girl that was having makeup and/or a manicure. This was a bride who was impressed with our organization because *she* was organized! This is a businesswoman who respects

details and expects attention to them, as well. She chose us because we represented what she felt was important: She wanted a competent salon to take care of the beauty part of the wedding. Price is usually not an issue for the bride who is service-oriented.

Having a wedding department with a solidly defined image does not attract the do-it-yourself bride. Having and marketing a wedding department attracts busy professional women who are willing to pay for a well-executed service. A bridal department does not involve major remodeling, nor does it require a ton of money. What it does involve is a lot of planning, preparation, and a desire to be the best in your area!

I like best what Paul Hawken, author of *Growing a Business*, says about money and growth:

"*In a business, money does not create anything at all, much less ideas and initiative. Money goes where those qualities already are. Money follows, it does not lead. As a businessperson, you foster money with thought, strategy, demeanor, and deed.*" [4]

Take this thought to heart. *The Business of Bridal Beauty* will give you guidance from my experiences over the years, but I cannot make you do it. Read, take it all in, and digest the information in this book—then plan and execute it!

"You have to set goals and be absolutely unashamed about working toward them," says Ruth Roche, former artistic director for Trevor Sorbie and an artistic consultant who works as a national performing artist with Redken.

Money follows, it does not lead.

Roche suggests women set yearly objectives for themselves.[5]

This is the mindset needed to plan and develop a bridal department and its image. I truly care about your success. I want you to succeed.

I've discussed the salon's image and its importance. You are prepared to conduct your survey. Let's look further into what makes a successful bridal specialist. (Here's a bonus: what makes a successful bridal specialist also makes for a successful stylist.)

PERSONAL IMAGE

For the stylist who wants to be successful with the bride there is one very important quality you must develop: *A positive personal image.*

Everything I have to share in this book all works together for a successful launching of a bridal department in the salon, whether you are an individual who wants this for yourself or you are an owner. You need to look at each section as a piece of a puzzle—you can't leave one piece out and expect success. This section on developing a positive personal image is one of the corner pieces you must include. The importance of a positive personal image is key to success, period.

Who You Are

Do you like yourself?

Yes, no, sometimes. So many of us are so easily influenced by outside factors and popular opinion that we have come to believe what has been said, creating an untrue image of a flawed self, even if what has been said is untrue or someone else's "truth." The problem may be that those who did the judging did not like themselves very much to begin with. In order to elevate themselves, they had to lower you a few notches. For some of us this can be devastating, while others seem to persevere. Some people rise above their adversities in life while some are scraping the bottom. Many just float along with the waves of life, crashing now and again, feeling hopeless. Some strive for success. A fortunate few have experienced enough healthy encouragement along life's road to balance out the negative.

In the article "15 Ways to Get More Confident," in the September 1996 issue of *McCall's* magazine, many professional women shared their strategies. Allison Davis, a public relations firm partner in Glen Rock, New Jersey, said,

Having grown up with a mother who was very shy, I resolved to always try to look confident on the outside, even if I was a bundle of nerves on the inside. If I'm at a cocktail party at which I don't know anyone, I stand tall, give a firm handshake, and ask open-ended questions. Everyone believes I'm the most confident one in the room!"[6]

Don't measure yourself against someone else who *seems* successful. You will always fall short in your own eyes. Strive instead for your personal best. Use that person as an example not as a standard of measure, and always be yourself.

The importance of a positive personal image is key to success, period.

How you dress, speak, and present yourself is your personal image. A healthy self-image will transcend into loving your neighbor, your friends, respecting your coworkers, and satisfying your clients. The personal image you present to your clients will have more bearing on your success than just doing great hair.

Consider the following:

- 85% of why a client comes back to you is based on how they enjoyed the experience

- 15% is based on your technical skills

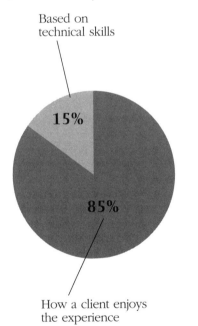

Based on technical skills

15%

85%

How a client enjoys the experience

Read that again and let it sink in!

What constitutes an enjoyable experience? Clients have told me over and over again, it is when *they* come first. They are paying us to meet their needs. The tricky part is that everyone has different needs. Your reasons for giving an enjoyable and well-executed service has to match the client's needs. You are one person. What counts is your personal image.

Everyone knows of a stylist who is busy, yet may not even be a talented hairstylist. What is the secret to their success? It's their image that is attracting clients. Remember the definition of *image?* You have the power to create an image in the mind of the client.

Some hairstylists spend more time on education and less time on fine-tuning their image. Try to strive for equal balance in both.

Do you need an image check?

Take a few minutes right now to stop and think about those clients and people in your life whom you respect. I mention clients and associates because we see them regularly and we tend to see their good and bad sides. Maybe you could even write the names of those who come to mind. (Someone famous is not a good choice because they only show their best qualities in a controlled setting. We may admire them but we never truly know them.)

Ask yourself these questions about those clients, coworkers, or friends who you thought of.

- What is it about them you admire? Write down those qualities next to their name.

- Is it their "look" or their sense of style?

- Is it their generosity? kindness?

- Is it their positive attitude?

- Is it their physical appearance?

- Is it their financial success?

- Ask them how they became successful.

You have the power to create an image in the mind of the client.

We don't have control over everything, but we do have control over our choices and actions. Begin to emulate those people whom you admire. When I first decided to come back into this field, I did so by emulating and following others whom I respected: John and MaryAnne McCormack; Eric Fisher; Ginger Boyle; Noel deCaprio; Sam Broccato; Michael Cole; the Chadwicks; Jeanne Braa; Michele DeLamar; and my closest mentor, Paul DiGrigoli. I followed these people and the careers of many others. I took seminars from them, read about them, and did what they did.

Some examples of their influences are: from Ginger Boyle and her husband I learned how to get my work published. At the time Ginger Boyle co-owned B.O.B.S. in Beverly Hills, California, with Clay Wilson. Ginger's husband is a talented photographer; they make a great team. I followed what they taught and said at an IBS seminar in New York City. My work has been published in *Coiffeur Q* magazine and *Men's Passion* magazine. Michael Cole's input helped me to be one of the first salons in town with a computer to take care of every detail. There are many role models to whom we can look.

Always be open to learning. When a client who got her hair cut by Frederic Fekkai, in New York City, sits in my chair, I study it like it is a piece of artwork! Of course I can cut her hair to please her, but how does he get almost $300 for a haircut? Being French and good looking is a start, but his professionalism and consistency are also part of his image. Don't be intimidated or defensive. You have to admire someone for their success. Now look closely with whom you associate. Ask yourself these questions:

- Are you in a social rut?

- Have you done anything new or gone anywhere interesting lately?

- Do your outside activities benefit your career?

- Do you solicit new clients when you are out socially?

- Are you a proactive person who takes action toward success and solutions?

- Or, are you reactive and feel everything is out of your control?

- Do you continuously react to problems, and always seem to be putting out fires?

Ginger Boyle has some great advice to add to this.

"*Nothing can kill your will to take risks and succeed like negative remarks. This may be easier said than done, but avoid involving yourself with friends and romantic partners who make you feel unsure of yourself and your talents. If you want to be great, you need people who believe in you, people who give you the strength to go on.*" [7]

It can be hard to be objective about yourself. Changing something about yourself or a situation is very hard and takes time. Set small realistic goals for yourself. Brook Wainwright, an at-home mom and freelance illustrator in Rumson, New Jersey, gave this advice to McCall's magazine,

---

Are you a proactive person who takes action toward success and solutions?

Things To Do

1. _____
2. _____
3. _____
4. _____
5. _____
6. _____
7. _____
8. _____
9. _____
10. _____

> *At the beginning of the week, I make a list of everything I want to accomplish in the days ahead. One day I might pay bills, return calls, bring the car in to be inspected, and send a client an estimate for a freelance job. I feel great when I've crossed off everything on my list."*[8]

Getting a handle on the day-to-day stuff will give you encouragement to face more important issues.

Write down all of your challenges and difficulties. Don't be discouraged and never give up. Make your life one long career of learning.

Is your personal image what you want it to be?

What came to mind? What did you write down? Tackle one thing at a time. It's said that it takes doing a new task every day for 21 days in a row to create a new good habit. It may be as simple as smiling more. Susan Fignar, an image consultant in Chicago, says, "A sincere smile will make you more approachable. When you're approachable you'll get more information out of people—information that can help you in your job."[9]

Smiling, courtesy, information. Better communication, a positive personal image, a kind word, loving yourself, and more success with your clients. Let's see how a positive personal image transcends into your professional image.

PROFESSIONAL IMAGE

The one thing that affects your career more than any other is your professional image. Your personal image equals your professional image.

Cynthia Hanson wrote an article for the *Chicago Tribune*, "Professional Image Might Need a Boost." She states,

> *Image counts, regardless of your title. Your image—based on your communication style, interpersonal skills, body language, and visual appearance— will play a major role in your success, whether you're in an entry-level job or on the fast track to a vice presidency."*[10]

Clients will judge you in the first six seconds upon meeting you based on your personal and professional image. That goes for the salon as well. And this is even before they can see what you do!

> **Y**our personal image equals your professional image.

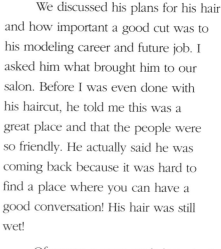

There is a lot you can do for yourself, your career, and your professional image.

The other day, I had a young gentleman in for a haircut. He was extremely handsome and all of the younger girls were eyeing him. We talked about college and how he wanted to be a middle school teacher. We talked about a car accident from which he was still sore. I asked if he was a model, which he was. He had modeled Brooks Brothers suits, Structure underwear, and Champion athletic wear.

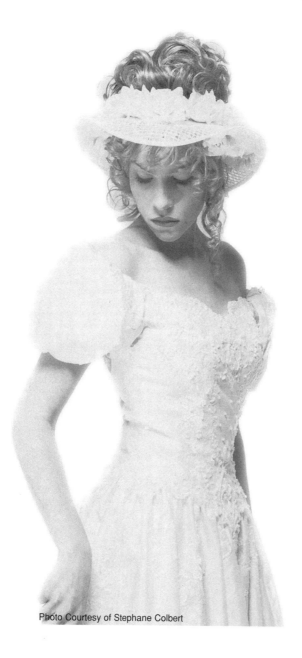

Photo Courtesy of Stephane Colbert

We discussed his plans for his hair and how important a good cut was to his modeling career and future job. I asked him what brought him to our salon. Before I was even done with his haircut, he told me this was a great place and that the people were so friendly. He actually said he was coming back because it was hard to find a place where you can have a good conversation! His hair was still wet!

Of course a great cut is important, but it was the general good feeling that he got out of his service that day that will make him become a regular salon client.

Notice I said "salon client" because they are only "yours" when they are in the chair. You hold the power with your personal and professional image to make them come back again and again. And when you can please a bride on the most important day of her life, she will be back as a regular client.

Professional Image—The Good Times and the Bad

Think back to a situation where you had a pleasant experience. It may have been a great meal, or a nice stay at a hotel. That is an easy situation in which to behave professionally. Now think back to a difficult time you had. I remember one of my first horrible experiences I had with a salesman. I ended up screaming and yelling on the phone. I was a wreck when I hung up. He had no integrity whatsoever. He did not care whether the service I bought from him even worked for me. He only cared that he got his money. (Since then I have a very hard time believing any salesman and, consequently, I do a lot of research on my own before I buy anything that is a great "deal.") This was a situation when I did not handle myself professionally.

I had another situation with a very difficult client. To make a long story short (and not dwell on the negative!), I ended up mailing back this client's check, suggesting that perhaps her services would be better met somewhere else. Polite, professional, and to the point.

We are only human and never perfect, but my point is, there is a lot you can do for yourself, your career, and your professional image. Think about the following:

- How do you handle problems with a client?

- Do you send thank you cards to your clients after holiday gift giving?

- How do you dress for an educational class on a Monday morning?

I work with a young woman who is always dressed impeccably. She always looks professional and neat. She is well groomed, in style, and makes this a part of her life. She knows the importance of her professional image. I have seen her go from a kid of twenty fresh out of school to a well-respected woman of twenty-nine. She has been an educator and platform artist for close to six years. Her appointment book is always booked solid. She owns a new car and just bought a condominium. It is her whole package that keeps the clients coming back:

quality work, professionalism, a polished image, and consistency.

At a recent hair show near Boston, I witnessed the exact opposite. I was shocked by the lack of professionalism at a student competition. Many of the participants were in casual leggings and tee shirts! Yes, it might have been a small hair show but there was no excuse. I could pick the winner just by looking at the participants. The winner did not only win because she had the best hairstyle there, but because she paid attention to details. She and her model presented themselves as winners from the beginning. She showed a great professional image. Whether you go to a hair show or take a class on a Monday morning, invest in yourself!

Gerrieann Murray, who owns Classic Occasions, a bridal consulting business in Grand Rapids, Michigan, says: "The number one thing is by dressing and looking professional. It seems to make a major difference."[11]

If you are serious about success and making money you need to be committed to caring about your professional image, whether you are an owner or a stylist.

As a former salon owner, when I had to deal on a business level, I had to present a professional image in my speech, manner, and dress.

As a stylist, I can be more trendy while still presenting a positive and professional image.

As a platform artist, I need to be genuine to the audience, on top of the newest movements in the field, yet fun and relaxed.

If you are serious about success and making money you need to be committed to caring about your professional image.

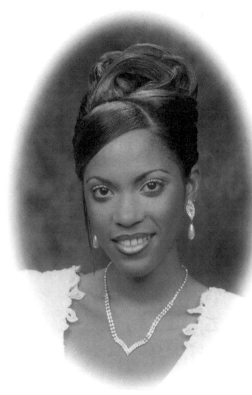

Take two classes a month if you must," advises Ruth Roche.[12]

Associate with other professionals and grow as a person. Read your trade magazines! Here is a list of the magazines I read every month:

- *Modern Salon*
- *SalonOvations Magazine*
- *American Salon*
- *Salon News*
- *Time*
- *Vogue*
- *Seventeen*
- *Town and Country*
- *Sassy*
- *Spin*
- *Elle*
- *Rolling Stone*
- *Top Model*
- *House and Garden*
- *Elle Decor*
- *Inc.*
- *Harper's Bazaar*
- *W*
- *Modern Bride*
- *Brides*

As an educator, I must be able to reach my students where they need me most. I have to be approachable, sincere, and positive. When I am in the classroom, I tone down my dress from the platform.

Which "hat" do you wear most?

Change is difficult, whether it is a new look, behavior, or job. But—challenges will grow you as a professional. List your personal goals then "grow" yourself one day at a time.

CONTINUING EDUCATION AND PERSONAL DEVELOPMENT

"The industry is changing at lightning speed and to stay competitive, you must learn every new [advancement].

I rarely watch television. But this is me and I enjoy my research. I look for emerging trends in clothes, hair, makeup, photography, and home decor. I try to keep up with the teen trends because of my prom clientele. I watch the fashion and headpieces in bridal magazines for my brides. I like to read about the ethnic artists and see where they are taking fashion. I look and see which models designers are using. I study makeup application, modeling poses, photography lighting, and marketing trends. Maybe by now you may think I'm a little eccentric, but one thing I *am* is honest and sincere about sharing. If you were to ask any of the top people that you admire in the industry, their lists and drives would be longer and stronger. Ruth Roche also has this to add: "Ask others how they did it, take classes like crazy, read, go to trade shows even if you hate crowds." [13]

Making the Most of Continuing Education

Your education *of* the industry does not always have to come *from* the industry. Also try going outside of the salon industry for seminars and education. Business seminars are great to attend. (By business seminars, I am referring to those outside the industry.) If you are a stylist, take the initiative to research this subject. Bring the information about seminars back to the salon to share with others and the owner. Even if you do not get financial support to attend, go anyway! Do it for yourself! If you don't invest in your career, who will?

If you are the salon owner, let me say you cannot force feed seminars to anyone. I have been to enough seminars and workshops to see well-spent dollars wasted on employees who sit in the back or skip out early. Offer education to them, but do not push it. Then you will see who the team players really are. I even suggest

not to pay for all of the cost, or tie it into an incentive program. It will mean more to the stylist if she or he has to work toward education. If someone is not being a team player consider whether that person is worth keeping. As they say, one bad apple can spoil the whole bunch. Denise Pereau, owner of Salon Pereau in Cherry Hill, New Jersey, recently faced the difficult task of firing her star colorist. "Firing my colorist was difficult—I liked her as a person and she was bringing in top money, but she wasn't a team player." Pereau says to put the good of the business and staff first, "no matter how unpleasant." [14]

Having a staff meeting before and after a seminar is a good way to share what each person got out of it. It is a method of holding those who attended accountable for what was offered. And owners, *you* set the example! I have seen owners skip out to the bar early for a drink, leaving the staff behind like they are dropping kids off at day care. You can never hear good information too many times.

Personal Development. Everyone is at a different place on the ladder of success. Some are happy hanging out around the bottom. You have to decide if that is what you want for your salon. Some want to climb up. Some climb slower, some jump to the top. But a calculated, steady ascent will provide sure footing, knowledge, and experience to stay on top.

A great resource for seminars on personal development outside of the salon industry is Career Track, Inc. Here

Try going outside of the salon industry for seminars and education.

are some of the seminars which I have attended from CareerTrack, Inc. over the years:

☞ "How to Deal with Difficult People with Tact and Skill"

☞ "Assertive Communication Skills for Women"

☞ "Image and Self-Projection for Women "

☞ "Self-Esteem and Peak Performance for Women"

☞ "The Manager as Coach"

(For information on seminars coming to your area call them at 1-800-334-6780. They are also offered on cassette tapes and some are on video.)[15] These seminars have not only helped in my personal development but they have helped me to become more confident and business minded as well.

There are also many great books and tapes at your local bookstore or library. Dust off your library card! Another resource for business and personal development books are office supply stores.

The next time you attend an International Beauty Show or any educational event check out the classrooms. Sit up in the front. Even as a stylist you will benefit from the owners' classes. For over two years before I opened my salon I studied the business and personal development side of the industry. I was a kitchen hairdresser looking to better myself. I sat in on all the owners' classes and I sat up front taking notes. I read business magazines, books, salon industry trade magazines, and listened

to tapes. I highlighted, ripped out pages, and kept files.

Think successful, act successful, and you will become successful!

Paul DiGrigoli, whose success as a multiple salon owner, as well as owner of Paul DiGrigoli's Advanced Training Center in Easthampton, Massachusetts, says, "I firmly believe in the immeasurable power of education to uplift the mind and spirit of the individual. Once an individual possesses the burning desire to learn and constantly improve, no doors will remain closed. Continuous education is not contained to one class, or to several, but involves committing oneself to a way of life."[16]

Now that is a piece of information all of us should take to heart. A way of life is truly personal development, and Paul does live this way. He is one person with a strong conviction and a burning desire to see his goals come to fruition. For the readers out there, you can do the same. Here are some words of wisdom from salon owner Denise Pereau: "Well, often men reach the top and we don't simply because their wills are stronger; women often let things crop up—a baby, a break-up of a marriage, [and] money problems become excuses to blow off dreams. Men experience the same problems, but they don't let dilemmas become more important than their goals."[17]

As I said before, this chapter is a corner piece of the puzzle. I hope you are encouraged to take all of this information to heart and become your best. Create the best bridal department in town. I'm still learning. New ideas and situations constantly arise.

Now you have a better understanding of the impact of the salon's bridal image, as well as the importance of your personal and professional image. Following are some reminders that sum up the best information from this chapter.

One last thing—with the invention of video we have become a generation that has access to much more information, information that is right at our fingertips. You know how when you see a movie for the second time, you see things that you missed the first time? It goes the same for reading a book. Reread *The Business of Bridal Beauty* every few months!

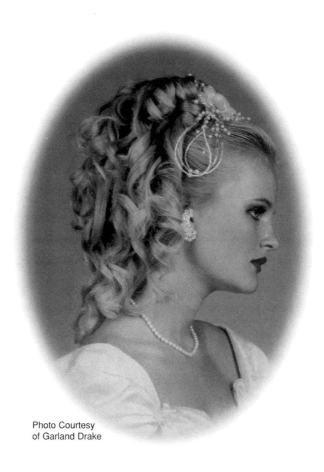

Photo Courtesy
of Garland Drake

TIPS

🖋 Define your salon's current image.

🖋 The salon image will set the tone for the bridal client the salon will attract.

🖋 Be organized and have a plan.

🖋 Interview your current and past brides.

🖋 Remember your personal image equals your professional image.

🖋 Smiling more allows for better communication.

🖋 List your personal goals.

🖋 Look outside of the salon industry for education and seminars to grow yourself professionally and personally.

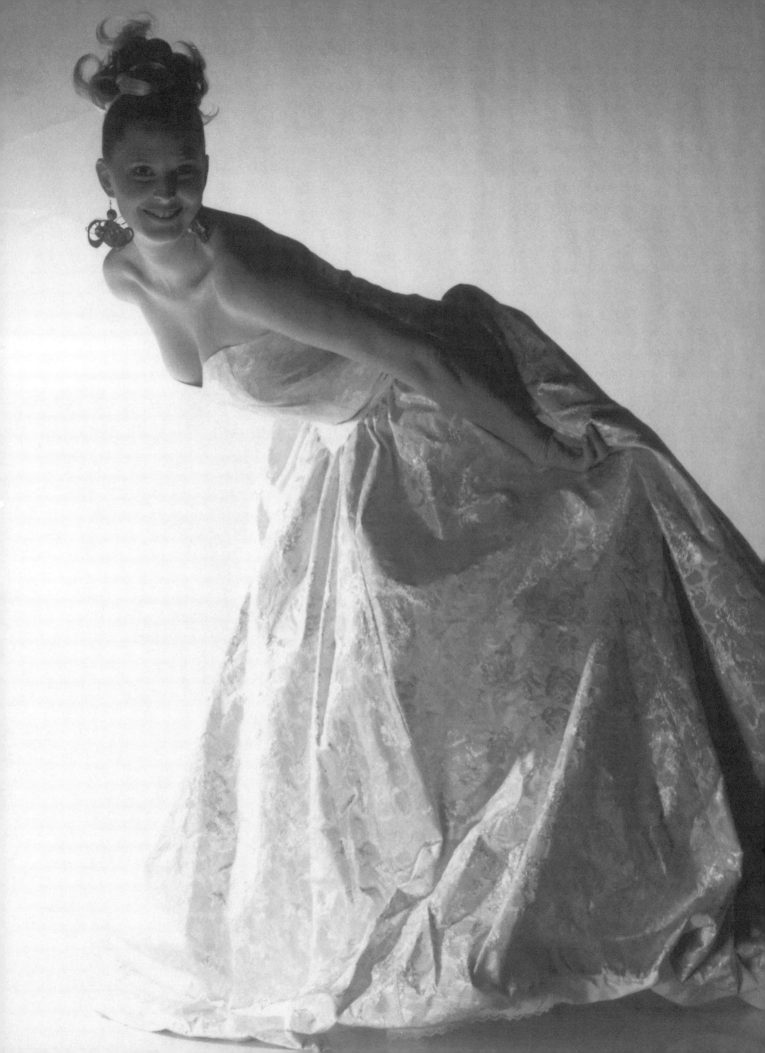

CHAPTER 2

Getting Your Salon Bridal Ready

*O*rganization coupled with effort, action, and follow-through is the path to success to anything in life. Anything worth having takes effort and commitment. Be it a well-toned body, discipline in food choices, a good marriage, or a successful career. There is a choice involved.

🖎 *The Business of Bridal Beauty* will supply you with the information you need to develop your own bridal department within the salon—*It's up to you to make the commitment.*

🖎 *The Business of Bridal Beauty* will show you the steps necessary to get your department off the ground—*It's up to you to initiate them.*

🖎 *The Business of Bridal Beauty* will provide you with the insight to keep it running—*It's up to you to keep this book in sight while you're moving ahead.*

Whether you are an owner, stylist, or booth renter you need to be Bridal Ready! The brides are coming! Many fifty-year-old adults have children approaching marriage. The baby boomers "babies" stand to provide brides for the next twenty years!

In preparing to get your salon bridal ready you must understand the bride is unique. She is different from any other client. This is her most special day. And it is a day where she gives extra attention to herself, a day when she wants the best!

🖎 93% of brides-to-be will make a personal care change during their engagement

🖎 78% will hire a professional to do their wedding day hair—many will be looking to you and your salon for help[1]

These are results of the Health and Beauty survey conducted by *Modern Bride* magazine. This survey showed that brides consider the following subjects in the bridal magazines "extremely" or "very" interesting:

🖎 Wedding day hairstyles (88%)

🖎 Tips for keeping your hairstyle looking great all day (88%)

🖎 Choosing the right hairstyle for your headpiece (84%)

🖎 How to keep makeup fresh all day (82%)[2]

These statistics should send chills up the spine of every salon professional who has yet to market the bride. The bride is more concerned about her beauty on her wedding day then she is concerned about other things. As long as she feels beautiful who cares if the ice sculpture fell over. In preparing to market the bride you have to get your salon bridal ready with the organization of a bridal team.

By having an organized bridal department with a specific bridal team of stylists ready to meet the needs of the wedding party, you will ensure a salon client for life.

*B*y having an organized bridal department you will ensure a salon client for life.

Let me share an example of what happens on a regular basis with my brides. A bride who I had done a year before has become a regular client. Besides referring new cut clients to me, she is now getting highlights, her sister is getting highlights and two of her friends are also getting highlights. (Actually, the bride and her sister are models in this book.) Getting your brides turned on to color ensures a more loyal client. Even if they are leery of you cutting their hair they may be willing to try color. Having gone to our colorist, they went from bridal clients to salon clients. The spillover into the salon is tremendous. Two or more of my clients—daily—are spillovers from the wedding department.

I have heard the argument, "Don't brides just go to their regular stylist for their wedding services?" Don't let this deter you. Begin by presenting an organized department. Create an image in the mind of the bridal consumer that you are a specialist. You will attract "new" clients into the salon. How many stylists have lost a client because her wedding day was a disaster? A bridal department also keeps your bridal clients in the salon. If a stylist who does not do bridal hair has an upcoming bride, she refers the bride to the bridal department. Just as if it were a color department or you were sending someone over to get a facial. Clients remain in the salon.

THE BRIDAL TEAM

A bridal department should consist of a separate and specific bridal team. This bridal team consists of specific individuals who are talented with long hair and the dressing of hair. They are individuals who set aside time, energy, and creative juices to be available when a wedding party is coming into the salon. Our bridal team consists of one of our top colorists. Some on our bridal team only do blow-outs. It can be anyone who is interested. As an owner you need to ask who is interested in being a part of the bridal team. The team works together with an entire party.

Team Leader

There also needs to be one person who is the team leader, who becomes responsible for the department as a whole, keeping it organized, clean, and training others. This person is responsible for supervising scheduling of the wedding parties. If you have a large receptionist staff there could also be one receptionist who will work with the bridal team leader.

The team leader position may also be a rotating responsibility, with someone being the leader for a year at a time. The team leader is not necessarily the one who always does the bride—if a bride requests someone from our team, that team member does the bride's hair—but the team leader still makes sure everything is scheduled properly. Follow the system laid out in this book and every wedding will go smoothly.

As our bridal department's team leader I am responsible for every wedding that is booked at the salon. I am in contact with the bride and call her with any questions the salon may have. This works for us at our salon.

> *Getting your brides turned on to color ensures a more loyal client.*

> The bride will be much more relaxed if you can get her out of the chaos.

Just as everyone is unique so is every salon. *The Business of Bridal Beauty* is here to help get you started. I am sharing my system, experience, and what makes our bridal department successful. You are free to follow the systems in *The Business of Bridal Beauty* or adapt and create a system to meet your salon's needs.

The Bridal Team's Responsibilities and Commitment.

There needs to be a commitment to the bridal team and all that it entails. Creativity, patience, and flexibility are essential. Some stylists are creative but not patient or flexible. Some are young and technically good, but do not yet have the interpersonal skills to consult with members of the wedding party. With these stylists the team leader should do most of the consulting. The team leader can then guide the junior stylists in how to get started with the client, but the leader must be allowed to lead. It works out best this way since the team leader has already spent some time with the bride and this enables the more-junior stylists a chance to see how to handle the consultation. This department incorporates a team atmosphere. The leader needs the team members and the team members need someone to keep the party on schedule. The emphasis must be on the team. As our salon's team leader, I always thank the team members for their support and compliment their work.

Every team member must understand that many times the bridal party will need to be seen before regular salon hours, especially if the ceremony is at 10 A.M. The bridal team may be needed at the bride's home or hotel or in the salon as early as 6:30 A.M. for a 10 A.M. wedding. Sunday weddings also demand flexible hours.

Many brides come to our salon simply because we offer flexible hours. Offering this option in all of our print material does encourage more brides to call our salon for services.

At first many brides think they want the bridal team to come to their home because it will be easier. I explain it may be hectic at home the morning of her wedding, with a lot of friends and relatives interrupting her. (I have been interrupted by bridesmaids asking the bride when they should take a shower! I had another bride called away to a long-distance phone call from Japan! One bride even fought with her brother over cooking bacon and stinking up the kitchen!) If they do not live too far away and the wedding party needs to be done during regular Saturday salon hours I encourage the bride to come to the salon.

The bride will be much more relaxed if you can get her out of the chaos. I have some brides who bring the whole party and *make* a party out of the preparation. Some brides come alone on purpose to relax quietly. Even in a busy Saturday atmosphere you can create a calm for the bride with exceptional service and the systems in this book.

Sunday weddings are also encouraged to come to the salon.

However, if the bride wants us to travel to her home or hotel we are more than willing. I have had some lovely experiences doing hair at a cozy inn and in elaborate country clubs. Be prepared to work from kitchen counters, bedrooms, cramped country club "Bridal" rooms and old inns with very few outlets. Be prepared for pets, half-dressed attendants, family members, and squabbles. (In Chapter 9, Going the Extra Mile, I will go into detail on how to pack and be prepared for these trips.)

Always be prepared to be asked to do more heads than was planned for when traveling to a home. And charge for them! Inevitably when someone who was skeptical about having her hair done sees your work, she will want her hair done as well. I had a bride on a Sunday who was having a very small and simple wedding. I was only supposed to do her hair. Her sister ended up asking me to do her hair as well. As it turned out this sister was getting married in two months. She was planning a large and elaborate wedding and wanted me to do the hair. She works in Manhattan for a plastic surgeon and sees many of the top models. Who knows where this connection could lead?

Along with traveling, bridal fashion shows and participation at bridal fairs may also be necessary commitments of the bridal team. Bridal fashion shows are discussed in Chapter 9, Going the Extra Mile. Bridal fairs are discussed in detail in chapter 4,

Networking and Advertising. Being a part of the bridal team is rewarding, fun, and exciting!

My clients know my specialty is weddings. Wedding parties are booked well enough in advance so that regular clients can work their appointments around them.

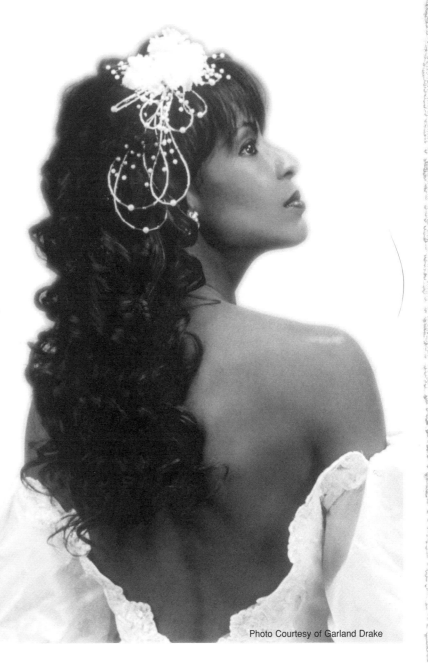

Photo Courtesy of Garland Drake

TRAINING

The bridal team of stylists must be trained. Of course I suggest you come to the source and take my updo classes! (My class schedule and any information you need can be found by calling DiGrigoli Academy at 413-527-5100.) I am also available to come to your salon, either to help you get a department up and running or to train your staff.

Let me share two true stories of what can happen when the salon is not properly trained.

I had a bride who came to me two weeks before her wedding day. She was desperate. She had spent six months working on a style with another salon close by. She was unhappy. This bride had fine hair as well as a very high forehead. The other salon was making her grow out her bangs which she was uncomfortable with. Every time she went for a trial run she ended up with a French twist and hated it! She asked me why they did not try anything else. She wanted softness and curls. I explained, in a professional manner, that they may not know any other style. She was shocked, assuming, as the general public does, that being "stylists" we should all be able to do any style they throw at us. I ended up recutting her bangs and giving her a soft, loose, curly updo. She was thrilled.

On the day of the wedding, the bridesmaids, who chose to keep their appointments with the other salon, came over to pick up the bride at our salon. They all had French twists. One bridesmaid's twist was already falling out. I quickly redid her hair at no charge.

On another occasion, I had a client in for an updo for a fancy dinner party. As we were talking she told me about her wedding day horror. She went to her salon and had a trial run of her hairstyle. It was great and she liked it. But the stylist did not record what was done. (I always take a Polaroid photo of the style, make some sketches, and file it.) On the day of her wedding the stylist who did the trial run was unavailable. This bride was told that the other stylist could put up her hair just as well. The bride had to explain the hairstyle all over again. It took five times before the stylist got it right. Now you can imagine the butterflies in everyone's stomach! The bride was now running very late, and she was hungry.

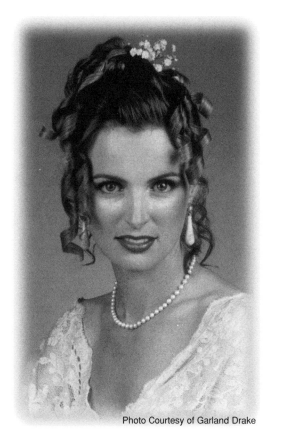

Photo Courtesy of Garland Drake

On the way home she had to stop for food. No sooner was the food down than she ran into the bathroom and threw it all up. What a horrible way to start your wedding day.

Both of these episodes, and many others like them, could have been avoided with the information and systems provided in this book. Make sure your salon is bridal ready! In today's market you can't afford to lose one client. Practice the styles in this book.

Attend as many updo classes you can get to. Many shows are now featuring more long-hair looks. There are also videos available. Check out a Milady/SalonOvations catalog for other great books and videos.

12 IDEAS TO GET STARTED

You may wish to start out with a full bridal team or just yourself. Here are some ideas to get your bridal team trained and excited:

1. Bring in an educator who specializes in styling hair.

2. Expose the salon to continuing education, and encourage participation.

3. Organize training evenings with models to try out the styles in this book.

4. Have each stylist responsible for bringing in a long-hair model to practice on.

5. Incorporate a photo shoot with these training evenings to build a portfolio.

6. Call a local camera shop to see if they know of any photographer who would like to photograph beautiful models for their portfolio.

7. Post a sign for the clients asking if any of them know of a photographer who would be willing to shoot for the cost of the film and developing. Or maybe a haircut and massage!

8. Many bridal salons have used and older headpieces they will let you borrow or barter for—or practice placing sample headpieces from a local bridal shop on hairstyles. It's a good idea to be able to get your hands on some headpieces and become comfortable with how to attach them.

9. Stress patience, understanding, and being a good listener as important qualities for anyone who wishes to be on the bridal team.

10. Use role-playing and pretend your model is a real bride. Practice the consultation. (The importance of these interpersonal skills are addressed in Chapter 6, Relating to the Bride and Her Party.)

11. Include the salon's makeup artist on the team. Maybe you don't have one now, but you will need one if you're going to be doing a lot of weddings. This is a great opportunity for someone from the salon to become trained in makeup. Or you can bring in someone on a freelance basis.

12. Collaborate on ideas for packages and brochures.

Make sure your salon is bridal ready! In today's market you can't afford to lose one client.

The team members need to be comfortable in all areas of styling hair of all lengths. The most important piece of information I can give you, which I will repeat many times in this book, is *the client must be comfortable with how she looks from the front*, even if that means you suggest she do her own bangs. During one trial run I had with a bride who had naturally curly hair. I could not do her front in a way she liked. Remember patience and flexibility? I suggested she come in the day of the wedding with her front done the way she likes it. Then I would put up the rest. She was relieved. No harm done, no professionalism lost. Understanding accepted, trust established!

All team members do not have to have equal ability. The stronger members can take the challenging clients with very long hair, while leaving the "easier" clients for those less experienced. I find naturally curly clients and hair with body to be the easiest to work on and pass those along to the other team members.

Some team members can act as assistants by doing the setting and prep work. This is very helpful to me and a great place to use someone who is in training. When I have a large party of five or more, I work on two or three at a time, each one in a different stage of updo development. An assistant, who is in training for the bridal team, can be a great help with large parties.

Here is how we work together as a team. I already know what the bride wants and do her myself. With the rest of the party, I see who has the most "needy" hair. The longest and thickest heads get set first. After I do the consulting, I may have an assistant set them. We may set up to three heads in a row. Some go to our makeup artist after they are set, some get their nails done. Then I start combing out the first head that was set while number four is being set, and so forth. Sometimes the bride is done first, sometimes later. It all depends on the hair of the individual. We also work our proms this way. This is how money can be made in this department.

BRIDAL MARKETING IN THE SALON

An attractive bridal display area lets the clients know the salon is bridal friendly as well as bridal ready! Remember the importance of presenting your professional bridal image.

The first thing that lets our clients know we are bridal friendly is a glass display case we have in the waiting room. It is topped with a beautiful gold mirror hanging above it. An artistic client decorated the mirror with a cherub, strings of pearls, antique jewelry, and a big plume. Below the mirror is a glass display case filled with lace, tulle, bridal jewelry on consignment, and custom bridal hair clips. You can also bring in accessories such as gloves, bags, or premade hair ornaments. We also have a lovely coffee table wedding book in the case and wedding "cake" sculpture. On top of the case is a Lucite frame holding my certificate stating that I belong to the Association of Bridal Consultants. Along

You have the power to create an image in the mind of the client.

with that is a holder containing our separate bridal department menus.

Always be on the lookout for new and different ways to market the bridal department and keep it interesting. I constantly read the trade magazines. I am not necessarily looking for new ideas, but when I find one I rip it out for future reference.

In 1989, in *American Salon,* I saw a very nice bridal display that caught my eye. It was in an acrylic case hung on the wall in the reception room. It was small but very target specific. Bargas Design of Cleveland, Ohio, did the display. They had taken a hair spray can and conditioner bottle and dressed them like a bride and groom. It was very simple, the groom just had a bow tie and a boutonniere flower. The bride had a small headpiece, veil, and bouquet. Then they used gel, mousse, and shampoo bottles for the wedding party. At the bottom of the case was a bouquet of lipsticks wrapped in a lace doily with ribbon colors that matched the product colors. They displayed a travel package for the honeymoon. Also in the case was a magazine picture of a wedding couple. It was framed and edged in lace with ribbon color that matched as well. There was a little sign inside that said "FOR THAT SPECIAL DAY" and another said "GIFTS FOR THE WEDDING PARTY."[3]

One other idea that I found in a trade magazine was very profitable for me when I owned my own salon. It is not for brides but the story is an example of how taking an idea you found in a trade publication and following through on it can be profitable.

The article was about hairstylist Robin Weir in the Washington, D.C. area who at that time did Nancy Reagan's hair. His salon also offered a child's first haircut package. Mr. Wier took an ordinarily special appointment and made it extra special. The baby's First Haircut package included the haircut, a lock of hair, and a certificate with a photograph. He was able to charge extra for this service because it was presented as something special.

With that inspiration, I went to a printer and had Baby's First Haircut certificates made up. I ran an advertisement in the children's section of our local newspaper. A major newspaper for our area saw the ad in the local paper. They contacted me because they thought it was a different idea and wanted to run a story on this service and my salon. I was to call them when I had a child on the appointment book for this service. They wanted a real life story, to interview the mother and take pictures. Of course I hustled and tried to find someone who I knew to get them in right away. I got a friend from church whose daughter was the perfect age. The newspaper came, took pictures, and interviewed the mother and myself. They ran the photo in full color. I got a huge spread and front cover of the Living section of the Sunday paper. It was also mentioned with a small photo on the front page! We got a lot of babies from this. As the children became repeat cut clients we eventually got the mothers and fathers to become clients. Seven

Always be on the lookout for new and different ways to market the bridal department and keep it interesting.

years later I now do their siblings and family members and friends as well. Did all this happen because I am the only one who cuts kids? No. It came about because I followed through on a great idea. Remember, you hold the power to create success for your salon. A little effort goes a long way.

Bridal marketing in the salon must be ongoing. Consistency is key. Don't you expect every time you go to your favorite restaurant that the service be perfect? Don't you expect the food to be just like you remembered it the first time? Aren't you impressed when the rest rooms are neat and clean? Aren't your hard earned dollars worth a great experience? You must constantly put yourself in your client's place. There is no rest for the weary. The point of this book is to help you put in place a system that will help the bridal department run smoothly.

9 IDEAS FOR DISPLAYS

Here are some other ideas for marketing in the salon:

1. Cut out pictures from bridal magazines and put together an album with hairstyles neatly and attractively displayed for the clients to look at during the consultation. Brides appreciate this. Many times I have neatly arranged on a display the same pictures that the bride is trying to find crumpled up in her purse. Don't neglect to put up pictures of short- and medium-length hairstyles.

2. Subscribe to a bridal magazine for the salon. If the salon won't cover the cost, pay for it yourself and keep it at your station. I believe my career is in my hands. I have personal goals for me that many times require I invest some money.

Photo Courtesy of Salon Pereau

3. Incorporate salon products such as nail polish, makeup and hair products in your bridal displays.

4. Check out your local malls and see how the big name companies display their products.

5. Have small signs printed and placed throughout the salon announcing the new bridal team department.

6. If you don't have a computer find a client who does and is willing to make the signs for you. Treat every thing as a business deal. Don't ask for favors. Always respect someone's time, talent, and experience. Offer discounts or services of equal value in return.

7. Regularly read all the trade magazines for ideas.

8. Drive to top salons in other towns and look at their windows.

9. Better yet, get inside and receive some of their services.

THE BRIDAL CORNER

The way our bridal department evolved was out of necessity. I was doing all of my wedding party clients at my regular station. Also, anyone who was helping with the party was working at their station. Our materials got spread out all over the place. Bobby pins were everywhere. Regular clients were getting choked by all the hair spray. Bridesmaids traveled in a pack. Everyone from the party wanted to watch whoever was getting their hair done. Add cameras flashing and loud

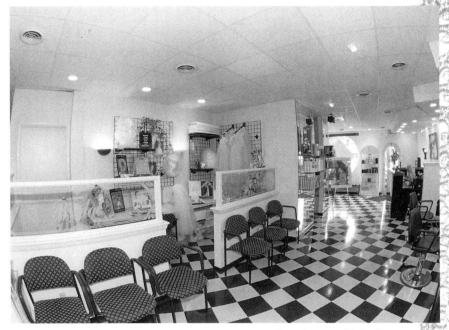

Photo Courtesy of Salon Pereau

talk to an already busy Saturday and it equaled chaos. The salon got very crowded and other stylists were cramped. One of our stylists suggested that an area of the salon away from the regular clients be created to service the wedding parties. This was a great idea.

The way our salon is set up, we had an area devoted to nails, makeup, and skin care. It was quiet and away from the regular hum of the main salon floor. In this area we added a long counter along one wall. A mirror was put up making the space look even larger. It is basically a wide hall area of dead space where our clients entered

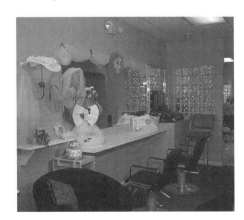

the pedicure and facial rooms. At one end are three nail stations, the other end houses our makeup area. This provided enough space for two styling stations. It also provided a congregating area for the parties. They could watch each other get their makeup and nails done. This captive audience idea has created an increase in wedding parties and proms getting extra services from the nail and makeup department. The clients feel special and they have a lot of fun.

The two styling stations are for dressing hair. We use them for weddings, proms, and anytime a client needs her hair dressed. Under the counter we store all materials needed for dressing hair. Extra hot irons, curlers, hot rollers, and Velcro rollers. All of our pins, brushes, and combs that we need are also stored here. This saves running all over the salon looking for the proper tools and accessories. Even a nonwedding client who needs her hair dressed is escorted there

because everything is in one place. They always comment how nice it is. It also shows our regular clients that we cater to weddings, adding up to more referrals.

An empty corner is also a great place to set up a simple working bridal area. Depending on space and budget a bridal area need not be large nor elaborate. Its purpose is to show that weddings are special at your salon—and your special area is set up to prove it.

Keep the accessories in that area white, cream, gold, and silver. You can add a complementary color as the seasons change. Green or yellow in the spring time, purple and red in the winter, blue in the summer, orange and yellow in the fall. A great way to get some decorating ideas is to shop local bridal salons. Also many specialty gift shops have a bridal area set up. I always keep my eyes open for new and unique ideas. My favorite idea I "borrowed" was from a bridal display at a lovely silk flower shop in Vermont.

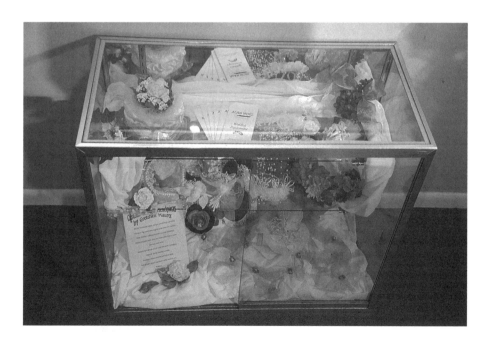

They had a wedding "cake" made out of Styrofoam covered with tiny rose buds. I made a similar cake out of ropes of white Chinese silk with green leaves dipped in gold leaf glued to the top.

Having a bridal room is for the salon that can afford the extra space or one that can set aside maybe a skin care or massage room for changing. Visit high-end bridal shops and lovely gift shops for ideas for decorating the bridal corner or bridal room. It is important that the bridal area reflects the image of the entire salon; it will flow better. Unless of course the bridal area is totally separated from the commotion of the salon's main floor, then it can have a feeling all its own. Music should be soft and soothing, much the same as one would play in a massage room or spa.

GIFT BASKETS

- ✎ Make up pretty wedding gift baskets. Vincent Farracielli of V. Farracielli in New Haven, Connecticut, makes up a gift basket of travel shampoos, conditioners, and body wash. The products bear the salon's name and the basket is presented to the bride as a gift on her wedding day.

- ✎ You may wish to add gift certificates and market these baskets as gifts to the bridal party from the bride.

- ✎ Make up some sample baskets.

- ✎ Offer customized baskets with coordinated makeup and nail colors.

- ✎ Look in the phone book for basket wholesalers and paper companies to get your fillers and plastic shrink wrap. All you need is a business tax number.

BARTERING

Barter for anything you want. Bartering is a great way to get the services you need from someone and then give them your services as payment. My employer, is getting some cabinets redone in a new color of Formica. He, in turn, will offer salon services to the workers' family. I barter a dollar amount in services for any models I use for hair shows and for the models in this book.

Here are some other ideas for bartering:

- ✎ Barter with a florist for a weekly wedding arrangement. Offer to hand out their business cards to your clients.

- ✎ Ask if you may display your brochure in their flower shop. Many brides are interested in fresh flowers for their hair now.

- ✎ Use this as a connection point between you and the florist.

- ✎ Also remind the florist of the prom business and the connections there to your clients. Clients are an endless supply of birthdays, and wedding and anniversary occasions; a relationship with your salon should prove very beneficial for any florist.

- ✎ Barter for the services of a professional window dresser or artistic client to create a lovely display. Your clients are a rich resource for talent and networking.

> *It is important that the bridal area reflects the image of the entire salon.*

❧ Barter with someone who wants to make wedding accessories to sell. Barter for their wholesale cost and sell them at retail.

Elaine Howe of Elaine's Nail Boutique in Laredo, Missouri, bartered nail services for her nail technician's chair, her client's chair, and reupholstery of furniture as well as matching drapes and some plants.[4]

Renee Ruder of Italienne Salon at the Oaks in Bakersfield, California, bartered services for a housekeeper, art classes, a math tutor for her son, weekly massages, and even had her house painted![5]

Denise Pereau of Salon Pereau in Cherry Hill, New Jersey, has taken bartering to the next level. Without bartering she would not have grown her business of 2½ years as fast and successfully as she has. She calls herself the barter queen. In speaking with her recently she shared a great bartering story. A local newspaper approached her to advertise weekly in their beauty section. It would have cost $300 a month to run a weekly ad. Denise's budget allowed for $75 a month. Her suggestion and solution was this: Denise offered to write a 250- to 300-word weekly article for the paper. She would interview other salons and beauty-related businesses such as plastic surgeons. They in turn would purchase ad space to run alongside the article she had written about them. Denise has now become identified as an expert in beauty among the readers in her area and is in print every week! This has also afforded her many contacts with other professionals, some of whom she

has invited to run health care/beauty-related seminars in her salon.[6] There are so many ways of bringing in new clients. It just takes a little thought and follow through.

THE INDEPENDENT STYLIST

Booth Renter

Personally, I feel the most financial rewards garnered from a bridal department come from a team atmosphere. Only a team can handle large wedding parties. I am talking about parties of over six attendants. I have had quite a few parties of twelve or more. However, there are many talented professionals who prefer to work renting a chair. This niche would not have evolved if there was not a force pushing it. Many stylists went from salon to salon and gave up on the employers. Many are happy making their own choices and hours. If you are one of these individuals, and you love to dress hair, then listen up. *You, too, can attract the bride.* It just takes some thought and planning.

Market the bride alone. Do not market full bridal parties. I have had plenty of brides who let their parties fend for themselves elsewhere. These brides want a quiet time and prefer having me all to themselves. If you are an independent stylist this is the bride you want. You can be as aggressive in marketing her as you wish to be. You can market the bride just as successfully as marketing others. For the individual stylists or the booth renter who wishes to target the bride without the help of the salon here are some ideas to get you started.

- ❧ Write something about why you enjoy doing brides and how you plan to service them.

- ❧ Use wording to let the reader know you want small intimate parties.

- ❧ Mention any classes that you have attended.

- ❧ Mention that you offer free bridal consultations.

- ❧ Contact a local nail salon or skin care salon and see if you can work up a referral plan—work together on offering packages.

- ❧ List your prices.

- ❧ Have all information professionally printed on one side of a sheet of paper or have it done in calligraphy.

- ❧ Display it in a beautiful wedding-type frame on your station.

- ❧ Have copies readily available to pass out to clients.

- ❧ Make a bridal and service menu just for you.

- ❧ Let the other stylists in the salon know that you will be specializing in weddings and brides. Not everyone enjoys dressing hair and may be glad to send their brides over to you.

- ❧ Market heavily that you are willing to make house calls. There is a lot more money in doing wedding hair this way.

- ❧ Market Sunday weddings.

- ❧ Use the same marketing and networking ideas listed in Chapter 4.

- ❧ Invite other stylists in the salon to be on call for large parties.

- ❧ If you are crafty make sure you read about custom headpieces. Offering headpieces is a beneficial way to increase revenue.

Non-Booth Renter

What should you do if the salon does have a strong team and the owner does not seem interested in reaching brides? If you wish to create a bridal department and you are not the salon owner, don't feel it is impossible. This is a business matter and it needs to be approached as such. You need to show good professional business qualities with follow through. Just as an owner needs to present a business plan to the bank, you as the stylist need to be just as professional.

Establish your own business plan:

1. Plan out how you want to approach the owner.

2. Try to have the creation of the department broken down into steps or small goals.

3. Make an appointment where you will have the owner's undivided attention.

4. Stress that this department can be created with minimal investment.

5. Utilize all the information in the first four business chapters to get started.

6. List all the benefits the salon will receive as a result of reaching the bride and her party.

7. Don't just show the owner pages from this book.

If you wish to create a bridal department and you are not the salon owner, don't feel it is impossible.

8. Put your personal touch and creative effort into this project.

9. Demonstrate, in your presentation, what you are trying to sell to the owner. Show how creative and business-savvy you are!

You need to earn the owner's trust. You must establish in their mind that you are responsible. This is done by follow through and not just talk. Your presentation is a start.

I have been running a bridal department for a little over a year at this writing. Because of how it has been specialized and presented, along with a well-trained bridal team, we are seeing a tremendous amount of weddings. One, two and three weddings are booking every weekend in the heavy wedding months, mainly March through November, with heavy times in May, June, September, and October. Some are also booking for a year ahead. Just think what you can do!

CREATING PACKAGES AND PRICING

A good idea is to create a separate bridal services menu. This again defines our salon's image as one that specializes in weddings. This menu is also a mailer and it is what we send out to prospective brides in our area. This marketing information will be covered in detail in Chapter 4, Networking and Advertising.

Most of the brides I see purchase one of our packages. Most of them purchase the most expensive package. As the statistics pointed out earlier,

brides are willing to try more services. When it comes to their big day they are willing to spend more money. They will spend it at your salon in a greater sum if you present your services as something special. Remember, I am not the salon owner but I am allowed this responsibility with creating the bridal menu because I am the department head. When it comes to creating a package you need to gather some information first. Here are some great ideas to help you get started in creating packages for your salon:

- Call at least five salons in your area, posing as a bride.

- Ask them what they have to offer you, the bride, and your party.

- Write down any package information they offer or have them mail a brochure to your home.

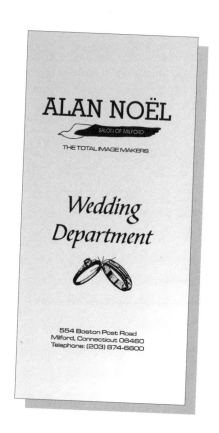

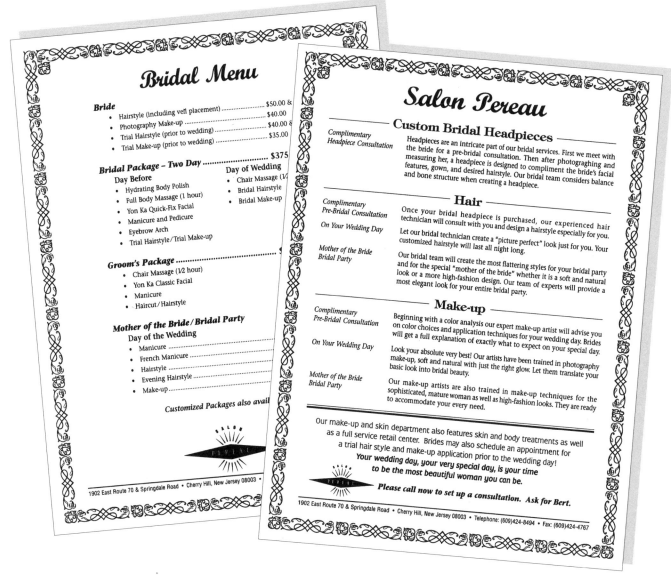

Bridal Menu

Bride
- Hairstyle (including veil placement) .... $50.00 &
- Photography Make-up $40.00
- Trial Hairstyle (prior to wedding) .... $40.00 &
- Trial Make-up (prior to wedding) $35.00

Bridal Package – Two Day $375
Day Before   **Day of Wedding**
- Hydrating Body Polish   • Chair Massage (1⁄
- Full Body Massage (1 hour)   • Bridal Hairstyle
- Yon Ka Quick-Fix Facial   • Bridal Make-up
- Manicure and Pedicure
- Eyebrow Arch
- Trial Hairstyle / Trial Make-up

Groom's Package ....
- Chair Massage (1⁄2 hour)
- Yon Ka Classic Facial
- Manicure
- Haircut / Hairstyle

Mother of the Bride / Bridal Party
Day of the Wedding
- Manicure
- French Manicure ....
- Hairstyle ....
- Evening Hairstyle ....
- Make-up ....

Customized Packages also avail

1902 East Route 70 & Springdale Road • Cherry Hill, New Jersey 08003 •

Salon Pereau

Custom Bridal Headpieces

Complimentary Headpiece Consultation

Headpieces are an intricate part of our bridal services. First we meet with the bride for a pre-bridal consultation. Then after photographing and measuring her, a headpiece is designed to compliment the bride's facial features, gown, and desired hairstyle. Our bridal team considers balance and bone structure when creating a headpiece.

Hair

Complimentary Pre-Bridal Consultation

Once your bridal headpiece is purchased, our experienced hair technician will consult with you and design a hairstyle especially for you.

On Your Wedding Day

Let our bridal technician create a "picture perfect" look just for you. Your customized hairstyle will last all night long.

Mother of the Bride Bridal Party

Our bridal team will create the most flattering styles for your bridal party and for the special "mother of the bride" whether it is a soft and natural look or a more high-fashion design. Our team of experts will provide a most elegant look for your entire bridal party.

Make-up

Complimentary Pre-Bridal Consultation

Beginning with a color analysis our expert make-up artist will advise you on color choices and application techniques for your wedding day. Brides will get a full explanation of exactly what to expect on your special day.

On Your Wedding Day

Look your absolute very best! Our artists have been trained in photography make-up, soft and natural with just the right glow. Let them translate your basic look into bridal beauty.

Mother of the Bride Bridal Party

Our make-up artists are also trained in make-up techniques for the sophisticated, mature woman as well as high-fashion looks. They are ready to accommodate your every need.

Our make-up and skin department also features skin and body treatments as well as a full service retail center. Brides may also schedule an appointment for a trial hair style and make-up application prior to the wedding day!
Your wedding day, your very special day, is your time to be the most beautiful woman you can be.

Please call now to set up a consultation. Ask for Bert.

1902 East Route 70 & Springdale Road • Cherry Hill, New Jersey 08003 • Telephone: (609)424-8494 • Fax: (609)424-4767

🖎 Use the information in it to create packages for your salon.

I did this and used the information I gathered to create the packages we currently use. I presented myself as a bride, with four attendants, who was getting married in four months. I explained that I am trying to find a salon that can handle my wedding party, and am calling for prices and to see if they have any wedding packages. A couple of times I was put on hold while someone went to check. This helped me learn a very important lesson for my own bridal department: It is very important to have all the answers for any question a client may ask. That is why a system is so important to use and follow. Remember how important and strong your image is. You are leaving an image behind in the mind of the bridal client or any client who is calling.

Two of the five salons I called had nothing prepared to say over the phone to a prospective bride. Noelle Spa for Beauty and Wellness in Stamford, Connecticut, a world-renowned leader in day spas, and

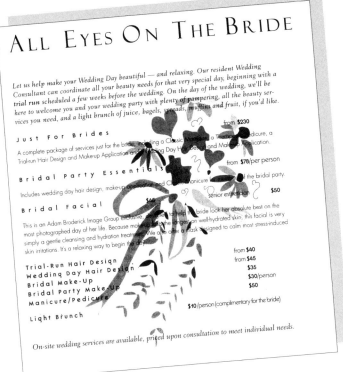

ALL EYES ON THE BRIDE

Let us help make your Wedding Day beautiful — and relaxing. Our resident Wedding Consultant can coordinate all your beauty needs for that very special day, beginning with a trial run scheduled a few weeks before the wedding. On the day of the wedding, we'll be here to welcome you and your wedding party with plenty of pampering, all the beauty services you need, and a light brunch of juice, bagels, spreads, muffins and fruit, if you'd like.

Just For Brides from $230

A complete package of services just for the bride, including a Classic Manicure, a Thermal Pedicure, a Trial-run Hair Design and Make-up Application and Wedding Day Hair Design and Make-up Application.

Bridal Party Essentials from $78/per person

Includes wedding day hair design, make-up application and Classic Manicure for the bridal party.

senior esthetician $50

Bridal Facial $40

This is an Adam Broderick Image Group exclusive, designed to help the bride look her absolute best on the most photographed day of her life. Because make-up looks the longest on well-hydrated skin, this facial is very simply a gentle cleansing and hydration treatment. We also offer a mask designed to calm most stress-induced skin irritations. It's a relaxing way to begin the day.

Trial-Run Hair Design	from $40
Wedding Day Hair Design	from $45
Bridal Make-Up	$35
Bridal Party Make-Up	$30/person
Manicure/Pedicure	$50
Light Brunch	$10/person (complimentary for the bride)

On-site wedding services are available, priced upon consultation to meet individual needs.

Courtesy of Adam Broderick Image Group

> **I**t is not so important that the packages are fancy, it is the fact that they are offered.

Adam Broderick Image Group in Ridgefield, Connecticut, who won Modern Salon's Salon of the Year, 1996, sent me their salon menus. They are an example to all of us of the very best. Another salon had packages to offer and read them over the phone. But they did not offer to send me a brochure.

Here are some more things to consider:

1. What should a package include?

2. How many packages should we offer?

3. How much of a savings should there be?

4. How should it be worded?

5. What will cost the bride extra?

If you are not comfortable with writing, look for a client who is and could help you. After I had all of my information I started to put together some packages for our salon. I typed up the information for the packages I wanted on my computer, then I transferred it to disk. The disk was then given to a friend who does desktop publishing. He laid it out to become a three-fold flyer, and also added some computer graphics.

Someone, somewhere, has a computer who can do this for you if you do not have one. There are also computer stores and large copy centers which have computers you can use for a small fee. They also have desktop services to offer. The cost is minimal compared to the return you will see.

What should you do if your salon is not full-service? Create simple packages. Stress things that you can offer like conditioning treatments and foot massages with pedicures. *It is not so important that the packages are fancy, it is the fact that they are offered.* As many salons became full-service in the eighties, day spas began emerging. As day spas grew, full-service salons felt the pinch in their spa services. Salon owners are looking at that skin care room sitting empty. Many are contemplating a decision as to whether they should add more hair and nail stations. Don't let not having spa services stop you from marketing brides.

If you have a skin care or nail salon nearby, you can work with them on a referral basis by adding their services to your packages. Victoria Wurdinger, former Eastern States editor of *American Salon* and now contributing editor for *Modern Salon* says, "Show interest in their business, not just yours, so they see that it's a mutually beneficial relationship. Exploring who they are also gives you clues as to what direction your services will take."[7]

Before you contact any business you think you want to be related with go get a service or two from them first. It is also not so important that you have an expensive three-fold brochure. It *is* important that you are organized. This shows the bride you are service oriented toward her specific needs. You may also wish to devote some space in the salon's general menu specific to brides instead of having a separate menu. Whichever you choose, it is important that it is readily available to give to the bride during the consultation.

PRICING

Pricing for services is based on what your area can afford and what you are comfortable charging. But don't get *too* comfortable. Wedding-day work is specific and specialized, so charge enough for it.

For wedding-day work, hairstyle prices should *start* at the price of a haircut. If you get $25 for a haircut, then updos should start at $25 and go up from there. If you get $15 for a wash and blow-dry, then a wedding-day blow-dry should start at $20 and go up. Maybe you will add some hot rollers to the blow-dry. The price may go up based on the detail and amount of hair. I generally charge the bride ten to fifteen dollars more than I do the bridesmaid. This is because I have designed a style to complement her dress, her features, and headpiece.

If the bride or anyone in her party are interested in hair additions, the price starts at $50 per track of wefted hair added to the client's hair (up to 16"). Price starts at $60 per track of wefted hair that is 18"–24" in length. (An average full head of weave takes approximately three to four hours, including the cut and style.)

As Charlotte Jayne, of Garland Drake International, says,

Hair addition services are considered the fourth dimension of the professional beauty business. A licensed professional cosmetologist offers services that involve: curling, coloring and cutting hair. Professionals who have advance training that qualifies them as Hair

Dear

On behalf of Salon Pereau, I would like to thank you for choosing us to provide y
with services to enhance your beauty on our wedding day. We appreciate your
confidence in us and look forward to helping you relax and to enjoy your day.

We would like to reserve an appointment time for you and/or your bridal party.
to do so, I have enclosed a contractual agreement. Please sign one and return it
and keep the other copy for yourself. This will receive your appointment on yo
wedding day.

I will call you one month prior to your wedding day to confirm all arrangeme
you should have any questioned in the meantime, I'll be glad to help you in
Please feel free to call at any time.

Again, thank you for choosing Salon Pereau.

Bert Ostroff
Bridal Coordinator

1902 East Route 70 & Springdale Ro
Cherry Hill, New Jersey 08003
Telephone 609 424-8494 Fax 609 42

WEDDING DATE _____
LOCATION _____

NAME _____
ADDRESS _____
CITY, STATE, ZIP _____
PHONE-HOME _____
_____WORK_____

CEREMONY TIME _____
PHOTO TIME _____
LOCATION: Church _____
RECEPTION _____ Synagogue _____ Other _____
PHOTOGRAPHER _____

NUMBER OF CLIENTS _____
       # FOR HAIR _____
       # FOR MAKE-UP _____

$_____ TOTAL CHARGES FOR SERVICES
$_____ 50% DEPOSIT - UPON SIGNING OF CONTRACT
$_____ BALANCE DUE UPON COMPLETION (Day of wedding)

*If there are any changes in the schedule please notify us immediately.
*We suggest you call the salon two weeks before the wedding to confirm all the arrangements.
*Payment Policy-a 50% deposit will hold the wedding date. If the services are cancelled 30 days
prior to the wedding day we will refund the deposit in full. The balance is due in full upon
completion of the services on the wedding day.

_____
Purchaser

_____
Bridal Co-ordinator

_____
Date

_____
Date

Please sign and return one copy to us along with your check payable to Salon Pereau and keep
one copy. Thank you.

1902 East Route 70 & Springdale Road
Cherry Hill, New Jersey 08003
Telephone 609 424-8494 Fax 609 424-4767

*Addition Specialists offer this fourth
dimension of services: adding hair.*

*The reasons that hair addition
services are an important part
of hairstyling include: fashion,
convenience, and hair loss issues.
Whatever your client's needs and
their fashion desires, there is usually
a solution. Hair addition services can:
add hair to increase volume, add hair
to increase length, add hair to create
a different style, add hair to replace*
*missing hair. These services can
include any one or a combination
of the above."*

In Chapter 3, The System, I go
over specifically, from the first phone
call to the wedding day, how to handle
the bride. At this point, I want to
discuss just the pricing. For pricing of
the consultation here are a couple of
ways to do it.

Vincent Farricielli, of V. Farricielli
in New Haven, Connecticut, has a

bridal department. Vincent charges for the bridal consultation. He then credits the bride the price of the consultation toward her next appointment if she chooses to use his salon for her wedding day. This is a great idea! He is known for doing the hair of every Miss Connecticut for the last thirteen years as well as being an active member of Hair America.[8]

Denise Pereau goes a step further. She has the bride sign an actual wedding-day bridal contract. She also encloses a letter with the contract which is sent to the bride's home.

At our salon we offer complimentary consultations. Everyone likes to hear the word *complimentary.* This works for us and I have had every bride book for a trial-run appointment from that initial meeting. Consultations do not include any hairdressing, just talking and helping the bride to feel comfortable. However, there may be an out-of-town bride who comes home just once before the wedding. In this case, we combine the consultation with trial-run appointment and charge for it. Also, some of our very busy corporate brides like to combine these appointments because of time constraints.

Trial-run appointments are priced per half hour. Pricing can start somewhere between the price of a blow-out and a haircut. Some brides want a few styles tried, most are happy with the first. The tricks to getting it done right the first time are discussed in length in Chapters 5 and 6. Chapter 5, The Total Bridal Look, and learning about personality types in Chapter 6,

Relating to the Bride and Her Party, will help you to "read" your bridal client. You will know what will work before you even begin.

Believe me, if you create a feeling of value by your presentation, and commitment to detail and service, clients are willing to pay any price.

Joy Gray-Miott who operates Joyous Occasions in Fort Washington, Maryland, and co-wrote a book of wedding locations in the greater Fort Washington area, says, "They [the bride] want to make a statement, even if they don't know what the statement is."[9] Gray-Miott notes today's bride finds atmosphere important and is willing to pay for it. The same goes for her hair. Do not underprice your creative work.

Working with brides can be emotional and lead some stylists to feel sorry for the bride with all her expenses. We develop a relationship with them that the florist and photographer never do. I have met many stylists at the hair shows I do for DiGrigoli Academy. They tell me they make headpieces for free because the bride is a "friend" or has been a good client for many years. When you work at the salon there are no "friend's" prices. If your friend works at K-Mart do you get stuff for free? If your friend is a receptionist at a dentist's office do you get your fillings for free? To gain respect for your talent and grow in your career you cannot afford to have "friends." Real friends will pay for services in the salon. My friends all pay for services at the salon.

Kate Kelly, who wrote *How to Set Your Fees and Get Them,* offers this

If you create a feeling of value by your presentation, and commitment to detail and service, clients are willing to pay any price.

Tailor your menu, packages, and pricing to your area and your salon's image.

tactic to get your price: "Use the words, 'In order to do this...I will charge such and such amount.' Be direct, and use a convincing tone of voice; it works."[10] I received this information from Kate when she spoke at an Association of Bridal Consultants meeting.

Think business, be professional, and charge what you deserve. They are willing to pay for a great experience.

Packages sell because they are a package and the bride has less to think about. If she sees all the services she wants in a package it makes it simpler for her. Pricing for packages is usually a little less

than if all the services were purchased separately. Add up the fee for all the services in a package and subtract 5 to 10%. Our packages are only a couple of dollars less than if purchased separately. Because they read nicely and are offered as something specific for the bride, the brides purchase them without a second thought. Packages encourage the bride to try more services, such as nails, skin care, body care, and waxing. They also can be sold as gift certificates for shower gifts.

Tailor your menu, packages, and pricing to your area and your salon's image.

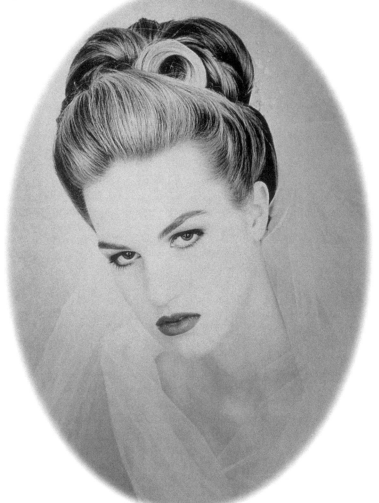

Photo Courtesy of Geri Mataya

Here are some reminder tips for this chapter.

TIPS

- Organization + Effort + Follow-Through = Success

- Establish a bridal team of committed members.

- Practice, Practice, Practice!

- Have a bridal consultation area set up at all times.

- Make creative bridal displays.

- Market the bridal department within the salon.

- Barter.

- Plan your approach to the owner about creating a bridal department.

- Have your prices and procedures in writing.

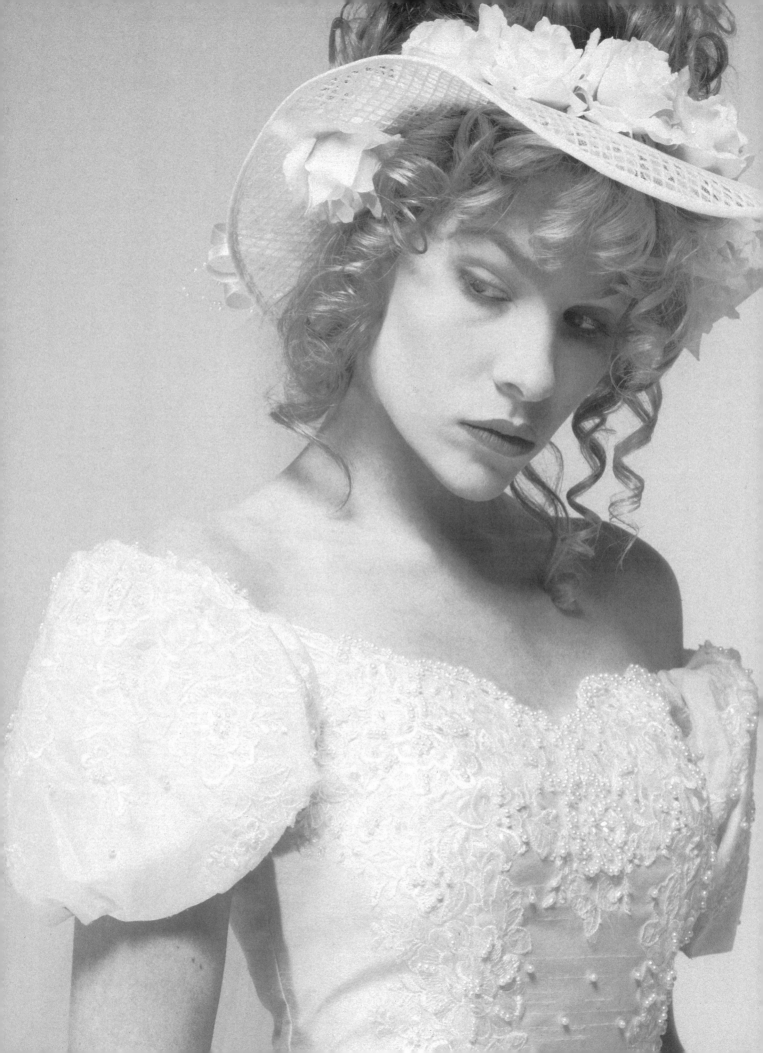

CHAPTER 3

The System

Photo Courtesy of Stephane Colbert

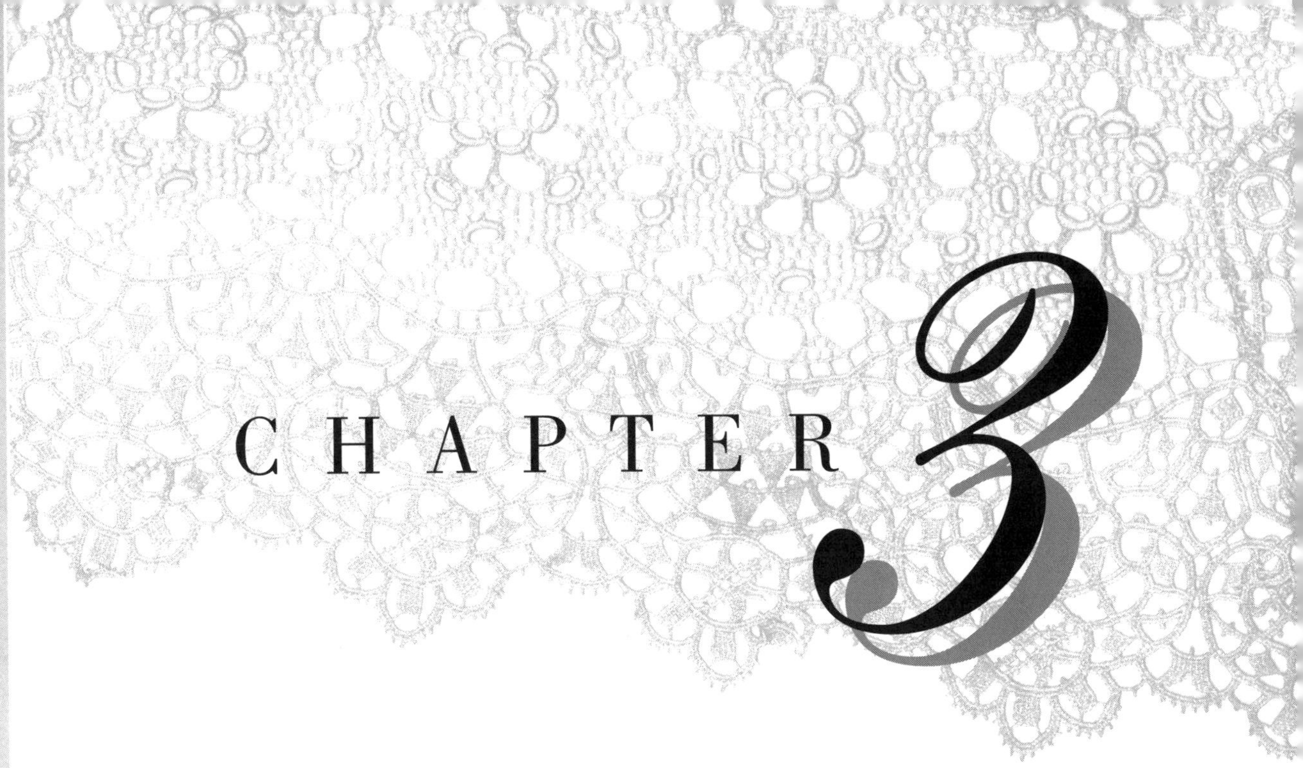

*L*et's see what Webster has to say about the word *system:*

System: Arrangement of things so related or connected as to form a unity, a set of facts, principles, rules, etc., arranged in orderly form to show a logical plan. A method, procedure, orderliness.[1]

Sounds great doesn't it? But why is it so hard for many of us to create a system and stick to it? Because organization does not come naturally to many of us with creative minds. Some feel it is beneath their creative thought process or that it will hinder their free-flowing ideas. Quite the contrary! The thoughts and ideas will always come, and being organized will help many of them to become a reality. And great ideas becoming a reality will bring more profits. Having a system in place allows us the time to keep our ideas flowing. We see how systems work over and over again in everyday situations. Just look at McDonald's. There is a system for every thing that needs to get done. From the ordering of supplies to the method of cooking and serving the food. Also success stories from others in our field should encourage us all to be our very best.

As I researched this book I spoke with many successful people. Every one of them started out the same. With an idea, a dream, and goals for their lives and careers. What sets the successful apart is taking that burning desire and feeding the fire—not putting it out with negative thoughts. That burning desire

is fed with fuel, fuel such as ambition, drive, goals, and organization. Each and every one of them did not do it alone. They will all tell you of someone whom they watched; someone they copied and followed, someone they admired and mirrored.

Visit any multimillion dollar salon organization and you will see a system in place that everyone must follow. The teaching staff at DiGrigoli Academy in Easthampton, Massachusetts, (myself included,) decided to do just that. We took a visit to New York City to visit top salons. Now, Paul already has a system in place for each and every aspect of his company, from how to answer the phone and take a message to how and when he evaluates the progress and assesses the goals of each individual stylist. But his ambition does not stop there, he does not get "comfortable."

We were very impressed by the organization of some of the companies we visited. We were unannounced, had no appointments to meet anyone specific, and were well received.

I was very impressed with Bumble and bumble, an award-winning salon on East 56th Street. We were shown the entire salon from the sky-lit color department to the basement staff room. We saw their marketing and editorial departments, their new staff training room, and their appointment booking room, as well as their product distribution area and their retail areas. They even demonstrated their computer system.

To be the best you need to learn from the best. If you only compare your company or self to those doing worse than you, then you will never improve. Your salon may not have lofty goals for being huge, but whatever your goals and dreams are you need to put a system in place to get you there.

THE IMPORTANCE OF A SYSTEM

Paul DiGrigoli knows the importance of having systems yet he also knows the importance of always improving. He has even taken two trips out to Minnesota to see the operations of Diane and Rocco Altobelli. Diane and Rocco were featured as Super Heroes in the October 1996 issue of *American Salon*. Together they own nine salons, have an advanced training school, 320 employees, and a product line. Altobella International in Eagan, Minnesota, is the product company they created. They personally work with their own chemists to develop their products. Their nine salons and day spas range in size from 2,500 to 6,000 square feet. Their company services 22,000 clients a month. They have over 65 haircolor specialists and one salon alone has 12 receptionists. On Paul's last trip to see Diane he brought his salon coordinators.[2]

Make the choice to learn from those who have something going for them that you admire. Utilize this book to its fullest for your bridal department. Read your trade magazines. Order books and tapes from Milady/SalonOvations' catalog. And get systems going for your salon!

Most people are flattered when you approach them to see how they became successful. And if they are truly successful they will not worry in sharing what they know. Even if your goals are not as lofty as those whom you contact or admire, you can still learn from them. Strive to be the best in your area.

On your quest to improve yourself you will run into someone who does not share your desires or goals. That person may be a coworker, a business partner, a staff member, or, if you are the stylist, it may be your employer. Don't let circumstances or pessimists stop you, but, at the same time, don't expect everyone to be enthusiastic. And if you are trying to instill a new system they may not understand it or its purpose right away. Give change a chance.

The bridal client is a unique client with separate and specific needs, needs that are different from her everyday appointment. This is the most important day of her life! And having a system in place to handle emotional wedding parties is a must for any salon considering a bridal department.

Here's an example of how not having a system in place can ruin a bride's start to the most important day of her life. Judy Rockwell, owner of the Bridal Loft, a bridal salon in Hamden, Connecticut, and owner of Jose Bridal in Westport, Connecticut, has graciously lent me all the beautiful gowns for this book. Judy also has a story of the horrible experience she faced on her wedding day. She decided to have a trial run appointment of her wedding-day style. The stylist did a good job but failed to make any record of what she had done at the trial run. Come the wedding day the stylist had completely forgotten what she had done to Judy's hair and kept asking Judy if she was doing it right! (It is *not* the bride's job to remind us.) Because the stylist forgot what to do to Judy, the stylist started to run late. With Judy half done, the stylist made her wait while she did someone else! This was Judy's wedding day.

Hundreds of people are involved in a wedding and the most important one is in your chair. There is a schedule to keep. This is why a system is so important for a salon to follow. You better believe customer service and communication are a big factor when purchasing a bridal gown from one of Judy's bridal salons!

With your salon's bridal image defined, a department organized, and a bridal team in place these problems and many more are avoided. This chapter covers all you need to know to get started.

THE RECEPTIONIST'S ROLE

Just as the bridal team needs to be committed to servicing the wedding party the whole salon needs to be bridal friendly and bridal ready. This starts with the front desk and that first important contact the bride has with the salon—the phone call. Every bride must call the salon to see if it can accommodate her wedding party. It is right here that you can impress her or lose her.

Some salons have one person who handles all the scheduling of wedding parties. DeniseLor Cerullo of Adam Broderick Image Group in

Ridgefield, Connecticut, is the salon's bridal consultant. DeniseLor answers all the questions the bride has and also does all of the scheduling for the salon's bridal team. When I asked her what her main duties were, she said, "Selling services." She also asks the bride to consider services for the whole party as well as the out-of-town guests. DeniseLor and her system are key to the success of the Adam Broderick Image Group's wedding department.[3]

When the bride calls the salon for a consultation appointment the receptionist needs to ask specific questions. You can lose 30 percent of your business through poor phone skills and by not being prepared to consistently answer a client's question. The bride is even more particular when it comes to her wedding day.

Consider an article that ran in *Modern Salon* in the September 1996 issue. It featured one of New York's brides who was looking for that perfect salon to handle her wedding. The article highlighted her numerous trips and trial runs at various New York salons. The first salon made her wait for 45 minutes at her consultation appointment. They were immediately dismissed. Another salon needed an "attitude adjustment." The bride, Samantha Fox, said everyone from the receptionist to the coat check person to the stylist acted as if the she were lucky to be there. They were dismissed. The third salon did a horrible job on her hair. Dismissed. The fourth salon was great and she loved her hair, but Samantha was uncomfortable with a man doing the wedding party's hair.

Her reason was that everyone would be in different stages of undress while having services in the salon's preparation room. Chalk one up for women stylists! So that salon was dismissed, reluctantly. The fifth salon sped through the trial run, even though Samantha liked her hair. Dismissed, *maybe*. Samantha had one more salon appointment to keep. Stylist Nikki Albino of Minardi Salon got the job.[4]

This article was great. I encourage you to order reprints for the salon. It shows the readers how much importance the bride puts on how she looks for her wedding day.

Bridal Consultant, Bridal Department Head, or Bridal Coordinator as Bert Ostroff is called at Salon Pereau in Cherry Hill, New Jersey, a front desk person with one of these titles is vital to a well-run bridal department. Answering the phone and saying, "Wait a minute let me go ask someone that question," will make the bride dial elsewhere. The entire salon needs to be versed in the system and how it works.

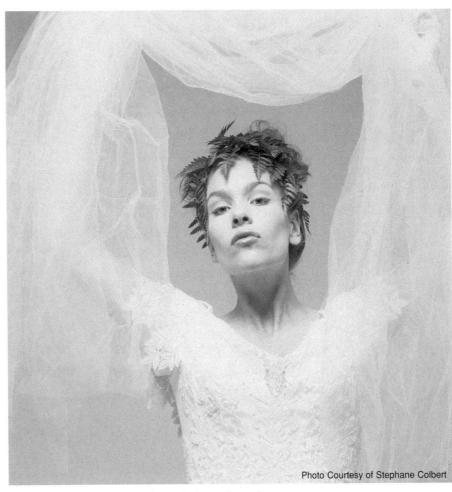

Photo Courtesy of Stephane Colbert

At our front desk is a big white notebook called "The Wedding Book." The first sheet inside has four key questions anyone answering the phone needs to ask the prospective bride. Each following page is a month where all the brides and their weddings are listed. (See sample on page 53.) When the client identifies herself as a bride the receptionist pulls out "The Wedding Book" notebook.

FOUR KEY QUESTIONS

1 When is your wedding date?

The first thing to find out is if we are available on her wedding date. She is then penciled in to hold that date and time. Some brides call eight months to a year in advance and cannot give detailed information about the entire wedding party's needs at that time. But we do hold her date. If another bride requests the same day, we then get specific times from everyone so we can be sure to accommodate more than one wedding. Some brides call only a few weeks ahead of time.

2 How did you hear about our salon?

The last page of the book has a space for recording this information. The bride is either a salon client, a referral from a salon client, someone who saw us at a show, a guest who was at a wedding we did, or a bride who received a brochure from us in the mail. This allows us to measure which marketing or advertising strategy works best for us.

3 Do you have a headpiece yet?

We offer custom headpieces and many brides call us specifically for this service. If she is unsure she is told I can help her with a decision. If she has one already she is instructed to bring it to the consultation. Some brides do not have their headpiece for their consultation. This is when you can help her choose the correct style for her total look.

4 "May I book a complimentary consultation appointment for you? At that appointment our wedding specialist will be better able to listen to you and answer any further questions you may have." (This is the actual script our receptionist uses.)

These four questions are asked when the bride calls our salon. This system of consistent questions lets the bride know up front that our salon is in control and competent to handle her wedding. This system also helps the receptionist get off the phone quicker. If I need information right away I call the bride back to discuss specific things, like times and how large the party is. If not, I will meet her at the consultation.

Sometimes the brides want to speak to me before they book a consultation, especially if they have any questions about a headpiece. As I mentioned before, sometimes I already have a wedding booked on their day and I need more detailed information as to the times involved and the size of the party. With this information I sometimes can do two or more parties in a day. If the bride really wants me to service her and my bridal team is booked, the bride will come alone so I can fit her in. One time I was booked with two morning parties and had to turn away a third bride, yet she wanted me to make her a headpiece. I still had to do a trial run on her as part of the headpiece consultation. In the end I got paid for the trial run and made her a $300 headpiece. This is without even having to do the bride on the day of her wedding! Chapter 5, The Total

Brides

	(fill in month here)

NAME	PHONE	WEDDING DATE	CEREMONY TIME	# IN PARTY

Bridal Look, will go into detail regarding custom headpiece work.

Once the bride schedules a consultation, the receptionist instructs her to bring in a magazine picture of her dress or a Polaroid picture of her in it. Many bridal salons have posted signs asking there be no picture taking. This is to protect them from a bride taking a picture of her dress and going to another bridal salon and trying to get a better price. If the bride has already purchased the gown she just needs to ask if she can take a picture for the hairstylist. The bride is also encouraged to bring along with her any other information or pictures she would care to show the stylist. If she needs a custom headpiece then that is written in the regular appointment book next to her consultation. If she has one already she is asked to bring it along with her to the consultation.

By following this system, or any system, consistently, the department will run smoothly. By doing this you are also giving the bride permission to relax and know in advance that she will be listened to. With a little inward sigh of relief the bride can now look forward to her consultation. I have had many brides say, "Well, that was easy. I was nervous about my hair." The bride is relaxed and confident and we haven't even done her hair yet!

The system becomes the ace in the hole, the key to success. And will help in building a larger client base for the entire salon.

See how it all works together? Follow the information in this book and see your bridal business take off!

- 🕊 You must be prepared by practicing your craft.
- 🕊 Train your eye to see differently and your hands will become more creative.
- 🕊 You must get outside of your comfort zone and try new ways of doing things or you will never grow in your profession.
- 🕊 Never stop learning.

THE CONSULTATION

Guaranteeing a successful wedding day for your bridal client begins with a successful consultation. Lisé Padron of Weddings by Lisé in Honolulu, Hawaii, gives this advice: "I work in advance to have consultations and establish relationships."[5]

This information is so very important and cannot be stressed enough. In any relationship, be it a parent/child, student/teacher, or husband/wife, predicaments always stem from communication problems.

The bride is now sitting across from you. She is either armed with folders, photos, and her planner or she is waiting for your input. In Chapter 6, Relating to the Bride and Her Party, I go into detail about different personality types and communication skills to help with the consultation process. But regardless of personality type the first step is to actively listen to your client. You must listen with your eyes as well as your ears. Your eyes will be watching her body movements and her hands. Your eyes should be studying her body type and her face shape. Look how she is dressed. Your ears may hear a strong personality or a quiet, unsure person. You will be listening for clues that tell you which personality type she may be. Also look for clues that will tell you about her bridal image type. Her choice in clothing will reflect her wedding gown style. Bridal image types are discussed in Chapter 5, The Total Bridal Look.

16 QUESTIONS TO ASK THE BRIDE

Here's how my system works:

⚘ For my system I have a 5 x 8 index file box.

⚘ My files are separated by months, not alphabetically. That way each month I can see who is coming in.

⚘ On the card I write the bride's name, date, and phone numbers across the top.

⚘ The cards are also used for sketches or notes I may wish to add.

Following are some questions you may list on a sheet of paper to be used with each bridal consultation. Do not have the bride fill it out. Ask them yourself. Eventually these questions will become a part of you. Write down her answers or notes as she speaks.

1. What time is the wedding?

2. Where are you getting dressed?

3. How far away is that from here?

4. How far away is that from the ceremony?

5. Are you having photos done before the ceremony?

6. What time does the photographer want you ready?

7. Where is the reception?

8. What time of day is the reception?

9. Tell me about the kind of wedding you want to have. (A morning or garden wedding is less formal than an evening wedding. Listen for key wording like romantic, traditional, or elegant and opulent.)

10. Will you be having your makeup done at the salon?

11. Will we be doing the entire bridal party?

12. How many are in the party?

13. How many want updos? Blow-outs? Makeup? Manicures?

14. Do you want to talk about the option of a hair addition or sections that can be added to your veil?

15. Are there any out-of-town guests who need our services?

16. Are the bridesmaids getting a style you want them to have or is it their choice?

I staple any information such as pictures of hairstyles or the dress to the back of the index card. If she does not have a picture of her dress then I ask her about the style of her dress. Sometimes they can find one comparable to theirs in a wedding magazine. If they cannot find one similar then ask about the neckline, the bodice or waistline, the shoulder area, and the flow of the skirt. How to match her hair to her dress is also discussed in length in Chapter 5. If I am designing a headpiece I will write notes pertaining to that as well and take measurements.

> "*Tell me about the kind of wedding you want to have. Will we be doing the entire bridal party?*"

During the consultation it is also important to discuss the condition of her hair. Haircoloring, cutting, and perming need to be scheduled accordingly. It is also another way to increase your revenue from the bridal client and hopefully turn her into a regular salon client. You are doing your bride a disservice by not offering to get her hair in its best possible shape prior to her wedding.

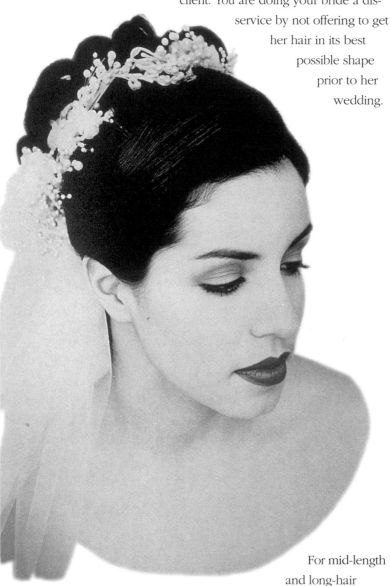

Photo
Courtesy of
Geri Mataya

For mid-length and long-hair brides, once they get engaged they just start growing out their hair. Many of them suffer with too-long bangs and more-than-enough length necessary for an updo. During the consultation advise a shaping, a much-appreciated suggestion for the shaggy bride, but do not push services on her at this time. When she comes back for the trial run, when you have your hands in her hair, that is the time to lead her to make some additional appointments. The majority will end up becoming salon clients. When the bride is handled correctly and you make her wedding day special, a trust is formed and that trust enables her to keep coming back.

When recommending services to the bride here are the guidelines I usually go by. Of course you know your clients best so please use your professional judgment.

Pre-wedding Service Guidelines

Three months before the wedding:

- ❧ Have the consultation now so you can decide on the course of action for her hair (growing it, new cut, color, perm, etc.)

- ❧ Begin conditioning treatments up until the wedding on damaged hair

- ❧ Regular manicures

- ❧ Try out a new hair color

- ❧ Try out a new haircut

- ❧ Begin tanning

- ❧ Begin facial series

One month before the wedding:

- ❧ For long hair that needs a perm, do it now

- ❧ For long hair that needs a good cut, do it now (trim layers or bangs the week before the wedding)

- ❧ Trial run of wedding-day hairstyle

- Trial run of makeup (order makeup the bride will need for her wedding and honeymoon)

Two to three weeks before the wedding:

- Haircut on short and mid-length hair

- Perm or body wave

- Soft highlights

- Give last facial

One week before the wedding:

- Haircolor

- Heavy foil highlights

- Bang trim

A few days before the wedding:

- Artificial nails

- Waxing

The day before:

- Manicures for the entire party

Most of the brides I see come to me just for their wedding-day styling. This is through word of mouth and our marketing. When the bride sees that we have thought of things about her wedding day beauty treatments that she hasn't given thought to, she is impressed. She then becomes more confident in trying out all of our salon services.

Having grown out her hair for an updo, many brides want it cut off shortly after the honeymoon—or sooner. I had a bride ask me if I would come in on the Monday after her wedding so she could have her hair cut off before her honeymoon! I told her I didn't work on Mondays. I suggested it would be better left long to be able to put it into a ponytail on her tropical vacation than having to deal with a new cut. She agreed and came back right after her honeymoon and got it cut short. Sometimes you need to think quickly on your feet.

Pilo Arts, a salon in Brooklyn, New York, takes the idea of getting the bride *and groom* back into the salon after the wedding a step further. They give out complimentary haircut certificates for the bride and groom to use after their wedding.[6] A great idea!

After the consultation you need to give the bride any salon literature or bridal menu she may not have seen. Explain all of your packages. Mention any gift baskets, bridal breakfast, or anything special you have to offer her. Show her around the salon if she has never been there before.

Finally, walk her to the desk and have the receptionist schedule a trial-run appointment. Instruct the bride to come in with clean, dry hair for her trial run. "Day-old hair" is what DeniseLor Cerullo of Adam Broderick Image Group calls it. It is easier and less time-consuming to work on hair this way. Most brides go along with it. Also have her bring in her headpiece again.

THE TRIAL RUN

When the bride comes in for her trial appointment, I take out the file card on her that was recorded at the consultation. It is a good idea to look it over before she comes in to see what was previously discussed. If this is my first

> After the consultation you need to give the bride any salon literature she may not have seen.

time with her then I combine the system for the consultation with the system for the trial run.

Make sure the bride is asked to bring her headpiece in for her trial-run appointment. Sometimes they haven't gotten it in yet. In our bridal display area I have some sample headpieces. These are used as examples of the different styles that are available or when the bride does not have hers. They are also samples of those I can make. It would be a good idea to purchase some older headpieces to have in the salon. Most bridal shops have some hanging around in the back room. Thrift shops and tag sales are also a good place to look. I had one out-of-town bride who told me her stylist back at home wrapped her head with perm cotton to mimic her headband style headpiece. Be bridal friendly—get headpieces in the salon!

Helping the bride choose her hairstyle depends on her headpiece and sometimes they have purchased the wrong one to go with the hairstyle they had in mind. If there is time, she can take it back to the bridal shop and exchange it. Many times the bride comes to the trial run with a loaner headpiece from the bridal shop. This is great because it is already beat up and soiled and you are not afraid to handle it.

The first thing that needs to be done at the trial run is to ask the bride to put her headpiece on where she is comfortable with it. (I have seen three brides place the same style headpiece three different ways.) Or she may want your suggestions in placing it where it

would be best. Certain headpieces are to be on the head a certain way. Some can be worn different ways. Any reputable bridal salon should be more than willing to give you an education on headpiece placement.

Also study the headpiece placement in the bridal magazines. Here is a great idea for making up some visual displays for the bridal department.

- Cut out pictures of headpieces from bridal magazines
- Group many variations of certain styles in separate piles
- Put all wreaths in one pile, back pieces in another, headbands in another, etc.
- Cut out pictures and make groups of headpieces based on the length of the veil
- Put all fingertip lengths in one pile, elbow lengths in another, Cathedral lengths in another, etc.
- Cut out fun trends you may spot in the bridal magazines – colorful headpieces, floral wristlets instead of bouquets, fun shoes, etc.
- Take the cut out pictures and make a collage gluing these pictures onto poster paper or place in a photo album

I made several posters to hang up in the bridal department. One poster shows different headpiece styles grouped together. A few pictures of all backpieces can be put in one corner of the poster, wreaths in another, crowns in the center, etc. The second poster focuses on the different veil lengths. The third poster is all of the new bridal

Be bridal friendly — get headpieces in the salon!

trends. I use these posters to help the bride pick out a headpiece and veil length. I also use them when I am consulting to make a custom headpiece. The bride enjoys seeing that you are interested in weddings. If you want to be a considered a bridal specialist then you need to get involved with weddings as a whole. Once you and the bride agree on the placement of the headpiece then you can design a style around it.

Showing the bride hairstyle posters made up from the bridal magazines, as well as bridal hairstyle books, is also a good idea. Use this book for your trial runs, too!

When looking at pictures of hairstyles with the bride here is a tip: Tell her to show you *anything* she likes, even if it is the front of one look or the back of another. Then, when she points to a particular style, ask her what it is specifically about the picture she likes. It may be the way one curl falls by the eye, or the texture of the curls.

Remember to ask her if she will be keeping the headpiece on throughout the whole day. Many headpieces now come with detachable veils allowing the bride to remove the veil but keep on the headpiece. If she will be removing the veil you may want to adorn the hair beneath it with accessories or pearls. I make most of my headpieces with a detachable veil. Sometimes the bride does not want any veil at all, then the hairstyle becomes the focus of adornment. Many times the hair itself can become the "headpiece" and a simple veil on a comb can be added to the back. A long-hair bride loves to show off her beautiful locks.

Once we have settled on a hairstyle I say, "This is a *general* idea of how your hair is going to look on the day of the wedding. Of course, every curl won't be in the exact same place." The bride nods in agreement and this statement gets you off the hook with that perfectionist bride.

To record it so we both remember:

1. I take a Polaroid photo of the bride's hair.

2. I attach that to the index card from the consultation.

3. I file the card under the month of her wedding date.

4. Visually, she sees "herself" go in a box for safe keeping.

5. She is comfortable knowing that I will have a record of what to do the day of her wedding.

6. This alleviates any nervousness on her part concerning her hair.

This is the best part of the system, a sure-fire tip for keeping the bride calm and cool. The trial-run appointment assures you and the bride a successful wedding day appointment. It is a must for making the bride feel comfortable and confident. It is your chance to gain her trust. This way the bride can instill her confidence in you to the other members of the wedding party. When the bride expresses to me, during the trial run, that the bridesmaids are worrying about their hair, I make a point of having the bride tell the girls that I will listen to them and that I am skilled in what I do.

The bride enjoys seeing that you are interested in weddings.

Many times, however, skill has nothing to do with the success of a bride. There are many factors involved for a successful trial run. Take this following story for example. I had a bride with naturally curly hair just past her shoulders which I set on hot rollers to smooth out the curl. The first style I tried per her request was loosely up with a lot of softness and tendrils. Now this bride was close to six feet tall. Once the veil was on she thought she might like some of her hair down instead. Her neckline looked bare and being this tall with all of her hair up just

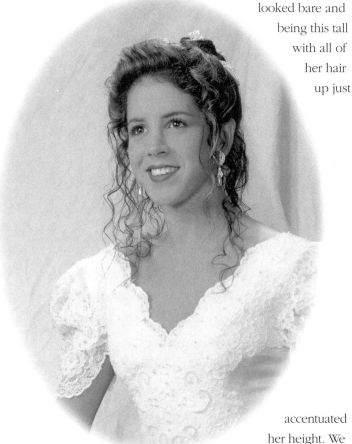

accentuated her height. We tried some of the hair up with some left down. In addition to her height this bride was a little older and didn't want to look too matronly or too cute. We took a Polaroid picture of this style I

attached it to her index card and filed it in my box.

During the trial run I brought our colorist over to discuss her hair. The colorist suggested to even out her hair with some color foil highlights and to cover some of her first grays. The bride then came in the next Saturday for color and also booked a trim with me. When she came over for her trim she loved her color, but I could tell from her way of looking at me that she wanted to talk about her wedding day hair. I sat down next to her and gave her eye contact and allowed her to fully express her feelings. She was still uncomfortable with what we had done at the trial run. She wanted to try her hair all down with her natural curl instead of the hot roller curl. Clients with naturally curly hair are so used to seeing it that way everyday that sometimes a change in texture is uncomfortable.

She happened to be my last client of that Saturday so I was able to work on her then. I diffused her hair to utilize her natural curls. I put some of her hair up on the sides and put a sample veil on her head. She liked it but was still unsure. This is when you have to separate yourself from the cause of her discomfort. She was not unhappy with my work. *She was unsure of what she wanted*. I did not take it personally. Too many times the stylist becomes threatened at this point and becomes defensive. She wanted my opinion. I asked her to describe her dress again. It was traditional with a full skirt. As I thought of her in her dress with her height, and her hair either up or down, it was painting a very vertical picture in my mind. My answer was, "I know you are comfortable with your natural curl, but at the same time you want to feel special. And leaving your hair the same way as everyday is too casual. Having it set and all of it up is too different. Let's try a more horizontal hairstyle, one that drapes across the back of your head, utilizing your natural curl and balances off the skirt of your dress." She loved it. We took another Polaroid photo for her file. And I got a really nice tip for my understanding. This is being a bridal specialist and I love it!

Keep on Top of Things

At the beginning of each month I go through my files and arrange them by wedding dates. I check over any headpiece orders. I see who is coming in and mentally prepare myself. This is especially important for my Sunday brides. Even with all my systems and mentally preparing myself, the unexpected can happen. I always worry I will forget my Sunday brides or that my alarm won't work.

My worst fears came true one Sunday morning in November. My family was at church and I was getting ready to go into the salon. (I always arrive a little early to plug in my utensils so they are ready to use.) I got in my car and it wouldn't start. The battery was dead. There was no way to call the bride because she had to travel further than I and was already on her way to the salon. There was no one at the salon to call to tell her I would be late. It was early and no neighbors were about. I had no choice but to ride my bike! So, I went back into the house. I got on my husband's leather coat and found some leather gloves. Remember—it was November in Connecticut! I rode like crazy. Thank goodness I live only a few miles away from the salon. I pulled into the parking lot at the same time as the bride. She thought I was some crazy exercise nut to be riding a bike in November in New England! We had a laugh over the whole situation. Today she is still a great client—one who knows I will go to any length to service her.

Let's recap the trial run:

- ☙ The trial run is a must for making the bride feel comfortable and confident. It is your chance to gain her trust.

- ☙ Separate yourself from the cause of her discomfort. She is *not* unhappy with your work.

- ☙ Don't take her indecisiveness personally or become threatened and defensive.

- ☙ She needs to bring her headpiece to the trial-run appointment.

- ☙ Take out the file card on her that was recorded at the consultation.

- ☙ Ask the bride to put on her headpiece the way she is most comfortable.

- ☙ Say, "This is a *general* idea of how your hair is going to look on the day of the wedding. Of course, every curl won't be in the exact same place."

- ☙ Take a Polaroid picture of the bride's hair and attach that to the index card from the consultation.

The trial run is a must for making the bride feel comfortable and confident.

🎀 Instruct the bride (and the bridal party) to wear button-up or zippered shirts. (You don't want them to pull clothes over their heads on the day of the wedding.)

🎀 File the card under the month of her wedding date.

🎀 At the beginning of each month go through your index card files and arrange them by wedding dates.

🎀 Secure and finalize all wedding party appointments.

Now you are both ready for the wedding day.

STRATEGIES FOR BOOKING APPOINTMENTS

Many brides begin planning the details of their wedding a year or two in advance. The basic appointment book many salons have do not allow for booking a year in advance. Here's how my "Wedding Book" works as part of a continuing system. The Wedding Book notebook I talked about earlier allows the receptionist to book a wedding a year ahead. Once the bride calls the salon and I have spoken with her, her wedding date is secured.

After the bride has her consultation, and this may be six months ahead or less, we book her wedding date into the regular appointment book. The wedding date has already been penciled into the Wedding Book. It is also on record on her card in my file box. The bridal team leader may also wish to have a personal record of all

weddings booked. A personal planner works best for this. You will learn to schedule your vacations and days off a year ahead so others on the bridal team can handle any parties when you will not be available.

So, there are four places the weddings are recorded:

1. the Wedding Book

2. the regular appointment book

3. in the file box system

4. in a personal planner

The bridal team leader, and bridal specialist or salon wedding consultant must then confirm all wedding appointments. This includes all the appointments of the entire party. If the receptionist is the only one allowed at the appointment book then the team leader needs to make an appointment with the receptionist to schedule and confirm the wedding parties. At the beginning of each month look one to two months ahead and try to confirm all appointments. Many brides do not know if everyone in the party wants an appointment. Trying to pin her down to specifics allows you to run the show and encourages her to be organized. Some brides have no control over their wedding party, some brides are right on. Some have an out-of-town relative making the appointments. Most people don't give it much thought from our perspective. *That is why the salon must have a system.* If we were to wait for the entire party to call us they never would. Then come close to the wedding day the salon would be trying to fit in attendants last minute.

Denise Pereau of Salon Pereau, in Cherry Hill, New Jersey, has come up with a solution to this dilemma. She goes as far as to have the bride sign a wedding contract. The bride is mailed a letter thanking her for choosing Salon Pereau. Along with the letter the bride receives a bridal contract. (See Chapter 2.) One copy is for her to keep. The other is to fill out and send back signed with a 50% deposit. The contract asks the bride to fill out how many people will be getting their hair done and how many will be having makeup. If the services are canceled 30 days prior to the wedding day they will refund the deposit in full. The balance is due in full upon completion of the services on the wedding day. The contract asks the bride to call the salon two weeks before the wedding to confirm all the arrangements.

"Most salons fall short in the area of salon management," says Pereau. Denise and her salon manager and bridal coordinator meet weekly to make sure things are running smoothly. Her wedding contract became necessary to protect the salon in the event of costly cancellations. Many times someone from the party gets cold feet, and changes her mind wanting to do her own hair on the day of the wedding. Sometimes they cancel their makeup or nails last minute. It is a good idea, as the number of weddings in the salon increases, to consider instituting some kind of wedding contract or cancellation policy.

Scheduling of the wedding party can be done as a block of time or as individual services. Some weddings are in the evening, some in the morning. Depending on the size of the bridal team and salon, two or more weddings can be booked for the same day.

When booking out-of-town bridesmaids for hair services it is best to just book a block of space. For example, just write "Smith wedding party" and not individual names. That way a team member who is strongest with very long hair or curly hair can do that particular client.

As far as computer systems go, and so many are different, you will need to make adjustments accordingly.

When scheduling the wedding party you must allow enough time for the following:

🎗 travel time home from the salon

🎗 travel time to the church

🎗 time for the bride to get dressed

🎗 time for her to apply her makeup if the salon is not doing it

🎗 time for the photographer to take pictures before the wedding

Remember most of these questions are asked at the consultation. A very important one to ask is, "Are you having a photographer come to your home for pictures before the ceremony?" If she says yes, then I ask her what time the photographer is coming. If she does not know I allow for two hours. Then I ask her how long is her drive to where she will be changing into her gown. Sometimes they are not changing at home and have not thought of the extra time needed to travel to where they are getting dressed. If she is doing her own

*I*t is a good idea to consider instituting some kind of wedding contract or cancellation policy.

makeup you need to allow for that time as well. Remember, the whole day is on a time schedule with you, the hairdresser, first on the list.

Think of the scheduling as a math equation. Let's use a wedding that starts at 2 P.M. and has a party of six, as an example.

First add up the time needed for travel, dress and photographer.

$$15 \text{ minutes for travel}$$
$$+$$
$$15 \text{ minutes for dress}$$
$$+$$
$$90 \text{ minutes for the photographer}$$
$$= 2 \text{ hours}$$

Take the ceremony time which is 2 P.M. and subtract the time needed for travel, dress, and photographer which is 2 hours. This means the bride must leave the salon no later than 12 P.M.

Estimate how long she and her party will need at the salon. I figure two people an hour including makeup. A party of six with three stylists and one makeup artist working will mean a total time of two hours needed to do their hair.

$$12 \text{ P.M. leaving time}$$
$$- 2 \text{ hours styling time}$$
$$= 10 \text{ A.M. starting time}$$

This exact timing is vital to her day running on time as well as your day running on time. It creates a stress-free environment for all involved. It is the unorganized stress of a wedding that causes many salons to shy away from doing bridal parties. But *The Business of Bridal Beauty* will see to it that this is not a problem anymore. You must be ready to handle all the weddings of baby boomers' babies that are coming your way in the next twenty years.

Will a bride refer friends or come back herself if the salon was unprepared to handle her wedding appropriately? Many late-starting weddings are blamed on the hairdresser who failed to take these things into consideration. I am very concerned with the public attitude toward our profession. Every time a wedding is messed up by the hairdresser, hundreds of guests, as well as many irate photographers hear about it. Following is a quote from G. Gregory Geiger, CPP (Certified Professional Photographer) of Gregeiger Co. Utd., Inc., located in Orange, Connecticut, regarding the importance of scheduling:

You, as the hairdresser, were hired for your talent. The bride is comfortable with your personality and confident of your creative abilities. Every wedding has a timetable or schedule, either printed or verbally established between the bride and the respective vendors. Most portrait-style wedding photographers want about two hours before the wedding to do photography. This time is requested to create all the different types of portraits and to allow for late family members, tardy bridesmaids, lost groomsmen, cranky ring bearer, shy flower girls, and weepy mothers."[7]

Gregory routinely does large, upscale weddings from coast to coast. He has learned the importance of scheduled time.

"When a makeup person or stylist runs past their allotted time, it creates a trickle-down effect. At some point one of the wedding professionals will have to cut short their needed time to get the wedding back on schedule. If it is the photographer ending early, then the couple could not receive all the family portraits they would enjoy having. From experience I know that it is next to impossible to get family members and all the wedding party together at the wedding reception. A good investment by the bride is hiring a wedding coordinator. This one person can be invaluable in keeping a wedding on schedule."[8]

If your bride is working through a wedding coordinator then you may be in contact with that person. But the wedding coordinator may assume *you* will have all of the beauty scheduling worked out. These tips from Gregory will put the importance of time and scheduling in perspective.

The importance of establishing a system from the first phone call, through the consultation, trial run, and the day of the wedding is the only way to bridal success.

TIPS

- Use a system

- Make your salon a "Wedding Book"

- Train the entire salon in the system

- Stress the importance of the system

- Don't take a bride's comments personally

- Record everything you do with drawings and photos

- Invest in a Polaroid camera (and always have film in the salon!)

- Eat, sleep, and drink the system

- Use the scheduling equation

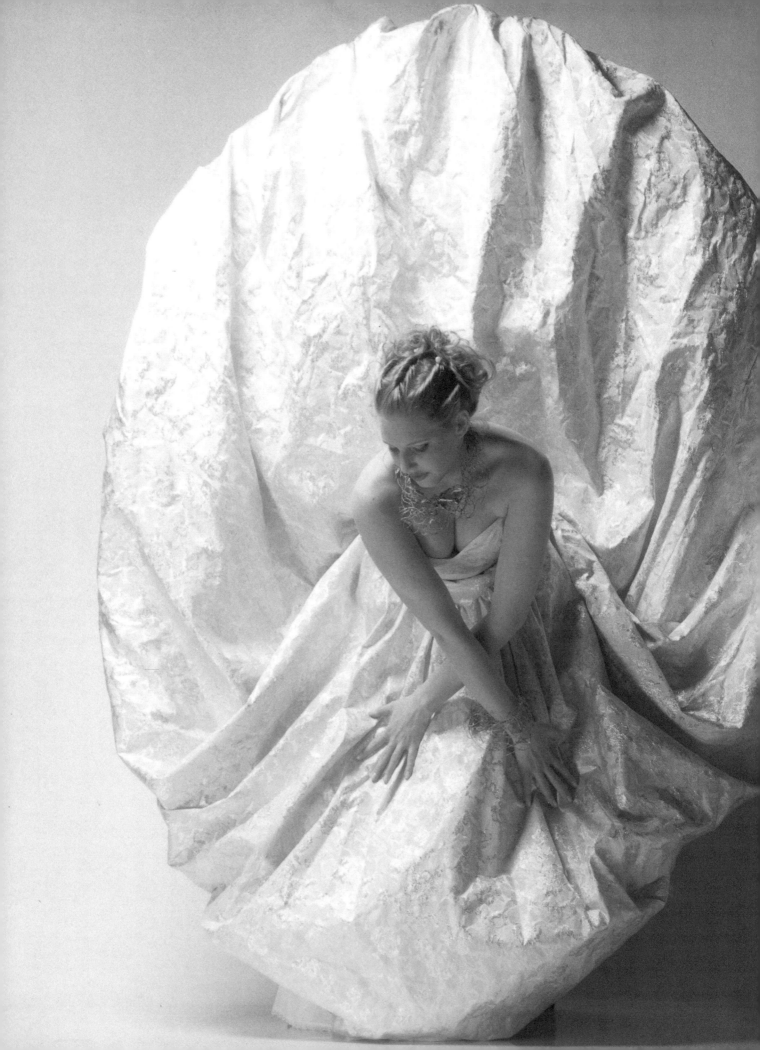

CHAPTER 4

Networking and Advertising

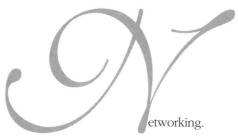

etworking.

I am sure you have heard of this term before but maybe you thought it just applied to businesspeople, or the salon owner.

Networking applies to you:

❧ if you have personal goals to improve yourself and your career.

❧ if you desire to have your own salon someday.

❧ if you own your own salon and are in a slump.

❧ if you want more clients in your chair.

❧ if you desire to be the best you can be.

❧ if you wish to become fully involved with the bridal industry.

WHAT IS NETWORKING?

❧ **Networking** is a state of mind. It becomes a mindset of thinking about your career even when you are not at work.

❧ **Networking** is when a group of people who share the *same* interests get together and exchange information.

❧ **Networking** is when a group of people with *varied* interests get together and exchange information.

❧ **Networking** can be as organized as a seminar or as relaxed as a dinner party.

❧ **Networking** can take place anywhere and everywhere, at all times.

TOOLS FOR EFFECTIVE NETWORKING

Networking means working the room (and I'm not talking about finding a relationship). Being visible and involved is key to successful networking. The following tools for effective networking will help you get started. These tools are a part of your image. Refer back to Chapter 1, Your Bridal Image, if necessary.

Tools for effective networking are as follows:

❧ A Good Firm Handshake

Never give a dead-fish handshake to anyone. I did once. When I was seventeen and I met my future husband's German immigrant grandfather, I gave my last dead-fish handshake. First of all I did not even offer my hand when we were introduced—at seventeen, I thought only men did that. Then, when he asked me to shake his hand, I got the best business lesson of my life. He grabbed my hand and shook it firmly. Speaking in a heavy German accent he told me what kind of a statement a good handshake makes and how important it was for me to do the same. He was a very successful businessman. He left behind a strong family business and instilled in his 11 grandchildren and

Networking is a mindset of thinking about your career even when you are not at work.

14 great-grandchildren (and one grateful granddaughter-in-law!) some important life lessons. Today when I meet someone I give a good, firm handshake. It's irrelevant whether it's my child's teacher, a new client, or a networking contact. If they give me a dead-fish handshake in return I secretly wish they had had the opportunity to have met Opa. Thanks, Opa!

Friendliness

When you network make sure you show genuine interest in the other person. Try to look for the good in people and situations. Do not use a person for their information and then dump them when you've learned what you wanted. It will not take long for your circle of "friends" to be able to see through your selfish insincerity.

Enthusiasm

Everyone loves to be around an enthusiastic person. Enthusiastic people give off an energy that is contagious. They inspire others and are not threatened by people using their ideas; they encourage others to strive for their own personal best. When networking you are giving as well as receiving. In researching this book I ran into a few professionals who were not interested in sharing information. I was either not worth their time or they felt threatened. It seemed like they were afraid I was going to steal their ideas and give others an "unfair" chance for success. On the other hand, the enthusiastic professionals who were generous enough to share were a great help and I thank them for the information they gave.

Knowledge

Remember the saying "Knowledge is power"? It most definitely is. I love to read anything on any subject because I know I am broadening my knowledge power. I want to be interested *in* my clients as well as interesting *to* them. I find it disheartening when a client assumes, because I am just a hairstylist, I must be unaware and uneducated. I noticed this attitude in a male client recently. His tone of voice and reluctance to communicate was evident. I asked him what his profession was. He replied, "Consulting." A one-word answer. Well, consulting takes place in many fields. Then I asked, "What field do you do consulting for?" He said, "Manufacturing." That also can be in any field. He could make toothbrushes or spaceships. Then I asked him, "What area of manufacturing?" Another one-word reply. "Semiconductors." Now we had common ground because I knew this was computers. Once he saw I had a brain he opened up and we had a good conversation.

Self-Control

Do you have it? In all situations, self-control is necessary to have when networking. If you do not know *what* to say, spend time *listening*. Listen and take mental notes. Or take real notes. But do not just jump in on a conversation. If others hear you

When you network make sure you show genuine interest in the other person.

talking about things you know nothing or little about or constantly gossiping, will they be willing to share information with you? Will they be willing to refer to a friend who may become a prospective client? Remember successful networking takes these skills. Do not try to impress people. Jim Smith, owner of Changes Salon in Greensboro, North Carolina, and president of ProManagement, had a list called "10 Ways to Keep Clients Coming." Here are a few that I feel are important to networking.

🖎 Always smile

🖎 Appear sincere

🖎 Never allow clients (or associates) see you upset

🖎 Never gossip[1]

I once had a problem at a hair show; I let down my self-control and possibly could have damaged my career. I had asked eight beautiful long-hair models, girls who were in high school, to do a show for me. It was the end of a long day. The girls were tired and I was so thankful they helped me out. Usually we give the models products for being in the show. Paul DiGrigoli brings them from his salon and we give them to the models. Plus, I give them their next haircut free. Well, this time we were using someone else's products on stage and they were to supply retail for the models.

When they placed a box of those small foil samples for the girls to take, I was personally embarrassed. We had used a lot of different products on stage and I told the girls they could take

whatever was opened. The manufacturer's representative, however, said I could not let the girls take the opened items and that they were being taken back to the supply house. I got very huffy and spoke to the rep in a disgusted tone. "You're taking back products that were opened and used? That is ridiculous!" I was professionally out of line and I knew it. I made sure I called Paul the next day and told him of the situation.

The person to whom I was huffy was the same person who sold tickets to promote our shows. I might have damaged my reputation in her eyes for good. At our next show I apologized to the woman and made sure I talked up the products that evening. Which brings me to the last tool for positive networking.

Admitting Mistakes

Stay away from the blame game. It is so easy to justify your mistakes and to blame others. This too is a transparent flaw that others around you will see through and should be avoided. If you do not take responsibility for your actions, regardless of the situation from your point of view, you can damage your reputation.

NETWORKING MEANS EVERYONE WINS

If any profession has the opportunity to use people skills necessary for small talk and networking it is the salon stylist. We have the chance to practice every day. We are not stuck in an office

> *If you do not take responsibility for your actions, you can damage your reputation.*

with the same ten people day in and day out. Networking can easily become second nature. Begin by networking with your clients.

Here's one idea to get you started:

- Get an empty binder at the office supply store.
- Purchase clear plastic sheets that hold business cards.
- Start collecting business cards from your clients who wish to network.
- Fill the pages with the business cards and start networking.

This binder can be placed in the salon waiting room or left at your station. I have also seen businesses use a corkboard where clients can pin up their business cards, but these can quickly become an eyesore.

When a client is new in town, you now have a book full of personal contacts you can share with that new client. Whether someone is looking for a florist, house painter, or a pretty boutique you have the resources at hand. My husband's employer is a real estate broker and I have given him some leads. He in turn sends any newly engaged couples to the salon for our bridal services.

In my personal planner I have a few pages for business cards. I collect cards from people whom I have met networking at various functions, classes, or meetings. I have one page of business cards relating to the bridal industry. They are:

- Wedding dress restorers
- Florists

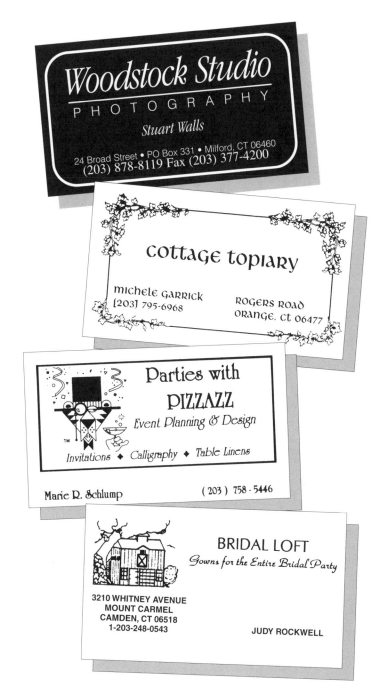

- Bouquet restorers
- Photographers
- Party planners
- Caterers/Reception halls
- Bridal salons
- Boutiques
- Lingerie shops

During the consultation I always ask the bride if she is all set with everything. If she still needs a florist or a photographer I have a few names to give her.

Networking sometimes allows you to be in the right place at the right time. Ask any famous person or any successful platform artist and they will tell you that besides always striving to be their best, they were in the right place at the right time, networking. I am constantly in a networking frame of mind. If I am scheduled to do a hair show I am prepared to do my best because I never know who is in the audience. Let me share what some of my networking has led me to do.

Networking Success Stories

My main areas of interest are the bridal industry and salon industry. This is where I network heavily. I started out with a love for dressing hair. I pushed myself out of my comfort zone and volunteered to do updos at a trade show back in 1991. My contact was an employee of a major color company. At that show my updos were discover by Paul DiGrigoli, a multiple salon owner, founder and director of DiGrigoli's Academy in Easthampton, Massachusetts. Paul is an educator in business, a superb haircutter, and a motivational speaker. Volunteering to do updos at that hair show allowed me to be in the right place in front of the right people at the right time.

When Paul called me at home the next day he asked if I would like to teach at his training center. I was shocked, but I welcome new chal-

lenges. As I drove to my first class I was so scared! The fear in the pit of my stomach lasted throughout the two-hour drive up to the training center. My stomach was in knots and my knees were like Jell-O. When I got up to speak, I literally had to bite the inside of my cheek to keep my teeth from chattering. But it was something I wanted to do. Don't let fear hold you back. (I tell my children, "A life lived in fear is a life half-lived.")

Fear can be good for networking. Susie Fields wrote an article for the *SalonOvations Magazine* in the September 1996 issue. It was entitled "Super Confidence and How to Get It." One of the subtitles was "Use Fear as a Signal to Grow." In it she tells how a friend went from fear*ful* to fear*less*. Lynette was shy. She would fidget and look at her feet when she spoke. What made her change to become one of the top real-estate salespeople in her city? "Fear," she replies simply. "I used to be afraid of everything. I vowed that anything I feared I had to do." Every day Lynette tries to do something she fears.[2]

I always feared New York City; I think it was from seeing too many movies. But I wanted to attend the International Beauty Show every year. At first I would go to the IBS with coworkers, but they just wanted to shop the show and then leave early to do more shopping. I wanted to go early and sit in on as much education as I could. I knew I had to start going by myself. At the train station in New York I had my first cab ride alone. I swore the driver could hear my heart beating.

Don't let fear hold you back.

Nevertheless, I kept going every year. Then I took my daughter to IBS. Last time in the city I took my mother and we used a map. We went to a bridal show and I learned how to navigate the streets. I plan on attending much more now. Let fear be a motivation to challenge yourself.

Another time it was networking through the mail that led me to many great opportunities. Being an updo specialist I have had many brides cross my path. In order to teach others how to handle the brides I decided to look into the bridal market further. I began to read bridal magazines to see what they were telling clients to look for in a wedding-day stylist. That is how I ran across professional photographer G. Gregory Geiger whom I quoted in the previous chapter.

In reading *Modern Bride* I ran across a story about a couple from California. They had won an all-expenses-paid wedding from the magazine. *Modern Bride* was sending photographer Gregory Geiger to California to shoot the wedding. Gregory's photography studio happened to be located in the next town over from where I live.

When I sent him a letter telling him I had seen the article in *Modern Bride*, I shared a little about my interest in brides and, at that time, information about my salon. I also mentioned that if he ever needed any help with a photo shoot or could refer any brides to me I was available. (It always pays to network and take chances like this.)

JOINING A BRIDAL ORGANIZATION

Gregory called me a few months later and we met. Subsequently he introduced me to the Association of Bridal Consultants (ABC), a national organization with members from every area of the wedding industry. I joined this organization and began networking at the meetings. Gerard Monaghan, president of the ABC, gave me this great quote: "Networking involves maximizing your return with minimizing your effort."

ABC member Karen Sauer, of Wedding Plans Plus, Fort Wayne, Indiana, offers another networking tip.

"*If you cannot approach another professional and ask them a question, how do you expect to ask a client for her business? To get ahead in the real world, you have to ask a lot of questions and do your homework. It was no accident that I took a seat next to one of the senior members at lunch or another senior member at dinner. I'm no dummy, I planned it that way. Business is no accident. You need to decide where you want to be and it's up to you to get there.*"[3]

These are insightful words of wisdom from a successful woman who believes in the power of networking.

I've been on TV twice thanks to networking. Our salon hosted a fundraiser at a local country club for a domestic abuse organization in our area. My employer, Noel, and I did

Join an organization and begin networking at the meetings.

most of the leg work for the show. She is a great networker and contact person. She was relentless on the phone and is great at following through on a lead. She secured Congresswoman Rosa Delora to speak and local newscaster Diane Smith to be the mistress of ceremonies. My input into the event was mostly creative. The entire show was designed with a bridal theme which was to showcase our new bridal department. The bridal team presented twenty models. I designed ten distinctly different brides, each with a custom headpiece. The show was presented like a hair show. The salon's bridal team even did hair live on stage for the audience.

I knew I would be meeting Diane Smith, the newscaster who also produced a separate news segment each week called "Positively Connecticut." It is a show that interviews people who are artisans or who offer unique services in Connecticut. I made sure I bought a new suit to be able to present myself as professionally as possible.

At the end of the afternoon I made it a point to speak with Diane alone. I did not hound her or take too much of her time. I knew my work spoke for itself, but I wanted to meet her personally. Our suits were very similar and I was pleased with my choice. I gave her a firm handshake, good eye contact, and an enthusiastic smile. She loved the presentation and said I was very talented, and that I should take my talent further, beyond the realm of the salon. I told her that was one of my goals and mentioned that I had this book coming out soon—

and I would send her a copy. She was pleased and said that she would be interested in doing a segment on her television show featuring my custom headpiece work. (I'm no dummy, I planned it that way.) And guess what? She did call me three months later. Her camera crew came to my house to videotape me at work in my headpiece workshop. Then we went to the salon and she interviewed me there as well. It was a lot of fun. I got exposure for my work and my employer got exposure for the salon.

You never know how things are going to work out and you must always be prepared in any event.

I encourage you to network. Join the ABC in your area. Their number is 203-355-0464. Tell them that Gretchen, the hairdresser from Connecticut, sent you. With always having to recruit new bridal customers, it is a good idea to get to know your local bridal-related businesses in town. An association such as the ABC gets them all in one room at one time, minimizing your efforts and maximizing your returns. And it puts *you* in front of *them*. This makes for a much more positive influence. (Remember, in situations such as these it is not the time to dress like you're going to a hair show. If I am attending a meeting where there are business-people of all kinds I make sure I dress stylishly because I am representing my industry. I keep my hairstyle current but I stay away from the strong trends. If I am doing a hair show I may dress a little more trendy.)

You may choose to contact some of these bridal-related businesses on your own:

- ✻ florists
- ✻ gift shops
- ✻ jewelers
- ✻ country clubs
- ✻ hotels
- ✻ banquet halls
- ✻ photographers
- ✻ wedding salons
- ✻ caterers

You can do this by sending out a salon brochure with a letter expressing your interest in working with them on a referral basis. Here are some tips for networking through the mail and over the phone:

1. Don't just call and try to explain what it is you want to do over the phone. Busy people do not have time to chat. Plus, you will need to speak to someone of authority.

2. The only reason to call the business in the first place is to get a contact name of the person to whom you should be addressing your material.

3. Make sure you have all of the spellings correct.

4. Ask when that person is available to speak over the phone. Explain that you wish to make a follow-up call at a later date.

5. Ask with whom you are speaking and write down their name and the date you called.

6. Save a copy of the letter you send out.

7. Make a note on your calendar of the date you need to call them back.

8. When you call back you can start by saying, "My name is…and I am calling in reference to a letter and brochure about…which I sent out on such and such a date. I had spoken to so and so and she said this would be a good time to call you."

9. Don't be discouraged. Some businesses will network with you and some will not.

When I had my own salon it was in a strip mall on a busy road. There was an established bridal salon in the same strip mall, but they had no interest in working with me. I had to go to another, newer bridal salon down the street. Newer businesses are more open to creative networking.

Here's a quote from Henry Ford's book, *My Life and Work,* from 1922. It still makes a valid point almost eight decades later.

Businessmen go down with their businesses because they like the old way so well they cannot bring themselves to change. …Seldom does the cobbler take up with a newfangled way of soling shoes and seldom does the artisan willingly take up with new methods in his trade."[4]

Think about this when approaching an established business. More than likely they have been burned along the way. And think about this when *you* resist a new way of doing a service that you have done one way for a long time. We are like the artisan Henry Ford is talking about.

Most business owners appreciate it when you are on the ball. They do

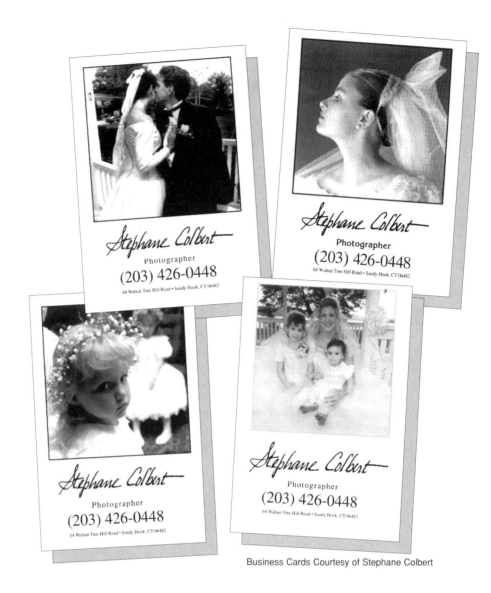

Business Cards Courtesy of Stephane Colbert

not have time for unprofessional people. Nor do they want to be associated with unprofessional businesses.

When networking on a professional level you must walk and talk their language. The material you present must look professional—that includes business cards, salon brochures and any letters you write. The best way to present a letter is on company letterhead. Not all salons have stationery. (If you or the salon do not have a computer, find someone who does or go to the library or copy center.)

When I first started corresponding with Milady Publishing I copied from the letters they sent me. I followed the same setup they used in their business letters to me. If you are unsure as to how to draft a professional letter, copy a letter you have gotten from a company or pick up a book on how to do it at the library. How your material looks and is presented equals whether it is read or put in the trash. Let me share a copy of an actual letter I sent out to *Passion* Magazine.

This is a simple, direct, neat letter. Remember: The people with whom you correspond do not have time for you to

September 16, 1996
Gretchen Maurer
My address
City, State, Zip Code
USA
Phone #

Editor Helen Moy
Dowa Planning Inc.
Dairoku Seiko Bldg.
1-31 Akasaka, 5 Chome
Minato-Ku,
Tokyo 107 Japan

Helen Moy:

Thank you for publishing past works in Coiffure Q and Men's Passion. This time I am sending you a more youth-oriented series of photos. I work on many youths in the salon. Since the baby boomers' children will be our next wave of clients I feel this is a timely campaign. Thank you for your consideration and for offering quality publications for the benefit and exposure of our industry.

Sincerely,

(my signature)

Gretchen Maurer (printed)

be anything but professional. Your work has to speak for itself.

I currently network with two bridal salons. One bridal salon holds open houses one evening every couple of months. They invite bridal-related businesses to come and set up in the bridal salon for a mini bridal show. There is a wedding cake baker, a florist, a manicurist, and myself. We all set up small areas. I set up a mini-station and do hair. I do hair on anyone who wants it done. The bridal salon does a mailing to its clients, and friends and family come, as well. A lot of brides have come to me as clients this way.

The other bridal salon owner and myself met when I was referred to her by a country club with which I network. She was doing a bridal show at the country club and the club events coordinator gave her my name. The events coordinator and the bridal salon owner both became clients of mine. Our salon also got a lot of brides from that show.

Not only did we do great hair for the show but we accessorized each look to go with the gowns the girls were wearing. We put flowers, feathers, jewels, and ornaments in the bridesmaids' hair for something different and beautiful. We stayed for the entire show and networked in the crowd right after the fashion show was over. We wore our salon T-shirts and handed out our business cards. I even overheard a group of women talking about the hairstyles, wondering who did it. I approached them and gave them our business card. I did one women's wedding, and her sisters and mother became clients of the salon.

Another way to network with the bridal salons in your area is to ask if you may display a small photo of your wedding work. I had a 5x7 bridal hairstyle photo and a business card matted and framed to be hung up at the bridal salons. If you get permission to do this take into consideration the image and the color scheme of the bridal salon. Keep the frame no larger than 8x10. A 5x7 photo and a business card fit nicely and look neat.

I also give the bridal salons stacks of my business cards. You may wish to purchase a lovely business card holder that matches the bridal salon so it can display your cards. The salon will appreciate your thoughtfulness. A pile of cards continuously falling over and being a nuisance will soon be tossed into the trash.

Don't forget to write thank you notes or purchase flowers to give to the businesses that help you to promote your services. This is especially important if you are working on a show or fundraiser together. Do as the big people do. When I was at a bridal show for vendors in New York City, flowers kept pouring in from *Modern Bride*. These huge beautiful bouquets of flowers were gifts to the vendors who had advertised in the magazine, a token of thanks from *Modern Bride*. (The vases were even printed with the magazine's name!)

HOSTING EVENING WORKSHOPS

You may also plan on hosting your own mini bridal fair workshops in your salon. Here are some ideas to get you started:

1. Contact a bridal salon to supply gowns for models for the evening. Two or three girls is plenty. Let the bridal shop decide which gowns they want to show.

2. Instruct the models to stop by the bridal salon for a fitting. The bridal shop will not make alterations so make sure the models are tall and around size eight or ten.

3. Invite bridal-related merchants to join your workshop.

4. Purchase a bridal mailing list (this will be discussed later in this chapter).

5. Take out an ad in a bridal section of the newspaper.

6. Share any mailing or advertising expenses with the participating businesses. This is co-op advertising. Co-op advertising is shared time and expenses with other bridal-related businesses.

7. Have a caterer serve hors d'oeuvres.

8. Have the bakery serve a cake.

9. Invite a photographer to set up a display.

10. Have the florist set out arrangements.

11. Invite a limo company to park outside and tie balloons to the car.

You may also invite a jeweler, a travel agent, or any other bridal-related businesses you can fit into your salon. Do this once a year after the holidays, during the doldrums of winter, or in early spring.

In time this mini bridal fair will become an expected event in your community. And every year that you do it, it will flow better and come together easier.

Do not neglect networking within your community. Becoming involved with organizations and service groups is a great way to network and grow your business. Ask your clients what groups they belong to. Here are a few to look for:

🕊 women's service groups

🕊 church groups

🕊 playhouses or theater groups

🕊 Girl Scouts

🕊 those who host annual fundraisers

🕊 civil service groups

This is also a great way to bring in new clients and brides. I cannot count how many fashion shows, school plays, and fundraisers in which I have involved myself.

"The more people in the community who know you, the more work you're going to have. And the more people in the industry who know you, the more renown you'll be. Go to all kinds of events, get involved with charities, do whatever it takes to get out there and meet people," advises Denise Pereau. Denise gave these words of wisdom to *SalonOvations Magazine* in the September 1996 issue.[5] These subjects and their benefits are addressed further in Chapter 9, Going the Extra Mile.

BRIDAL FAIRS

Bridal fairs are huge fairs held in coliseums, country clubs, or event halls. Every bridal-related business is there for the bride to see. Some salons get involved with bridal fairs. The Association of Bridal Consultants can give you a list of local bridal fairs in your area.

Attending bridal fairs is not for every salon, as they can be very expensive. The cost can be anywhere from $200 to $600 for a booth. The booth fee usually includes a copy of the mailing list of attendants. As long as you follow through and use the list for marketing afterwards it's worth the expense and time. Sending your salon to a bridal fair also requires having enough staff to be able to send stylists out of the salon on a Saturday.

Becoming involved with organizations and service groups is a great way to network and grow your business.

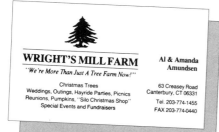

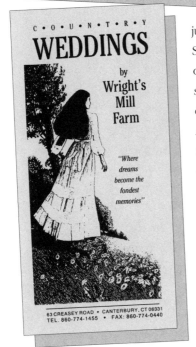

You can also inquire about sharing a booth space with another business. Also see if you can participate in the bridal fair for just one day on the Sunday to avoid the loss of business by taking a stylist out of the salon on a Saturday. At an ABC meeting one of the members said if you call close to the show date to see if there is any space left, you may be able to get it at half price.

If your salon is large enough and can afford to attend a bridal fair it can be great fun and a great opportunity to be very visible. Here are some ways to make the most of a fair:

1. First, inquire about doing the hair for the main bridal fashion show.

2. At your booth, set up a beautiful table and display in conjunction with your salon's image and colors.

3. Bring along accessories to sell; bridal menus, salon menus, business cards, and products.

4. Ask some beautiful clients to be models and give them fabulous hairstyles.

5. Have the models wear dresses from the bridal shop that is presenting the fashions for the show.

6. Instruct them to walk around and pass out information about your salon.

7. Put your salon name on a banner, beauty-pageant style, and have the models wear it. Instead of "Miss USA" across her chest it will say your salon's name.

8. Have a ministation set up and spin some hair!

Bridal fair attendees will line up to have their hair done. It does not need to be wedding-day perfect or so detailed that it takes too long. They will get antsy because they will want to see the rest of the bridal fair. Keep it fun and upbeat. Create the feeling of a hair show. Dress fashionably and in the image of your salon. Play music and have fun. This draws a lot of attention. The general public never sees us in this light and they love it!

Another idea I picked up at an ABC meeting is to put out a big candy dish at the booth. I also saw this done at a hair show. A products company knew how to get people over to their table—they passed out chocolate bars! Candy and free samples encourage people to stop and stand around those few extra seconds to grab their attention. Approach your distributor for hair products samples to pass out at the fair.

🕊 Start networking

🕊 Think beyond your chair

🕊 Get out from behind your chair

🕊 Mingle, meet and network regularly

🕊 Do not be intimidated

We all start off one step at a time, but where we end up is up to us. A turtle has to stick out its neck before it can take a step.

ADVERTISING

Advertising is very expensive. It costs about $50 to attract a single new client through advertising. I have heard many times that a prospective client needs to see your ad seven to twelve times before she will try your services. Basically, advertising is a shot in the dark.

Advertising in Newspapers

Advertising in the paper seems like the easiest and most obvious way to advertise but it's expensive. The uncertainty of reaching your brides is most times not worth the effort and expense.

The Bridal Line Network, a Division of Innovative Telecommunication Services, Inc., has this to say about newspaper advertising:

Often, businesses advertise in large metro papers because of their seemingly attractive circulation. However, if you are trying to target 3,000 brides, and your ad is being circulated in an astounding 600,000 papers, this presents two problems. First, 597,000 of the circulation is wasted to reach 3,000 brides. Second, not 100% of the brides subscribe or are even exposed to the ad. Metro papers are often pleased with 40% coverage. That could mean that even with your 600,000 circulation, 1,800 of the 3,000 brides will never even see the ad." [6]

Don't just wait for newspaper advertising to work—with brides it won't. They want something more personal. The only way newspaper advertising can be effective is to have it run every week. If you can afford this then use newspaper advertising.

Many larger towns have a local bridal magazine or a bridal guide you can advertise in. Also check out your local cable company for co-op advertising on TV.

How about advertising in a national bridal magazine? You can advertise in a national magazine and have your ad run only in the magazines that cover your area. The area or region, as it is referred to, is very broad. But just think how effective a marketing tool regional advertising can be. Not only will prospective brides see your ad but the prestige attached to having an ad run in a national magazine will boost your salon's bridal image. If you have the money to do this type of advertising, go for it!

Make the most of any exposure your salon receives. Have the ad framed and placed in the salon. Use a banner headline: "As seen in *Brides* magazine."

Launch an annual bridal fashion show and use the ad exposure as an anchor for a fundraiser. Tie that in with your ad running in *Brides* and secure local press coverage.

A turtle has to stick out its neck before it can take a step.

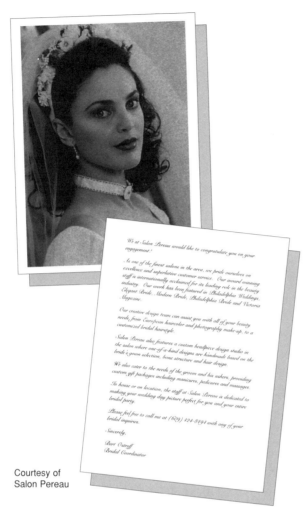

Courtesy of
Salon Pereau

BRIDAL MAILING
LISTS

Another beneficial way of reaching the
bride is direct mail. Bridal mailing lists
are available for purchase through
marketing companies. Look in your
phone book for marketing companies
and get some comparison prices. These
mailing lists are broken down by towns
and counties. What we do at our salon
is purchase a bridal mailing list through
Webster Marketing Co. in Atlanta,
Georgia. They can be reached at
800-543-8987. (We purchase from two
counties because our town is on the
border. Currently we are tracking our
brides to see what county is most
beneficial to us.)

Bridal mailing lists can sometimes
have a lot of duplicate names on them,
and some of the names may not even
be a bride. How these companies get
their names is through places like the
bridal fairs. Brides usually bring a friend
to these events and sometimes the
friends fill out a bogus wedding date
just for the chance to win a door prize.
But this is the chance you have to
take. A little time and effort with the
mailing list can help weed out double
names, as well as brides whose
wedding date is only a month away
(usually by this time the bride already
has made all of her arrangements for
her hair). We also delete any names
from towns more than one hour away.
Once our list is edited to our needs,
we then mail out a bridal brochure
(such as the one shown here) to brides
whose wedding date is three months
or more away.

To find out about advertising in a
national magazine such as *Brides,* I
called and spoke with Deidra Sirscusa.
Deidra is the regional advertising
contact person for Area 2, which covers
Metro New York City, Connecticut,
Northern New Jersey, and Eastern
Canada. Each area has a specific person
to contact for information. Look for
your region on the editors' page of any
bridal magazine and call for information
on your specific area. *Brides* magazine
has the largest circulation of any
national regional bridal publication.
This would be a tremendous boost to
the image of your salon. Also consider
carrying *Brides* magazine for sale in
your bridal department.

After our first mailing to three hundred brides we received ten calls within two weeks. A 3–4% return on direct mail advertising is average. Some brides held onto the brochure and some passed it along to others. Of the ten, who all scheduled appointments with our salon, eight asked for custom headpieces. The overflow into the cutting and color department has been tremendous for the salon.

SUPPORT FROM THE TOP

I am fortunate to have the support of my employers, Noel Direnzo and Alan DeMonte. Noel, co-owner of the Alan Noel Salon where I work in Milford, Connecticut, had wanted to tap into the bridal industry for several years before I came to the salon. She had a great idea and saw a huge potential market. As a partner in the Alan Noel Salon with Alan Delmonte, working behind the chair as a color specialist, pursuing college, and raising a preteen daughter, she just did not have the time or personnel to make it happen. When I came to work at the salon she allowed me the freedom and offered the financial support I needed to get the department up and running. If more stylists would take on responsibility, lay out a plan using the information in this book, and present it to the owner of the salon, I'm sure they would receive the support needed to get a bridal department started. Alan Noel Salon is living proof it can work!

Noel has this to say to the stylists and owners considering a bridal department:

First, be committed to the plan, look at it as a cooperative effort. The salon owner has to have the frame of mind to support a willing stylist or manager who wants to work to their full potential. An organized and detailed bridal department generates more money from wedding parties. By seeking mutual benefit it creates a win-win situation for all involved.[7]

Do your homework, plan some goals, sell your ideas to the owner of the salon. And for the owners out there, maybe there is already someone in your salon willing to take on the responsibility of creating and running a bridal department.

TIPS

⚐ When calling any business for information, have what you want to say ready, rehearsed, and written down.

⚐ Professionalism = First Impression

⚐ Realize networking is continuous

⚐ Get visible and involved in the community

⚐ Join the ABC

⚐ Plan a mini bridal fair in your salon

⚐ Purchase a regional bridal mailing list

> "*An organized and detailed bridal department generates more money from wedding parties.*"

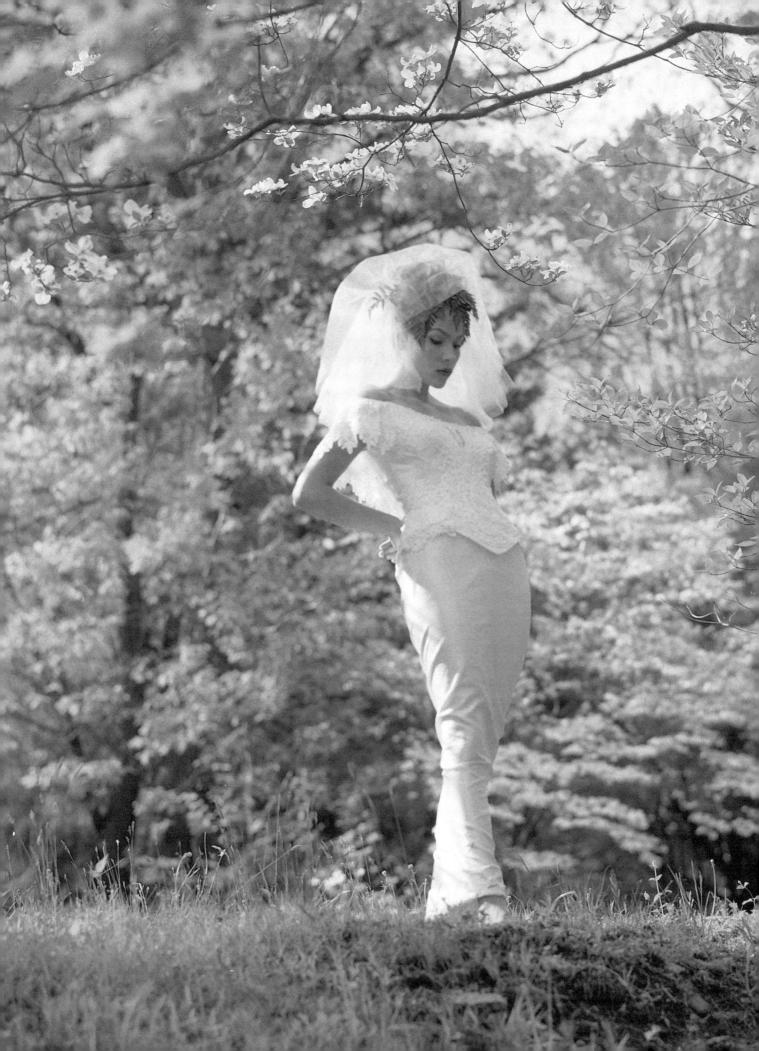

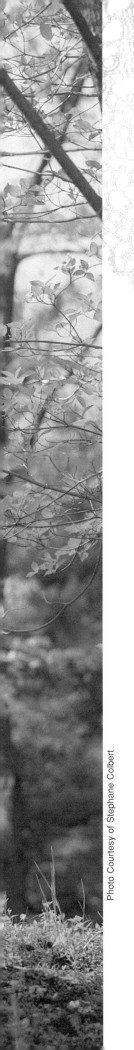

CHAPTER 5

The Total Bridal Look

_W_e are part of a wonderfully creative field. Creative people are all around to inspire and motivate us. We all possess the ability to become creative individuals, and creativity needs to be developed and continually fed. Creative people will tell you they are inspired by many different mediums. Hair, makeup, fashion, and the visual arts all feed the creative hairdresser. Creativity is the ability to put together pieces to form a finished look. Even when we put together an outfit or create a retail display, it is done by putting together different parts. These parts are called "elements."

Elements, when put together, become a total look. These elements can also create a certain mood and help define an image. Marketing specialists, who help a company sell and develop a product, try to create a certain "feeling" for the product in the mind of the consumer. This feeling attracts a certain type of customer. For an example, let's look at two different salon retail product lines.

The first product line we'll use as an example is designed to attract an environmentally aware client. A feeling and image for the product is created by using "elements" such as soft color tones, dried flowers, and smooth graphics in their ads.

The second example is a product line designed to attract a more youthful, upbeat client. Remember the original Vavoom line from Matrix? The ad campaign showed young, happy people full of energy with great, carefree hair. The black-and-purple packaging was exciting and bold.

I spoke with Vavoom's original creator, Dwight Miller, to find out how he came up with the idea. The word he keep using over and over again was _concept._

" _There were four or five lines out there at the time and they weren't selling. It was because they were too serious. My concept for the Vavoom line was one of fun. Bringing in the concept and element of fun into the product line was the reason for its success. It is so important for anything you want to create, even if it is a bridal department within your salon, to have a concept in mind and create from there._" [1]

Mood, concept, elements. The bride has one concept in mind for her wedding day. She needs you to bring it all together in her total bridal look.

The bride needs you to create a hairstyle that matches the bridal look she has in mind for herself on her wedding day. This chapter will help you to discover and execute her total bridal look. All the elements—her dress, hair, makeup, nails, and headpiece—need to work together.

ELEMENTS OF DESIGN

Let's take a closer look at the elements of design. Understanding them individually will make it easier to use them to your advantage.

> _The bride has one concept in mind for her wedding day. She needs you to bring it all together in her total bridal look._

The elements of design are:

- Line
- Size
- Shape
- Position
- Density
- Texture

You may refer to the appendices to get a better idea of these as we go through them.

Line

The line of an updo or a wedding dress is the direction it takes. Either horizontally across or vertically up and down. Horizontal lines broaden and shorten. Remember, the eye follows the width. Vertical and diagonal lines slim and elongate. The line within an updo may be horizontal or vertical. The line can be dramatic and sophisticated or soft and romantic. Picture an updo of sleek smooth curls dramatically drawing the eye upward. This added height creates a feeling of sophistication and elegance for your client. Picture a bride in a wreath headpiece with soft curls spilling out and lots of tendrils hanging. This line is horizontal and holds a soft romantic feeling for the bride.

Creating an updo equals selling a feeling. There is not a hair show that goes by where platform educator Paul DiGrigoli doesn't ask, "How many of you have made someone in your chair cry?" A few brave hands go up. Then he says, "Now tell the truth." A few more go up. Then he asks, "How many have done a new cut on someone, who then runs around the salon showing

everyone and the client says she wishes she did this five years ago?" Lots of hands go up. Then he asks, "What are we really selling?" The answer? "A feeling." And giving the bride the feeling she wants through her hair and total look creates a happy bride. And a happy bride becomes a client for life.

The dress also has a line and the line of the dress should match the hair. A long, slim-fitted wedding gown has a vertical line and is complemented with a narrow bob tucked behind the ears or a bunch of curls piled high on the head. The line of a traditional, full-skirt wedding gown is horizontal. Added to many full gowns of this style are off-the-shoulder sleeves which only enhance the horizontal line. This style is complemented by a softer, wider, more romantic hairstyle.

This is a general guideline for most brides, as for creative people and artists there are no rules. A bride with a flair for the dramatic and a strong personality can certainly carry off a total look that does not "match." This is why all things (personal tastes, coloring, personality, tradition, etc.) must be considered and why you need your bride to communicate her wishes to you.

Size

The size of an updo depends on a few factors. How much hair the client does or doesn't have. How tall or petite or full-figured she is. Plus, the overall line, size, detail, and length of her dress.

If the bride is in a slim suit for a daytime wedding it would be important to keep her hairstyle compact and

Creating an updo equals selling a feeling.

simple. If the bride is wearing a full skirt or bustled wedding gown, then she can have a larger headpiece and hairstyle. Again, try to match the overall size of the client and her head to her hairstyle. *This element of design cannot be altered because it is a matter of balance.*

I had a bride who was petite but wore a traditional full gown and chapel-length veil. She had a small head and young face. I created a smaller updo and made her a more-petite headpiece to be worn toward the back of the head. It allowed the horizontal line to flow but still worked with her proportions. If you have a petite client with a lot of hair you do not need to use all of the hair in the updo. Tuck and hide some of it inside a few of the curls. If you have a large client with little hair use a hair rat or hair additions. Or suggest a fuller headpiece and veil.

Shape

The shape of the finished updo or hairstyle needs to complement the shape of the face and head as well as the proportions of the client and her dress.

The shape is the outer line a hairstyle makes. Visualize a wide bob making the outer shape of a triangle. A shag or layered cut has the outer shape of a rectangle. A wedge has the shape of a diamond. Some shapes are reminiscent of certain time periods, like the full crown and flip of the 1960s. Many of the simple clothing styles from that era so popular today are complemented by the simple shape in the hairstyles adapted from that time as well. The feathered-back flipped hair worn by Farrah Fawcett in the 1970s was complemented by the flipped-out bell bottoms. The narrow shape and closeness to the head of the Roaring 20s bob was a visual match to the bound breasts and slim, body-hugging clothes worn at that time.

One of my bridal clients had a Gothic-theme wedding. The outer shape of her updo matched the shape of her wedding gown. Next time you see a picture of a Victorian lady in her bustled gown, notice that her hair is bustled up in the back as well.

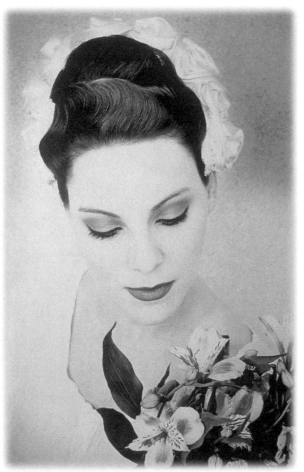

Photo Courtesy of Geri Mataya

Position

Let's go back to horizontal, vertical, and diagonal lines for a moment. A diagonal hairstyle must have something to balance its position. It may be a small wedding hat, a comb of flowers, or a headpiece designed to sit diagonally. I had an older bride who wanted a fun sexy look for her second wedding. She had a profile-style headpiece (the kind that sits along the side of the face). I had to position cluster curls in a pony-tail opposite it for balance. If you want to use a hair ornament for balance, first make sure the bride is not going to take it off after the ceremony.

A simple bun positioned on the top of the head can look like a child going to a dance recital. A bun posi-tioned at the nape of the neck can look matronly. If the bride wishes to have her hair placed at the nape because of her headpiece, make the style detailed and contemporary. An updo positioned vertically can be chic and dramatic. Placing the headpiece just under the design exposes the hairstyle, thereby showing off your work.

Is the back of her gown totally open? Suggest positioning one long curl to flow down the curve of her spine. Brides love your interest in them and welcome suggestions.

Density

Density has to do with the feeling and look of weight or thickness. If the bride is in a heavy satin gown and the brides-maids are in velvet, giving the party hairstyles of soft, wispy, flowing curls will not balance the total look. If the

bride is wearing a flowing tulle dress, the hair should also be flowing.

Many times I need to lead a client into an understanding of this element of design to produce the correct updo or hairstyle for her total look.

Density produces another set of challenges when the client's natural hair interferes with the style she requests. She may want a soft curly hairstyle but have heavy, stick-straight hair. In that case, if she is getting married in a few months, you may be able to sell her a perm service. Or the bride may have natural curl but want a smooth, sculpted look.

The first question I ask any special-occasion client, be it a wedding or a prom, is, "What are you wearing?" This gets the focus off her hair and allows you to listen for clues as to the appropriate hairstyle for her dress. You will get a feeling from her as she describes her dress. You can listen for density clues like "heavy satin" or "velvet" or "lace" or "chiffon." Allow her to get all of her information out; don't cut her off, assuming you know what she wants. She may use words like *fitted, soft, flowing, heavy brocade, lace, chiffon, elegant, romantic, chic, tradi-tional, unique, Victorian,* etc. Look at her face shape, and her body line and try to come up with something as she is speaking. When she is done, *then* make your suggestions.

Don't ask her what she wants for her hair before you know what she is wearing. Even if I have a client who begins to describe the hair she wants, I bring her back to talking about her

> **B**rides love your interest in them and welcome suggestions.

gown. That way, if what she wants contradicts the line, shape, and density of her gown I can point this out to her when we discuss her hair.

Remember, clients know only two words when it comes to long hair: *bun* and *French twist*. If you find that is all you are doing and you are bored with your work then this tip of asking about their dress will help. If all you know is bun and French twist, then get practicing the updos in this book. When something feels uncomfortable it means you are learning something new.

Texture

Texture has the ability to create a feeling with hair similar to density. Think about the daring strong statement produced by a head of glistening finger waves. Or the detailed, ethnic look created by small braiding. The smooth texture of a sleek bob is a classic.

Look for texture in the bride's dress and headpiece. Fabric can be braided, gathered, puckered, or smooth. Texture in the hair can be matched to the dress, or it can be done in the opposite direction to create contrast. Picture a bride in a long, slim, simple, fitted gown. Give this bride a head full of soft flowing curls and her hair is sure to stand out.

Now picture a heavily beaded and sequined gown. Complement this texture by adorning the hair with lots of pearls and crystals glued to hairpins. I had a bride that had a pattern of ribbons woven in her dress. I incorporated the same texture and pattern in her hair.

Pay attention to details such as these elements of design and you will become the bridal specialist every bride will want to use on her wedding day.

PRINCIPLES OF COMPOSITION

Now you have a better understanding of the elements of design. You are able to help the bridal client find her "total bridal look" by composing these individual elements together. The principles of composition are when you use these elements to create her "total bridal look." Now we will learn three key principles of composition as they relate to the bride's total look:

1. Emphasis

2. Contrast

3. Balance

Emphasis

What is to be the main emphasis of the bride's total look? It may be an antique headpiece or her mother's wedding gown from the 1950s. The bride may have beautiful, long red hair and want an updo to be the main emphasis. She may love the back of her gown and want the emphasis to be placed there. Ask the bride if she has a main emphasis to her look; she will appreciate the inquiry. Training the eye to look to the principles of design and composition will help you become more creative. When creating a custom headpiece I ask the bride what element(s) from the gown she would like me to emphasize in her headpiece. It may be the texture of the appliqué, the sparkle of the sequins, the bow in the back, or the flowers from the bouquet.

Contrast

Contrast reveals various shapes and lines. There can be contrasting textures in a dress, like a lace dress with a velvet sash. There can also be contrasting textures in a hairstyle. I had a young prom client and she wanted an updo that had curls, coils, and braids—all within one style. Contrast asks to be noticed. A shy person wants to avoid contrast.

Detailed contrast suggests clarity and density because it can be seen. A black-and-white wedding, for example, is detailed contrast. I have a bride who is having a black-and-white wedding and she also wants detailed contrast in her updo. The flowers for this wedding are a dense, detailed, round bouquet. Sometimes without even knowing it, brides tend to blend a theme throughout all of their wedding choices.

Subtle contrast creates a sense of vagueness, such as a floral pastel dress worn by the bridal party. When working with long hair remember to keep texture and contrast in harmony with the total look. In dressing short hair, contrast plays an important part as well. Curls made with a curling iron or Velcro rollers and then finger tossed are an example of subtle contrast. A pincurl set of deep waves is detailed contrast in a pattern.

Balance

Let me stress that a balanced look is the most important principle of composition. When composed together, all elements must be balanced. The bride's hairstyle and headpiece needs to look balanced to the dress and head form. The hairstyle should look balanced on the head. You don't want to create a style that looks like it is going to fall over.

Balance of the total look can be created with symmetry, meaning all elements are the same. For example, flowing dress, flowing hair, soft curls, and soft makeup. Symmetry also lends to a classical look. Think of the perfect bob haircut or the classic ballerina with a symmetrical bun. Picture a classic suit with a straight row of buttons.

A look may also be balanced *asymmetrically*. An asymmetrical look is created when different and unequal forces play opposite each other yet balance. This balance is called *counter-balance*. If a bride is to wear a hat tilted to one side the hairstyle should be fuller on the opposite side to counter-balance. If the bride has short hair, yet a full gown, suggest to her a fuller veil for balance of her total look.

If the hairstyle is to have orna-mentation, design the updo or hairstyle to use the ornamentation to create counterbalance. Balance is everywhere, in artwork, flower arrangements, sculp-ture, and architecture. Look for it.

FACE SHAPES

Not every client has a significant face shape that needs balancing by her wedding hairstyle, but you will run across some who do. All face shapes are defined by the outer shape the face makes. At the same time their features can be soft or angular within the face.

A balanced look is the most important principle of composition.

Let's look further into this important dimension of hairdressing.

The basic face shapes are:

🌾 Oval

🌾 Round

🌾 Oblong

🌾 Heart

🌾 Diamond

🌾 Square

🌾 Rectangle

🌾 Triangle

The first four face shapes are soft and curved. The last four face shapes have more angles and corners.

How many of your clients sit in your chair and say they have a round face? This is because they feel chubby. Someone can have full cheeks but it doesn't mean they have a round face. The face shape is determined by the shape of the outer edges of the face, not the fullness within it.

Following is a creative exercise to help you to determine someone's face shape. I suggest you put aside some creative time to learn how to find a face shape. First practice on the salon staff and friends until you are comfortable with the process.

To truly define a face shape you will need:

🌾 elastics, scrunchy, or headband

🌾 hair clips

🌾 brown eye liner pencil

Let's begin the exercise:

1. Put your model or client in a salon chair facing the mirror.

2. Pull all of the hair off their face and secure it out of the way.

3. Stand behind them.

4. Look at the outer edges of their hairline at the sides of the forehead. This area will either be curved or have corners.

5. With the eyeliner pencil, put a dot at the furthest outer edge or at the "corners" of the hairline. The dots must be visible when looking straight on at the client. See examples below:

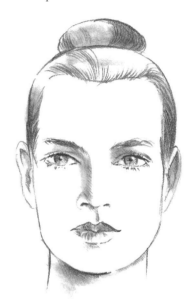

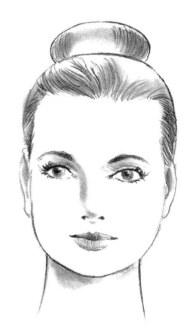

6. Next, look at the outer edges of their cheeks.

7. Place a dot on both sides at the widest point.

8. You must remain behind the model. Do not stand to the side of them.

9. You must be able to see the dots when looking straight into the mirror.

10. You will see either definite width in the cheek bone area, soft curves, or no width at all. See examples below:

11. Now look at the outer edges of their jawline.

12. Remain behind them, do not stand to the side of the person.

13. Picture the face as flat and one dimensional.

14. Place a dot at both sides of the edge of their jawline so that they are visible when looking straight at the person into the mirror. See examples below:

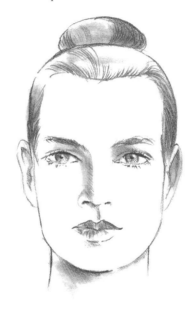

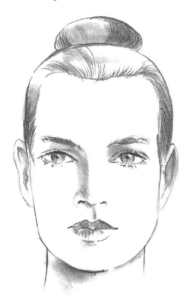

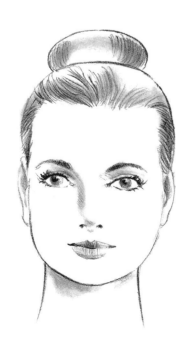

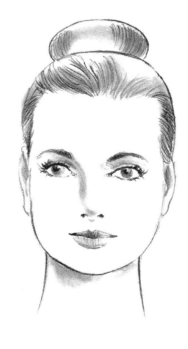

15. Now place a dot at the bottom edge of the chin. Do not put the dot under it or in the middle of the chin, but at the outer edge.

16. Again you must able to see the dot when looking straight into the mirror.

17. Think of the face as being as flat as a piece of paper. See examples below:

18. Now place a dot at the top of the forehead at the hairline. Use the nose as a guide to get the center.

19. This dot may be higher than the side hairline dots or it may be level with them. See examples below:

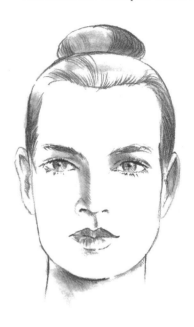

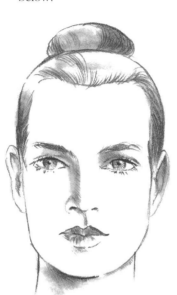

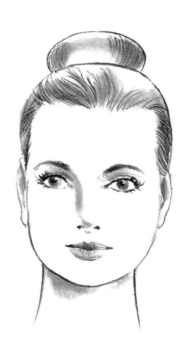

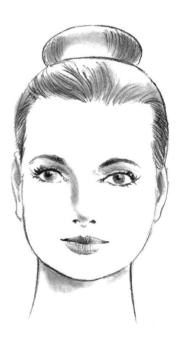

20. With all the dots complete, stand behind the person.

21. Look at them in the mirror.

22. Squint your eyes and mentally and visually connect the dots.

23. A face shape should emerge.

Which Shape?

❧ An **oval** face should be slightly longer than is it wide, with curved soft edges.

❧ A **round** face should have equal distance all around, with the nose as a center guide. It should be as wide as it is long, with rounded edges.

❧ An **oblong** face is an elongated oval shape. Many oblongs are mistaken for an oval, but placed next to a true oval you can see that they are oblong. Oblongs do not wear long hair well.

❧ A **heart-shape** is wider at the eye, temple, and cheek area, with a narrow chin. The edges are soft and curved. They look best in a bob below the chin to balance the width in the eye area.

❧ A **diamond-shape** face shape has edges or corners. The center hairline dot should be higher than the side hairline dots. From the chin dot up to the cheek dot should be a sharp angle. The cheeks should be the widest part of the face.

❧ A **square** face is when the temple dots and the hairline dot make a straight line across the forehead. The temple dots and the cheek dots also make a straight line along the side of the face. The jawline dots and the chin dot also make a relatively straight line across the bottom of the face. The chin may stick out a bit. When the distance from the top of the face to the chin matches the width, this is a square face. A layered hairstyle around the face softens a square face.

❧ A **rectangular** face, which I have, is similar to a square, but the face is longer than it is wide. I must have bangs to soften my broad forehead and lend curve to my face. With my bangs you would guess my face to be an oval. This is why you must pull all the hair off the face to properly determine the face shape.

❧ A **triangular** face is similar to a heart shape, but the lines and edges are sharper and more angular with a triangular face.

A face shape is not set in stone. Someone's seemingly oval face may look more round next to someone else's oval. Two people can both be square but one will be more square than the other. Do this as a group and compare face shapes. Eventually you will familiarize yourself with all the face shapes and will have found each one on someone. Then all you will need to do is pull a client's hair back and their face shape will be staring right back at you!

HAIRSTYLES FOR FACE SHAPES

With an understanding of balance and counterbalance, helping the bride choose a complementary hairstyle for her face shape is easy. Picture the face shape under the hairstyle.

Helping the bride choose a complementary hairstyle for her face shape is easy.

An **oval** face can wear any style but it must be in proportion to her body size.

A **round** face shape needs hair down along the sides to elongate it. I had a bride in for a trial-run appointment who had a very round face. She was not overweight but just had a distinctly round face. I tried her hair up several different ways and none of them flattered her. We had to do a style that was all down. I set her hair to create soft curls that blended with her soft features.

An **oblong** face needs width for balance. This bride looks great with a wreath-style headpiece. An off-the-shoulder gown also flatters an oblong face. The hairstyle should be wider at the sides of the face and not drawn back too severely. An updo of cluster curls looks best covering the width of her head and not piled too-centered or too-high.

A **heart-shape** or **triangular** face shape has width at the eye and cheek bone area. This bride needs width from the hairstyle at the bottom, or netting across the back of the head to balance a narrow chin. Also, a style that is narrow and higher balances the chin. A bob left down is a great look for this client, too.

A **diamond-shape** face shape is my favorite because it is usually accompanied by great cheekbones. I love to do photography and angular faces can be dramatic. If the bride is dramatic and strong, then accentuate her sharp features by pulling her hair off her face and doing dramatic makeup. A back headpiece will draw the eye up and back, exposing a beautiful diamond-shape face. If her personality is soft and her gown is traditional then soften her look with curls and tendrils. A diamond face shape is proportioned like an oval face and can wear most any style.

A very **square** jawline needs softness. Remember, softness, as in a tendril, can be detailed and smooth with a crisp, solid curl hanging down, or the curls can be fluffy and wispy. Let the density of the fabric in her gown and her features guide you as to what kind of tendril to choose.

A **rectangular** face can have a strong chin or a weak chin. There is more length than width, so widen the overall look with a wreath or a wider updo. Soften the rectangle with curls.

Face shapes are a lot of fun to learn about, but this is also very important for training your eye. Our profession is strictly visual. We are artists and all have a unique perspective. The "rules" of design are there to guide you; they are the basics. The basics must be mastered before you can bend and sculpt them. You do have a signature to leave behind, but remember there is a person under that head of hair. The bride's wedding day is not the time to bend the creative rules.

An artist's canvas does not talk back to the artist, have a budget to stick to, or an opinion. Neither can "it" get up and go to another studio because it wants someone who will listen to it. Our limitations with our creative work may be why we can become so frus-

The "rules" of design are there to guide you.

trated or experience burnout. Practicing on models or doing a photo shoot helps to curtail burnout. The brides are a real creative outlet for me; I enjoy them very much.

JEWERLY SELECTION FOR FACE SHAPES

To fully service the bride a salon may wish to carry bridal jewelry. There are many ways to do this. If your budget allows, you can purchase a line of wedding jewelry to have in the salon. The best way to find a line is to go to a professional bridal fair. Refer back to Chapter Four for fair information.

At our salon we carry a line of jewelry on consignment, so there is no cost or inventory for us to carry. Our bridal jewelry is separate from our regular jewelry and is displayed in our bridal area. I consider our jewelry consignor a part of the salon's bridal team. Michelle Popper, who carries a line of costume and semi-precious jewelry under her own name, will hunt down a particular style a bride may request. She also does jewelry consulting for bridal parties; she will pick out the perfect styles for everyone from the mothers to the flower girls.

If you wish to carry jewelry but your budget does not allow it, look for someone like Michelle who sees this as a win-win opportunity. Or you may wish to work with a bridal salon that carries jewelry. Ask them to provide your salon with a small display of bridal jewelry. It will work best if you can actually sell it at the hair salon, because of impulse buying. I had a bride that came in with a set of jewelry to put on after I finished her hair. She saw another set she liked better and bought it on the spot the morning of her wedding!

Call the Association of Bridal Consultants and inquire if they know of anyone in your area who carries bridal jewelry. Look in the phone book under "Jewelry." Most important, you are letting the bridal customer know you care about her *total* bridal look.

Before we begin discussing which jewelry is for which face shape, let's think for a moment about the difference between a diamond shape and an oval. Whether it is a jewel, a picture frame, or a face shape, there are distinct differences between a diamond shape and an oval.

🕊 A diamond has edges and corners.

🕊 An oval is soft and curved.

As in a face shape, a diamond, triangle, or square has edges, corners, planes, and angles. By "planes" I mean the surface, structure, and profile of the face. Are the eyes deep set with a strong brow bone, a sharp nose, prominent cheekbones, and a distinct jawline? This is an angular or sharp face. This face is best surrounded with jewelry with similar angles, sharp detail, or corners, like triangles, square-cut stones, or straight lines.

An oval, round, or heart-shape face has no distinct lines or edges. A soft face may be flatter. The eyes are closer to the surface of the face, the nose is rounder at the tip, the lips are fuller, cheekbones are less prominent,

> *Whether it is a jewel, a picture frame, or a face shape, there are distinct differences between a diamond shape and an oval.*

and the jawline is soft. This face shape is complemented by oval or round shapes and soft edges. A face may be a combination of both angular and soft lines, but have an overall feeling to it of being one or the other.

The jewelry itself will have its own lines. The outside shape the jewelry makes is similar to the types of face shapes. Jewelry also has soft lines, as in curves and ovals or hard lines, as in rectangles and diamond shapes. The lines need to match the lines of the face for balance. I did a photo shoot where the photographer had these great earrings. The earrings were so unique that they inspired me to create the same lines and texture in the updo (see Chapter 2 opening photo). The next time you look at photos of hairstyles in *Passion* study the jewelry and the clothes more closely. You will see how they bend, inspire, or contrast the hairstyle.

Most people are drawn to a complementary jewelry shape. You are used to looking at yourself everyday, subconsciously you are drawn to certain shapes. Many times stylists impose a look on a client complementing to *themselves* and not the bride. This happens without thinking. You are naturally drawn to what you like. As a specialist you have to learn to train your eye to see everyone for who they are.

The same guidelines for selecting a hairstyle to complement a face shape apply to jewelry. The neckline of the gown, the face shape, and the size of the bride all need to be taken into

consideration when selecting jewelry. The right jewelry will flatter the bride, the wrong jewelry will just stand out. To help the bride with her jewelry selection look to blending the lines of her face with the lines in the jewelry. To create counterbalance with the necklace and earrings look to her face shape and gown neckline.

Take these points into consideration:

🕸 Ask the bride what her dress looks like.

🕸 Pay particular attention to the bodice and neckline.

🕸 Is it off the shoulder?

🕸 Observe her face shape.

🕸 Observe her body size.

🕸 Is her face angular or soft?

Before you suggest a hairstyle ask the bride if she is planning on wearing any jewelry. If she hasn't thought that far ahead, then suggest a necklace and earring style based on her gown neckline and her face shape. You need to know her whole ensemble before you try out a hairstyle. If the bride is wearing an off-the-shoulder gown and is not planning on wearing a necklace then think of using some hair to fill in the space of skin that will be exposed between her chin and gown neckline. If she is secure in her appearance she may want the strong impact of her long neck and bare shoulders showing, minus any jewelry or tendrils.

Now that you have a better understanding of face shapes and jewelry shapes let's look to each face shape individually.

The same guidelines for selecting a hairstyle to complement a face shape apply to jewelry.

Earrings

- An **oval** face can wear any shape earring. Keep the size of the earring in balance to the size of the bride, whether she is petite or large. In keeping with the soft lines of her face, soft shapes such as pearls, teardrops, circles, and ovals are best.

- A **round** face needs earrings with length to elongate it. A drop earring works best in shapes that are also soft, like a teardrop.

- An **oblong** face does best with a button earring, drawing the eye horizontally.

- A **heart-shape** face needs earrings that are wider at the bottom to balance a narrow chin. Shapes such as teardrops, inverted triangles, or button earrings work well.

- A **diamond-shape** face can follow the same guidelines as for an oval, but this face shape can carry a more dramatic design. Corners, points, and harder edges complement the angular face. Cut crystals are nice with the diamond face.

- **Square** faces are complemented by a drop earring to create the look of length.

- **Rectangular** faces can do well with a button style, keeping with the lines of the face.

- A **triangular** face shape is similar to a heart shape but with more prominent angles. Balance this face with width at the bottom.

Necklaces

Necklaces should complement the neckline of the gown, the face shape, and the detail of the bodice. A very ornate gown and headpiece can carry a more ornate jewelry selection. Or the bride may choose simple jewelry so as not to compete with the gown. Let's look at each face shape individually with the necklace in mind.

- An **oval** face can wear anything. Match the texture and designs in her gown when choosing a necklace.

- A **round** face needs a necklace that adds length to her look. A longer or Y-style necklace complements a round face. Stay away from chokers or short necklaces. Also stay away from large stones or large pearls— you don't want to add any visual thickness to the neck with a round face. A deep-plunging neckline can carry a beautiful necklace and is great for a round face.

- An **oblong** face can carry a choker-style necklace well. This helps to break up the vertical line that is happening with an oblong face.

- A **heart-shape** face also looks great with a choker or a double or triple strand of pearls. With the heart-shape face the chin is narrow. Creating fullness at the neck with the right necklace balances the wider eye and cheekbone areas.

- A **diamond-shape** face is like the oval face shape but with corners. It can carry any style. Just keep it proportioned to the bride's size. Drops of crystals look beautiful with a diamond face.

🪶 **Square** faces need length and softness. A Y-style or a simple strand of pearls that hang a little bit longer is perfect.

🪶 A **rectangular** face needs softening and width. Shorter necklaces work nicely.

🪶 A **triangular** face is a heart shape with corners and angles. Remember, you can match the angles for impact or counterbalance them for softness. Stay away from necklaces that end with a point. A wider look balances the triangle face.

Brides will appreciate your knowledge. An educated bridal specialist should be educated in all areas of bridal beauty. The more you research the bridal industry the more knowledgeable you will become. The more knowledgeable you become the more confident you will be. You need to be able to address all the beauty needs of the bride. She will ultimately look to you to give her the total bridal look she is after. The bride eagerly looks to her stylist to make her wedding day personal and perfect. Let that stylist be you!

ORNAMENTING HAIRSTYLES

Ornamenting hairstyles is an area that is neglected in long-hair design. Or maybe you feel it is an area of design best left for hair shows. Let me assure you it isn't. If you are comfortable with updos or even bored with them, then you are ready to take your creative work a step further. Ornamenting your hairstyles is fun and it keeps the client interested.

Plus, it adds to your ticket price, and brings in many, many referrals.

With the bridal client, ornamenting the hairstyle may even replace the need for the bride to purchase a headpiece. With headpieces in the price range of hundreds of dollars you can easily charge the bride $150 and up for an ornamented wedding hairstyle. Here's how you can do it:

1. Ask the bride if she has looked at any headpieces yet.

2. If she says yes, then ask her what price range she has in mind.

3. Use that price range as a barometer to price what you want to do for her.

4. If the bride is thinking about purchasing a headpiece in a bridal shop that is $300 and you ornament her hair instead for $180 you are saving her money!

5. Pricing is based on the economic climate surrounding your salon and your image.

6. Basing your prices on what she had in mind to spend is always a good starting point.

When you become valuable to the marketplace you can set your own prices based on what you feel your work is worth. You are offering her something custom, unique, and beautiful. It is a win-win situation for everyone! Today's bride wants something different, something special and unique to her. Begin offering this service and your salon will draw brides like bees to honey!

What if the bride has already purchased a headpiece? Even if the

Shape	Characteristics	Hairstyle	Earrings	Necklaces
Oval	Slightly longer than it is wide, with curved, soft edges	Any	Any (keep size in balance to size of bride)—pearls, teardrops, circles, ovals	Any (match texture & design in gown)
Round	As wide as it is long with rounded edges, equal distance all around (with nose as center)	Needs hair down along sides to elongate it	Needs earrings with length—drop earrings, teardrops	Necklace that addes length — Y-style (no chokers)
Oblong	An elongated oval shape	Needs width for balance; hairstyles should be wider at sides and not drawn back	Draw eye horizontally—button earrings	Help break up vertical line—choker
Heart (Triangle)	Wider at the eye, temple, and cheek area with a narrow chin	Needs width at bottom	Needs earrings wider at bottom—inverted triangles, buttons, teardrops	Create fullness at the neck—double- or triple-strand pearls
Diamond	Has edges or corners, with cheeks as widest part of face	Any	Corners, points, and harder edges complement—cut crystals	Any (keep in proportion to size of bride)
Square	Distance from top of the face to the chin matches the width	Needs softness	To create look of length—drop earrings	Need length and softness—Y-style or hanging pearls
Rectangle	Similar to square but face is longer than it is wide	Needs softness and width	In keeping with lines of face—buttons for needed width	Needs softening and width—shorter necklaces

bride already has her headpiece, consider ornamenting her hairstyle. Use complementing pearls, crystals, or flowers that match her headpiece. This will "tie" together her hair and headpiece. Also consider ornamenting the hair under the bridal veil. This is especially important if the bride is going to take off her veil after the wedding ceremony. Many headpieces now come with a removable veil, allowing the headpiece to stay on. Some headpieces are very full with a lot of tulle. These cover most of the hairstyle. Many of the brides who wear these choose to remove the entire headpiece at the reception. Your hairstyle underneath needs to be perfect and ornamented. A bare updo will look unfinished when paired with the bridal gown.

I had a bride who wore a hat for her wedding headpiece. She wanted to be able to remove it at the reception. She wanted her hair in a horizontal roll that just showed under the brim of the hat. During the consultation I learned she had pearls in her dress, plus she had dark brown hair which is visually dense. I suggested to her that I drape strands of pearls on the outside of the roll. I also glued pearls of different size to hairpins and placed them along the seam of the roll. It looked lovely and even showed just under the brim of the hat. It created a beautiful, personal look and she was comfortable with removing her hat at the wedding reception.

There is a new trend emerging where the bride actually changes her entire wedding ensemble and has a different dress for the reception. I had one bride who was going to do this.

You need to think of her hair and how it needs to complement both dresses. An ornamenting style under the traditional headpiece is just right in situations like this.

The first step in ornamenting hairstyles is to have a creative desire to learn. Most craft shops, art stores, and local adult education centers offer a variety of art classes. The class that helped me the most in developing my creative eye and understand balance was a fresh flower arrangement class. A flower arrangement is the closest in design to an updo. It must look balanced and perfect from all angles. It has weight and texture and gives a feeling to the viewer just as an updo does.

Before I became a hairdresser I took sculpture in college. This and flower arrangement are both three-dimensional forms of design. A silk flower class would also be very beneficial for design purposes as well as learning how to use a glue gun.

If you would like a better understanding of color, a painting class would be very enlightening. I have also seen color analysis and French braiding offered as adult educational classes.

Why not teach a class yourself?

Call the board of education in your town to inquire about the classes being offered or how you might get involved teaching one yourself. Getting out from behind the chair and into the community will expand your mind. It will prevent burnout. It is fun. You may also get a few new clients out of it.

CLASSES TO CONSIDER TAKING:

- Flower arranging
- Sculpture
- Photography
- Drawing
- Painting
- Pottery

CLASSES TO CONSIDER TEACHING:

- Color analysis
- French braiding
- Mother-daughter braiding classes
- Face shapes and makeup application
- Skin care and makeup for teens
- Make your own hair ornaments

IDEAS FOR ORNAMENTING

Now is the time to go beyond threading pearls onto the ends of hairpins. Keep your eye open for beautiful buttons, old earrings, interesting pins, and beautiful beads. Look in consignment shops for old jewelry. Check out tag sales and yard sales for treasures. Look in fabric stores for buttons, beads, and jewels. Personally, I prefer older jewelry. The stones are of a better quality and will shine more brilliantly. Austrian crystal beads are much more beautiful than the plastic ones in the craft shops. Old buttons off old clothes are much cheaper than a new button in the craft shop. Since I have been making hair ornaments for a while, people bring me pieces of old jewelry and clothing. The owner of our local consignment shop

also calls me now and again when something interesting comes in the store. Talk about your new-found craft with your clients.

Here is a list of some of the things I have found:

- Old pearl necklaces
- Austrian crystal necklaces
- Colored glass bead and jewel necklaces
- Interesting earrings
- Jeweled pins
- Jeweled shoe buckles
- Feathers from old hats
- Anything rhinestone
- Old hair ornaments, combs, hair picks, barrettes
- Mirror-backed jewels from the craft store
- Dried flowers
- Silk flowers
- Small fabric flowers
- Beautiful small fabric or silk birds

To get started making hair ornaments you will need:

- to turn off the TV!!
- small bent-tip needle nose pliers from the hardware store
- straight-tip needle nose pliers
- regular- and large-size hairpins in bronze and black
- a small glue gun from your local craft shop
- extra glue sticks

- specific glue for gluing metal to metal

- a clean place to work

- patience

Preparation steps:

- Be sure to wash any old jewelry with a soft toothbrush and a mild detergent before working with the pieces.

- When cutting apart necklaces, do it over a small, mesh, handheld strainer. You can wash and drain the beads in it as well.

- You will need to pull off the backs of old earrings and pins. Use your pliers to do this.

- Glue the earrings and pins onto bits of combs or hairpins. To make a small comb, take a full size clear plastic hair comb and break it into two or three smaller pieces.

- To release stones from old pins and buttons use your pliers to bend back the prongs. The stones will come out easier this way. Glue the stones to the hairpins.

Display any ornaments you have made by sticking the hairpins into a Styrofoam dome or circle. Get creative and spray paint the Styrofoam first or cover it with a shear colorful fabric. By having these visible for the clients they will be more apt to purchse something for their hairstyle. You can also begin taking orders for specific colors and styles. For simple pearls or flowers, I add a few dollars to the cost of the updo. I always keep a few hairpins with blue beads glued on. I hide one of these into an updo for the bride who

forgot something "blue." She really appreciates the thoughtfulness.

Some ornaments are one-of-a-kind and priced accordingly. For any of my expensive ornaments that a client wants to use but not purchase, I require the client to leave a deposit. The deposit is always double the cost of the wholesale value of the ornament. When she brings back the hair ornament I give her back the deposit. If she chooses to keep it, it's the same as if she bought it. I also do this for any hairpieces that I add into an updo.

Don't forget to look in the bridal section of the craft shop. There are many things that are sold separately for the do-it-yourself bride to make a headpiece. You can purchase some of these packaged pieces and place them directly into the bridal updo. Look closely at some of the ornamented styles in this book. Bridal trim is sold by the yard. A heavily beaded trim can be snipped into sections and glued onto a comb or hairpin. Place these around an updo and it mimics an expensive headpiece.

CUSTOM HEADPIECES

Custom-designed headpieces can be a very rewarding challenge for the creative stylist. Making custom headpieces is the next step beyond ornamenting a hairstyle. Custom work usually costs more.

I am getting up to $300 a headpiece, plus the cost of the hairstyle for my wedding work and you can too! Marketing the department properly and

Custom-designed headpieces can be a very rewarding challenge for the creative stylist.

creating the correct image for the bridal client are very important factors in charging hundreds for your bridal headpieces. Go back and reread Chapter 1 on the bridal image. If the bridal gown salons can charge hundreds so can the hair salon. Get out and shop some of your bridal salons. See how they display their headpieces. What are the prices they are getting right in your own area?

At one of my seminars I had a women share that she had been doing wedding headpieces for a while but didn't "think" to charge the client as much as the bridal shops. I know a lot of you out there are doing it, too. Stop it! Charge as much or more than the bridal shops! You know hair, you know what will work best for your bride, and they will pay for perceived value!

I have always been a craftsperson and somewhat creative. Many of us are creative, that is why we went into this field. But creativity needs to be fed and challenged.

After spending many years asking the bride to take her headpiece back to the wedding shop for changes, I decided to begin making them myself.

It all started with a bridal updo I ornamented that was published by *Passion's Coiffure Q.* At that time I had my own salon and was in my second year of doing platform work with updos. I figured maybe other brides might like a non-conventional wedding hairstyle so I used this photo in a local country club's wedding advertisement book. I networked with this country club for bridal referrals. In my advertisement I mentioned that I do custom

wedding headpieces. I ran this ad with the photo and had never even "made" a headpiece before!

The first bride this ad brought in was a scientist who was marrying a marine biologist. She wanted simple fabric flowers attached to a French clip and no veil. Offering custom work usually brings in those brides who can't find anything they like in the bridal shops.

Right after creating my first headpiece my career halted a bit with the closing of my salon. At this time, after having my salon for five years and trying to do "it" all—marriage, children, teach, platform work, work behind the chair, sixty plus hours, employees, bills, and taxes—I had had enough. I weighed my pride against the needs of my family and my family won. I swallowed my pride and called an acquaintance salon owner one town closer to my home. Four of my employees and I and most of our clients all went to that salon.

Well, the rest, shall we say, is history. I kept doing what I love, teaching and platform work, and cut back to thirty hours in the salon. Time off and finally a paycheck! In the new salon I was able to develop a bridal department and pick up where I left off.

Right before I closed my salon I had booked us a bridal fashion show at the same country club where I had my headpiece advertisement. I was only at my new job a week. My previous staff and I put on our new salon's T-shirts and went and did the fashion show. I had no time to dwell on the changes and have never looked back.

Offering custom work usually brings in those brides who can't find anything they like in the bridal shops.

What made that bridal fashion show so unique was that we ornamented all of the hairstyles. Fashion shows move quickly, so we had many premade ornaments and stuck them in the hair as the model was getting dressed. I would see what she was wearing and have the piece ready, plus I helped the models organize and get dressed. There is always a ticket to hide, a strap to tuck, or a zipper that needs zipping. The ornamented hairstyles were a hit. Everyone wanted to know who did the hair. The wedding department at the new salon was off to a good start!

My next bride who wanted a headpiece was a woman in her forties. She wanted a simple wreath. She was having her gown made so I asked for some of the material and lace. It came out lovely and she was very happy. This was the slow beginning of my custom headpiece work and it has blossomed into a wonderful service.

Anyone can do it! It is more of a belief in yourself, confidence, and attitude that leads you to success. You can do it, too!

Usually the brides want something very simple. The complaints I hear most about the headpieces in the bridal shops are:

- The headpieces are too ornate.
- They are too big.
- They are too heavy.
- They are uncomfortable and don't fit right.
- They are all the same; they want something different.
- They are too expensive.
- I don't know what to get to go with the hairstyle I want.

SAMPLE HEADPIECES

When consulting with a bride, find out what she does *not* like about the headpieces in the bridal shop. Then meet her personal need! If the headpieces are

> *It is a belief in yourself, confidence, and attitude that leads you to success.*

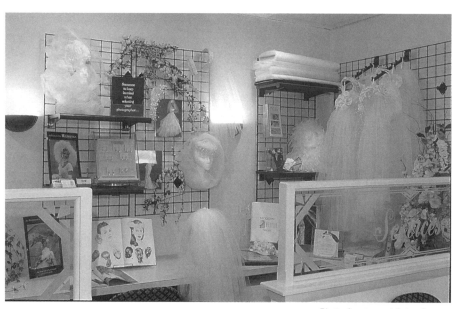

Photo Courtesy of Salon Pereau

too big make her a smaller one; if they are too ornate make her a simple one. Focus on meeting her need and solving her problem first; this allows her to love what you offer even more. There are books at the library and craft shops that tell you how to make fabric flowers and headpieces. If you can sew a straight stitch you can do it.

The safest and smartest way to expand into this area is to make some samples. Keep the samples simple and make at least three different styles. A crown or headband, a wreath, and a backpiece. From these the bride can choose something you are already comfortable making. Shop the wedding salons and look at how they are made. Look at the prices. You will not be making a headpiece for every bride who comes into the salon. I always have the bride shop for a headpiece first. This way she knows what is out there and what she does not want. Plus this also gives her an idea about the cost of a headpiece. Don't forget the bridal party will need some samples made up as well.

I make some of the veils myself using patterns from the fabric stores. Some I purchase premade from Paul's Bridal in New York City. Premade veils can be ordered from wholesale bridal houses in all lengths and styles. All of my headpieces have detachable veils (with Velcro) or separate veils on combs to allow for removal at the reception. This convenience for the bride also allows my updos to be better exposed for everyone to see. This helps with referrals.

NETWORKING WITH A MILLINER/ RESORCES FOR RETAIL

What do you do if you want to offer this service but do not have the time or desire to custom design?

Here are 9 options:

1. You can find someone who wants to make the headpieces for the salon. This person becomes part of the bridal team and needs to conduct headpiece consultations at the salon with the bride and the stylist. Ask around. Look in the yellow pages under "Seamstresses or milliners."

2. You may choose to order bridal headpieces wholesale and sell them in the salon. Keep samples in the salon for references. Have the bride order the headpiece from a catalogue. You will work with a sales representative just like you do with any other retail the salon offers. They can help you get started.

(Here is a tip concerning ordering headpieces. Many catalogues offer first communion headpieces. They are smaller than the bridal ones and can be used for a bride. You can also order a decorative clip or comb to add into an updo and make the veil yourself.)

To find resources look in the phone book under "Bridal wholesalers." Also call the Association of Bridal Consultants for information in your area. The markup on bridal headpieces is much greater than on a bottle of shampoo. If the salon does

T*he safest and smartest way to expand into this area is to make some samples.*

brides, the salon will sell headpieces.

3. Network with a milliner. A milliner is a person who makes just hats. Many also make headpieces. A visit to the millinery shop is in order to see if it is an establishment with which you want to be associated. If so, set up an appointment to meet with the owner. Have an agenda written up. Discuss percentages and have everything in writing, even if it is a friend. Conduct everything in a business manner. Networking is always a win-win situation for all involved.

4. Try networking with a gift shop that has a bridal section carrying unique hair ornaments.

5. If, in your travels, you come across a gift shop carring an accessories line you find interesting ask the manager or owner if they wouldn't mind sharing their resources with you. You can also purchase an item; call the manufacturer on the ticket and ask for the nearest distributor in your area.

6. Don't forget your salon industry distributor as well as trade shows as resources for hair ornaments. There are many beautiful premade hair ornaments on the market which, when added to the salon's bridal display, may generate some interest.

7. It is also a lot of fun to attend a jewelry or clothing retailers show. Both of these trade shows have hair accessories on display for orders to be taken.

8. Place a phone call to the convention center in your area for a schedule of events. Usually all that is needed to purchase a ticket is a business card, business check, or a business tax ID number from the salon.

9. There are also shops which sell only headpieces. Introduce the owner to the bridal department in the salon. Invite any establishment you associate with to the open houses and mini bridal fairs you plan on hosting. Hosting an event is a good way to see who is interested in working with your salon and what kind of attitude they have.

IMAGE TYPES

A salon that offers services to the bride beyond just doing hair offers her a total bridal look. A bridal department in the salon can be more than you ever imagined. To help the bride with her total look you need to "marry" what you have to offer her to her image. Her bridal image mirrors her tastes. You must understand the different bridal images in order to help her find her total bridal look.

Image type is defined by how a person chooses to dress. Many people are a combination of two or more image types. Here are some of the image types I have come across in my regular clients:

❧ Romantic

❧ Feminine

❧ Classic

❧ Preppy

❧ Earthy

❧ Western

A salon that offers services to the bride beyond just doing hair offers her a total bridal look.

- Trendy
- Contemporary
- Glamorous
- High-Fashion
- Modern (Mod)

I encourage you to seek out further resources about client image types. I have taken a few professional color analysis classes over the years and these have touched on image types. I have also spent some time reading up on the subject at the public library.

Remember back to Chapter 1 on the importance of your personal and professional image? You need to help the bride find and define *her* bridal image for her big day.

Brides sometimes like to break away from their everyday image type and sometimes they do not. I have had classic, suit-type clients who want to look like a princess on their wedding day, while other classic suit-types will wear a suit for their wedding. Tatiana of Boston, a wedding gown designer, understands the needs of each individual. She gave me these words of wisdom when interviewed by phone, "When I design a collection, I try to offer many different silhouettes from avant garde to sophisticated. This way, however the bride wants to look—innocent, sensual, or romantic—she'll find her personality reflected in my gown."

When having the consultation remember to listen to the wording the bride uses to describe her wedding. The following are the three image types I have defined for brides.

The Princess Bride

This bride is living out a childhood dream or fairy tale. She will have a lot of details and "stuff" going on with her dress—pearls, bows, ribbons, yards of tulle, and iridescent sequins will adorn the Princess Bride. They usually like to have a long veil and many have a long train on the gown. I had a Princess Bride who spent as much on her glittering headpiece as she did on her gown. She also had large glittery earrings and decorated shoes. The Princess Bride usually has a new dress. She also wants as much attention and detail to her hair—curls, tendrils, and an ornate headpiece all make up the Princess Bride.

The Town and Country Bride

Her look is understated elegance. Simplicity rules. She may have the traditional full-skirt gown, but the bodice will not be as heavily ornamented. She may have some lace and pearls but it will be elegant and "quiet." The Town and Country Bride will never have any iridescence. She will have more invested in the fabric of her gown. The fabric will affect the flow and texture of the dress. She may even wear a suit or a sheath. Her jewelry will be simple and expensive. When she describes her dress the first thing she mentions is the fabric and the second is the designer. Read the bridal magazines to keep abreast of the favored designers. She will also be more likely to want an understated hairstyle, but one that is definitly "in style." Older brides and second-time brides also tend to be

> *When having the consultation remember to listen to the wording the bride uses to describe her wedding.*

Town and Country Brides.

The Period Style or Ethnic Bride

Period styles are gown designs reflecting eras in history. The 1600s–1800s, the Renaissance, etc. Gowns may also reflect Greek or Roman times with draping and empire waistlines. The gown may reflect a decade, like styles from the 1920s, 1940s, or 1950s, etc. I had a bride who had a medieval style to her gown. Her daily image style was earthy/romantic and she was an art teacher. She did not want a veil to take away any focus from her hair. I did a beautiful, detailed medieval style with lots of curls cascading down. I incorporated fresh flowers throughout the style, which went along with the "Maid Marion-Robin Hood" feeling. The bridesmaids were in soft, flowing, floral dresses.

I have had brides who favor a Victorian style. The Victorian gown has a high neckline and a long row of bottoms down the back, it may also have a bustled back. I had a bride request an Audrey Hepburn style to her updo, complete with the chic little bangs. I incorporated her mother's headpiece which was from the early sixties into the style and she wore a slim sheath.

The Ethnic Bride may choose to reflect her heritage in her wedding ensemble. I did the hair for a bride from Pakistan who had come to the United States for an arranged wedding. The family gave me a videotape of the ceremony that took place previously in Pakistan so I could see what needed to be done. The makeup was fuchsia and Kelly green with gold glitter for her eyes and fuchsia for her lips. She wore rubies, emeralds, and diamonds in jewelry from her ears to her hair, and from her nose to her ears. Bracelets, ankle bracelets, and glitter covered this ethnic bride from head to toes. It was a fun experience! The Ethnic Bride may choose a certain colored fabric or cowrie shells to be added to her hair. Look at the Ethnic Brides that are in this book.

During the consultation you may put the bride in one of the three bridal image styles. However, do not tell her she is one of these types. People hate to be labeled. A great visual tool for you and the bride is to make up three posters.

- Cut out pictures of gowns from wedding magazines.

- Organize the pictures into three groups.

- One group is pictures of the Princess Bride.

- Another group is pictures of the Town and Country Bride.

- The last group will be pictures of Period and Ethnic styles. I also include unusual designs in this category.

- During the consultation show the bride the posters.

The bride will automatically be drawn to one of the posters and usually like a hairstyle on that poster. She will also be impressed that your salon is so "up" on the bridal industry and trends.

Use the information from this important chapter to create a total bridal look that is unique and special. Setting yourself apart as a bridal specialist is very exciting and fun! My creative work has led me to do updos for theme parties and balls, as well as opera singers and plays.

THEME WEDDINGS

Weddings can also carry their own special characteristics. Theme weddings can have a variety of styles. They can be ethnic in heritage, they can reflect a period of history, or they can be just fun, like having a western theme. I had a bride who had a nautical theme complete with lighthouse on top of the wedding cake. The reception was held at a yacht club. She wanted me to make her a beaded tiara and I tried to talk her into incorporating small white shells into the design.

A garden wedding would be perfect to suggest fresh flowers or ivy from the yard for the bride's hair. The consultation is the time to truly listen to the bride and ask many questions. She thinks she only needs to tell the stylist about her hair. When the stylist digs deeper to get a feeling for the entire wedding day the bride will feel very special.

Any particular period of history needs to be researched by the stylist doing the hair or the bride herself. If the bride wants a Renaissance look, having a book from the library on hand in time for the trial run will be necessary. A great book for any salon to have on hand is *Daring Dos: A History of Extraordinary Hair,* by Mary Trasko.[2]

TIPS

- Remember there is a whole person under that hairstyle.

- Consider line, size, shape, position, density, and texture of the hair.

- Remember emphasis, contrast, and balance is important to the bride's total look.

- Train your eye to be objective.

- Ask her about her jewelry.

- Communicate to find her image.

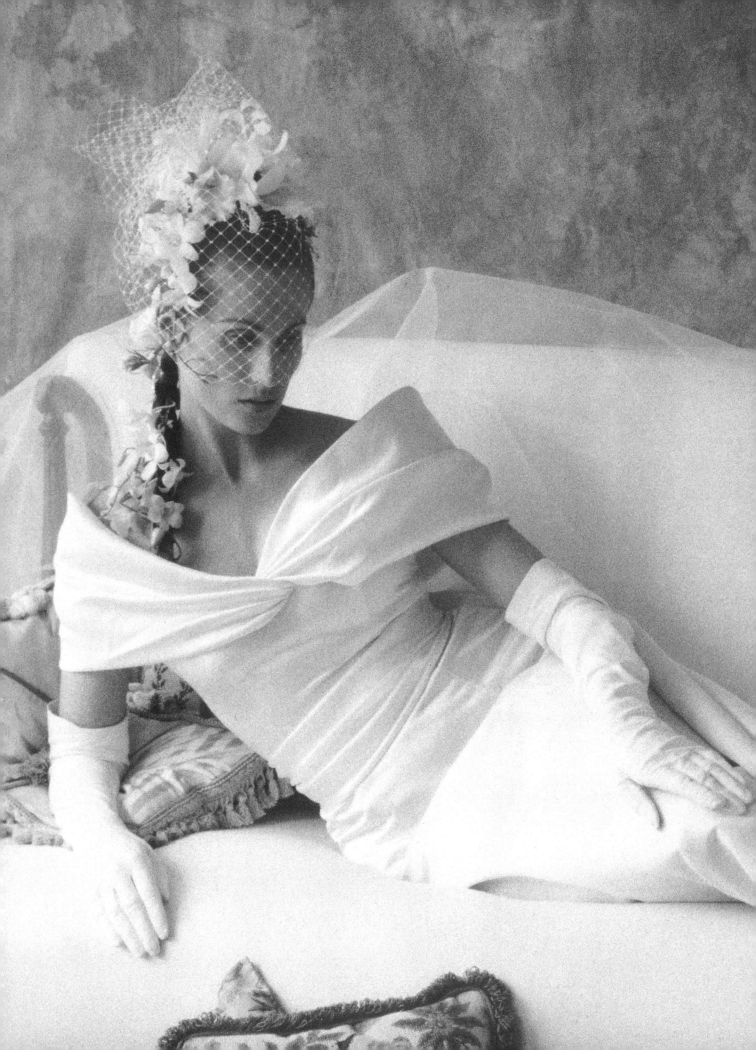

CHAPTER 6

Relating to the Bride and Her Party

This chapter will cover all the important topics having to do with relating to the bride and her party. Let me stress a very important fact again: 85% of one's success with a client is in how that client perceives their experience. Not how *you* perceive it, but how *she* perceives it. There is a big difference. Listening, understanding, recognizing personality and image types, touch, sensitivity, etc., constitute a major part of a successful appointment. Of that success, 15% comes from a technically well-executed service. This is a hard pill to swallow. We are professionals, we take classes, and we read and practice, yet the slightest undersight can turn a great service into a negative one. We are trained to execute a *service*, yet many of our clients are looking for an *experience*.

You all have had a client who, for one reason or another, is in your chair practically crying. Their stylist of twelve years has moved away and they had to change hairstylists. You are listening to her and looking at the worst haircut you have ever seen. Why did this client like a stylist so much who was so poorly skilled? The point is she did. That's the 85% factor. Yes, it is important to educate a client as to what is an "exceptional" technical service. However, if the bride walks out of the salon on her wedding day looking beautiful, but "feeling" rushed, stressed, and frazzled, then in her mind her experience was a negative one.

Every one of us is an expert at justifying a not-so-perfect experience.

> *We are trained to execute a service, yet many of our clients are looking for an experience.*

Who wants to take the blame? We tell ourselves is was the front desk's fault. Or you had a bad fight with your boyfriend. You were sick, but, "At least I came to work." When the client leaves upset because you were running late we say "Well, at least she looked good." They walk out the door. You have convinced yourself things are fine and you go on to your next client. You may never see that first client again and not know why. It is human nature to protect ourselves. If we don't acknowledge fault, then there is nothing to fix or change. We really are not helpless. We just need to look inward, to see a situation from someone else's side. We need to be in a constant state of fine tuning who we are and what we do. We need to care.

IDENTIFYING YOUR BRIDE

So here you are learning how to deal with the most emotional and stressful client of all—the bride on the day of her wedding. You can lose a bride emotionally if you do not successfully relate to her from the beginning. You must "figure" her out for a successful wedding day to take place. We have discussed all of the important factors up to this point: image, getting the salon and staff ready, systems, networking, marketing, design, styles, and image types. Now I will share with you the most important factors in the equation for making a successful wedding salon experience.

For a positive relationship with the bride to take place there are many factors involved beyond beautiful hair:

- The bride can *look* beautiful but not *feel* beautiful.

- Your job as a stylist is to make her feel beautiful.

- The best way to meet the bride's needs is to understand her personality and communication style.

The systems laid out in this book help tremendously to alleviate any wedding day rush or confusion, even though not all brides are fussy and nervous. With the business part of the service taken care of, you will now have more calm energy to direct toward the bride and her beauty needs.

There are "issues" with each bride that the stylist must confront. Many times these issues are not necessarily contingent on the stylist's hairdressing skills. Success now becomes contingent on interpersonal skills. Let me give you illustrations of two real brides to make this point more understandable. These two brides are very different. Each has her own issues for me to deal with. I have to relate to them both as individuals. I have to "meet" them where they are at the moment.

The first bride in this illustration is a second-time bride. Many brides today are getting married for the second time. They don't want their hair to be anything like it was the first time. This particular bride is actually carrying around a photo of her future husband's first wedding. She wants to make sure that nothing about her wedding will resemble his first wedding. She shows the photo to anyone who has anything to do with her wedding. She does not want her hair to look like his first wife's

hair. She does not want her dress to resemble his first wife's dress, nor does she want her flowers to look anything like his first wedding. This bride, who is beautiful, with long blonde hair, came to me ten months before her wedding. She already had a folder with cut out pictures and ideas of what she wanted for her hair.

In addition she also has bad memories of how *her* wedding day went when she got married the first time. She hated the way her hair was at her first wedding. She told me that hating her hair on her wedding day ruined her day, and feels it got her marriage off to a bad start. She remembers her wedding day with such disgust and how horrible she felt because she did not like her hair! As I am listening to this prospective bride I am taking mental notes as to what she will need of me.

So what is my objective? Being "better" than the first hairdresser? No. My objective is not to create the perfect hairstyle. My objective is to get her to communicate what she wants, and I don't necessarily mean what hairstyle she wants. My objective is to make her believe I am giving her what she wants. I have to make her believe I will be able to come up with something special for her special day. She wants me to understand her and I have to convey to her that I do. I must make her know that I am listening.

- Listening is an action.

- Listening is standing still and facing her.

- Listening is accompanied by eye contact.

> **Y**ou will now have more calm energy to direct toward the bride and her beauty needs.

> *When she feels listened to and understood she will want to know what I think is best. Not before.*

🎀 Listening is accompanied by verbally repeating back to her what she has said, but in my own words.

🎀 When she feels listened to and understood she will want to know what I think is best. Not before.

The problem in many cases is we tell a client what we think is best before they have given us permission to do so. They are not ready to hear what we have to say if they have not felt understood. Picture an argument. You have something to say. While the other person is giving their side you are not listening. You are just waiting for them to pause long enough so you can say what it is you have to say. People's heart's desire is to feel understood, to have their needs met—especially a bride on her wedding day, and especially one who has an agenda about what she wants.

This bride is welcome to as many trial-run appointments of the hairstyle as she wants. She needs to feel confident with *me,* not necessarily my work. For a client like this, an organized system for the bridal department is crucial. Properly relating to her and how to do it successfully is what this chapter is all about.

On the very same day that I met the first bride in this illustration I had a trial run with bride number two. This bride also came to me months earlier, but only for a haircut. She mentioned she was getting married, but did not want to make any appointments regarding a trial run or a consultation. She also thought she might want a custom headpiece but was not sure. At that haircut appointment I had time to try some of my sample headpieces on her but she never chose a specific one. I told her I needed a month's notice for the headpiece. I penciled in her wedding date to hold a space for her in the wedding book but we did not have a formal consultation. Consequently no index card was made up and filed. She was letting the wedding party handle their own hair appointments. She did not want to concern herself with their hair.

This bride is an FBI agent. She is a very busy woman and does not have time to fret over herself about her wedding day. She does her job and expects me to do mine. Two weeks before her wedding, she came in for color with the colorist. She walked up to me while I was doing a haircut and handed me some fabric to use to make her headpiece. I looked at her and did not remember who she was, though I acted as I did until my memory slowly came back. She said she wanted the simple, short veil she had tried on with some flowers to match her dress. She had a picture of her dress for me.

One week before her wedding I made sure she had her trial-run appointment. When her appointment time came she was on her car phone out in the parking lot. She came in very frazzled over a case. I tried to help her relax. I brought her some water to drink. I spoke to her gently with my hands firmly on her shoulders, assuring her that I would take care of her beauty needs. She visibly relaxed under the atmosphere of comfort and control I created.

This bride needed me to be in control, as opposed to the first bride whom I needed to let think she was in control.

Not only did my second bride not know what she wanted, she hadn't even thought about it! I tried to get some information out of her so I had some idea of where to start. When she didn't know what she wanted other than something "up and soft" we talked about her gown again. She loved the first thing I did. The bride's beeper went off twice during the appointment.

I went to get my camera to take a picture of the style. When I came back she was on the phone again. So I have a trial-run picture of her with the phone to her ear. The custom headpiece I made her was "just perfect." This was one easy bride.

Not only did I have to deal with these two totally different brides but I had to deal with them on the same day! Most brides fall somewhere in the middle of these two examples. Every bride is unique in her own special way and that is what you as the stylist have to find out.

The Bridal Line Network put out a list of the "Ten common reasons for insufficient bridal sales." Even though this list is designed for bridal consultants, salon professions will benefit from it as well.

Reason number two on the list is "Inability to establish a rapport with the bride."

...The Bride, more than the Groom, will look to feel some kind of connection with you. The most effective way to accomplish this is to separate her Wedding from any other. If she is under the impression that you sincerely believe that her Wedding is special, and you have a genuine interest in making her celebration unique, you will alleviate her fears of 'being among the masses.'" [1]

The dressing of hair for any special occasion comes down to creating a feeling. Bat mitzvahs for young girls, 8th grade dances, proms, ring dances, sweet fifteen and sixteen parties, graduations, and weddings are all very emotional events in the life of a young woman. Not only are you dealing with creating the perfect total look, you are dealing with some one just about to experience their first kiss, or a walk down the aisle to the man of their dreams. We have a tough job.

In the previous chapter you learned about bridal styles and image types. This chapter will tie in those individual qualities with personality types and how to relate to each one. I will show you how to meet the bride's wishes by understanding personality types and communication styles.

PERSONALITY TYPES

Personality types are as varied as people. We are all a mix of genetic tendencies with a lot of environment thrown in. There are cultural differences, regional differences, and age differences. We are the eldest, the middle child, or the youngest. We are spoiled, neglected, poor, privileged, or somewhere in between. Understanding personality types on a simple level becomes a helpful tool in dealing with the bride. Understanding personality types on a deeper level can help with life in general.

Understanding personality types becomes a helpful tool in dealing with the bride.

> *Whether at work, with our clients, or with family members, personality types are at the root of our interactions.*

There are many resources that specifically deal with personality types. It is a fascinating subject and it can be a lot of fun to take a personality test. I am sure many of you have taken one found in the magazines. Take the next step and go to the library or bookstore and research some books. We all experience the impact different personality types have on us and those around us. Whether at work, with our clients, or with family members, personality types are at the root of our interactions.

The salon industry has slowly been waking up to this fact. The corporate community has long been involved in educating their workers. If individuals can better understand themselves and those around them they will become better-producing employees. For the stylists and managers, understanding this subject will improve client-to-employee, employee-to-manager, and coworker-to-coworker interactions. There are scores of books on the subject. There are also seminars. I have taken many of these types of seminars over the years, some within the cosmetology field, some from the corporate business community. This subject is also addressed in child development books, marriage books, and relationship books and tapes.

One seminar I took was at the 1994 International Beauty Show in New York City called "People Reading." It was presented by DeAnne Rosenberg. DeAnne is a specialist in management education and supervisory development. She has written numerous magazine articles and film scripts concerning management, motivation, and performance improvement and has produced several cassette programs on communication skills. She does these seminars for many corporations, including Sebastian International, IBM, Anheuser-Busch, United Airlines, McDonald's, and General Motors, to name a few. Ms. Rosenberg had this to say:

A client's speech and behavior toward the stylist in the salon reflects her self-image in terms of one of the three personality patterns. A stylist or manager should first recognize that pattern, then use appropriate language that matches the client's self-image. Such 'personality matching' will increase rapport, harmony, and the client's satisfaction." [2]

Here is an overview of her seminar with some of my own notes added in from a hairdresser's perspective. Ms. Rosenberg describes in detail 3 types of clients.

1. The Achievement/Task-Oriented Client

2. The People-Oriented Client

3. The Power- or Influence-Oriented Client.

I am sure you will see some of your clients in the following lists.

The Power Client

- is impressed by upscale surroundings.

- will always challenge you.

- is manipulative; always looking for a deal.

- has the need to impress you.

- pushes limits.

- is a good negotiator.

- needs to feel she has the upper hand.
- objects to "red tape" and administrative rules.
- disappears if she feels you don't have "it" anymore.
- is impressed by one's status (*must* go to owner or specialist).

The People-Oriented Client

- is warm and friendly, and very communicative.
- talks a lot about personal experiences.
- is cooperative and personal.
- has a hard time leaving a particular stylist for a new one.
- is somewhat disorganized.
- needs a lot of personal interaction.
- needs input and compliments.
- dislikes change.
- is not impressed by a large, busy salon but prefers an intimate atmosphere.

The Business/Task Client

- makes decisions easily.
- likes a lot of power activity.
- does not like to wait.
- has high standards of excellence.
- wants the details and facts, like how her color works and why.
- comes across as unfriendly.
- at first communication seems cool.

- needs time to build trust.
- remains loyal, if you remain consistent.
- wants the best for her or the latest trend.
- understands systems.
- prefers time alone in a quiet place.

Do you see yourself? How about some of your clients? Please make a mental note or, better yet, photocopy these client type lists and pass them out to the entire staff. Use this information as the subject of your next staff meeting. Have everyone come up with a few clients to match each type, or as DeAnne says, "personality patterns." If you wish to get some of DeAnne Rosenberg's tapes her number is (617) 862-6117.

COMMUNICATION STYLES

Along with personality types we also have a communication style. Some styles balance each other and sometimes those which are similar may clash. Following are some communication styles I have categorized into 3 specific client groups.

1. The Quiet Client

2. The Know-It-All Client

3. The Uncertain Client

By recognizing communication styles and noticing body language you can help the bride have a successful wedding-day appointment. It is during the consultation when you need to pay close attention.

By recognizing communication styles and noticing body language you can help the bride have a successful wedding-day appointment.

After I describe each of the communication styles I match them up to two very different stylists. I will use an aggressive stylist versus a passive stylist as examples. The comparisons are extreme and humorous but their purpose is to shed some light on this subject in regard to the client-stylist matchup.

The Quiet Client

🖎 She needs you to draw information from her.

🖎 She needs you to suggest styles.

🖎 She needs you to look over pictures with her.

The passive stylist with the quiet client would be like the blind leading the blind. The passive stylist needs to

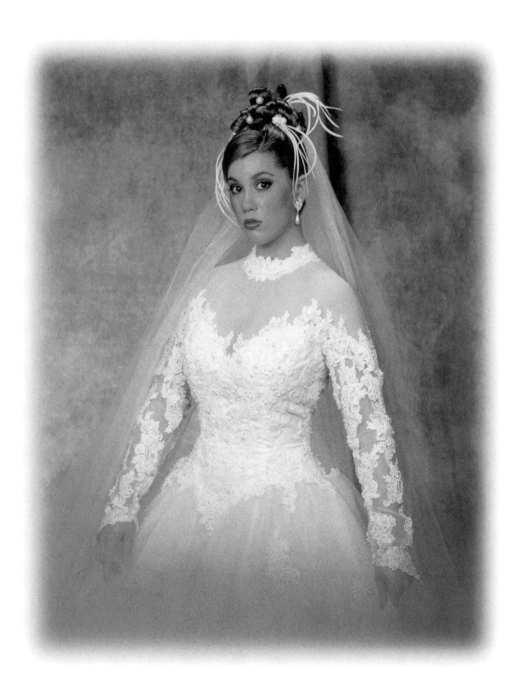

be told what to do and does not like to offer change. It is safer that way and all the blame for anything going wrong becomes the client's fault. "I just did what she told me to do." The passive stylist makes a great assistant who never wants to go on the floor. She becomes a salon fixture, leaning against the wall waiting for a client to appear in her chair.

The aggressive stylist with the quiet client is a dysfunctional marriage. The aggressive stylist will do what they think is best but may never see this client again. The aggressive stylist overpowers the quiet client and the quiet client never speaks up. She just leaves the salon. By lacking the skills necessary to draw out information from the quiet client the aggressive stylist becomes frustrated. A poor retention rate is an indication of this problem.

The quiet client is hard to read. An attentive stylist will recognize that she has a quiet client in her chair and encourage her to speak up. Look for body language clues that tell you she is unhappy. Some of these clues are lack of eye contact, looking in the mirror, sighing, and being unable to say whether she likes it or not. Or the quiet client may say she does like it, but her tone is unconvincing. A stylist may receive these clues but not act on them for a number of reasons including running late or being satisfied with what was done on her. Many times I have to give the quiet client permission to speak by saying, "It's OK if you don't like what I did, I won't take it personally, but in order to give you what you want and to please you, I need to

know what it is about this style you don't care for." Remember, this is her wedding day hairstyle, she has to like it and feel comfortable. This is also a good example of why a trial run appointment is so important. Once the style is settled on and recorded, the wedding day will run smoothly.

The Know-It-All Client

- ✍ She wants what she wants, when she wants it.

- ✍ She insists on your full attention and eye contact.

- ✍ She tells you how to cut or set her hair instead of telling you what she wants.

- ✍ She has her hands in her hair before you do, "showing" you what she wants.

The passive stylist will be chewed up and spit out by this client. The passive stylist will get burned out and stressed. The passive stylist will try to please this client but will never succeed. The passive stylist will quit the industry for a desk job somewhere.

The aggressive stylist, on the other hand, will start a war. They will be like two cats in a paper bag together, fur flying and teeth baring. The aggressive stylist must learn to back off, listen, and then gently "attack." When an aggressive client starts to tell me how to cut her hair I say, "Let's talk about what you want and how you want your hair to look. Then I can decide the best direction to take as to how the look will be achieved." With the aggressive client you must keep the

> *An attentive stylist will recognize that she has a quiet client in her chair and encourage her to speak up.*

upper hand or she will have no respect for you. Let her speak, listen well, then counterattack *gently,* with professionalism and confidence.

The Uncertain Client

🖎 She may know what she wants—but won't be able to describe it.

🖎 If she does have an idea, she is afraid to let you try it.

🖎 She usually is a nonvisual person— she can't picture your suggestion, her suggestion, or a magazine picture of a style on herself.

🖎 She's the one who gets a computer image of herself with ten new styles and cannot pick one out.

🖎 You see her looking through style books and when you ask if she would like something new she panics and say, "No, not this time."

🖎 She has no idea about current trends.

The passive stylist will listen patiently as this client talks, and talks, but she may never give the stylist the go ahead to try something new. When the uncertain client gets no help from the passive stylist, she finishes by saying, "Just do what you always do." And the passive stylist is relieved to be off the hook to make a decision and gives the client the same old thing. "This is really best on you any way," the passive stylist says.

The unknowing client will have to go to someone new to get a new style. She finally wants a change and goes to a different salon. She gets brave and asks for a complete makeover. The uncertain client is booked with an

aggressive stylist. Big mistake. The aggressive stylist loves makeovers.

"Something new? Sure, let's do this and this and color it this color; it will look fabulous. You will look ten years younger, trust me!" Remember, this client is uncertain and puts her trust in this new exciting stylist. Now this aggressive stylist lacks the ability to read this client's personal style. Plus, not enough questions were asked to find out what this person does for a living or what her styling habits are. And when the client is all done she doesn't even recognize herself in the mirror. The aggressive stylist thinks she looks great. The client believes the stylist because she's uncertain. That is until she gets back to her coworkers and husband. This is the client who leaves the salon loving her hair and then comes back two days later hating it.

When I run into an unknowing client who hints at wanting a change but is afraid to give me the permission to do so, I give her some homework to do before her next appointment. I ask her to pay attention to other people's styles, to hunt the magazines for style she likes, and to bring me something by her next appointment. Sometimes I will look for something for her and have it put aside to show her when she comes in.

When working with an unknowing bridal client I do the same thing. This is why I like to have a consultation appointment plus a separate trial-run appointment. At the consultation appointment the unknowing bride comes with nothing to show me and no idea of what she wants. She even has trouble describing her gown to me.

> **T**his is the client who leaves the salon loving her hair and then comes back two days later hating it.

So before the trial run I give her some homework. When the unknowing bride is given some direction, you, as the stylist, are giving her "permission" to pick something out. The unknowing bride has to be told what to do and usually has a dominate mother or maid of honor who is making most of the wedding decisions.

The unknowing bride may also come to the consultation with "helpers" from the wedding party who offer their opinions. Recently I was talking with a minister and discussing these "helpers" and he said this type of bride tends to make her wedding choices by way of committee. When you, as the stylist, are consulting with the unknowing bride and her "committee," you must immediately establish yourself as the expert as far as her beauty needs go. Encouraging the bride to come in alone for her trial run will relax her and give the two of you a better chance at coming up with a style.

I encourage you to look further into this subject of communicating and personality types to better understand yourself and those around you. It will not only enhance your career but your personal life as well. All of the information I have read over the years has helped in my career as well as in my marriage and in communicating with my children.

FOUR CLIENT TYPES SPECIFIC TO BRIDES

Since 1980 I have experienced all personality types in my bridal clients. Along with each personality type comes a communication style. I have learned to work with each one differently. I have taken personality types and communication styles and broken them down into four client types specific to brides. I am sure you will recognize some past brides. Utilize this information to help with future ones. These brides are a mix of personality patterns and communication styles. With each type I share how best to handle them.

The Verbal Bride

This bride is very verbal, describing exactly what she wants. She may be a task or power client. This personality type is assured and possibly demanding. She will only be demanding if she doesn't feel she is getting what she wants. The key word here is *feel*. What she wants is to feel understood, listened to, and respected. Subconsciously, feeling understood is more important to her than what she is asking for her hair. It is important that you give this client good eye contact. Let her talk and don't interrupt.

Verbal people or talkers are used to being interrupted. They talk fast to get it all out. Let her. As she sees you are listening, she will slow down. Show attentive body language—lean back on your station; look her in the eye, not in the mirror; fold your arms and tilt your head. When you have listened and she feels heard, you are now free to give your creative input and educated advice. Repeat some of her requests back to her. This will show her you have listened and do care about her needs. If this client is handled this way from the beginning many problems can be avoided.

Look further into this subject of communicating and personality types to better understand yourself and those around you.

The Nonverbal Bride

This bride basically sits there and does not offer much information. Remember the quiet client? You do not need to fill the conversational void, or she will never talk. Making her feel comfortable will allow her the courage to speak. Having the bridal questionnaire to read from during the consultation is very helpful in this case. She may have spent years being verbally shot down. In order not to "get hurt" emotionally, she keeps her opinions to herself. When she feels she can trust you and you have encouraged her to speak without interrupting her she will open up. Asking pointed questions will help with this bride.

If she cannot tell you what she wants, find out what she does not want. She will need your help in creating the perfect hairstyle for her. This bride needs encouragement to share her wishes, as well as reassurance from you that you have it all under control for her.

This bride may also be a task-oriented person and expect you to do your job quickly and without unnecessary fuss.

The Nonvisual Bride

This client can be verbal or nonverbal, but she is definitely nonvisual. Most artists are, however, visual. We can visualize a haircut on someone or a new color. We can visualize an outfit and then shop for it. The nonvisual client is the one who buys everything the mannequin is wearing. She also cannot visualize her wedding-day hairstyle. Even when you do a style on her she

keeps saying "I don't know if I like it," "I can't tell if it is right." This client may require a few trial runs of her hairstyle. You may suggest that she have a trial run on the same day she has a fitting for her gown. That way she can see the style with her dress and feel more comfortable about it. This client also needs others to tell her how great she looks. Having another stylist or the owner walk by and compliment her helps tremendously.

The Defensive Bride

This client can be verbal or nonverbal. She may also be nonvisual, but she is generally a pessimist. She seems to be a negative and unhappy person. And she is. She has decided even before you get started she won't like it. But you can win her over and have a successful wedding experience. If I am sensing this client being reserved and guarded then I know she may have had a previously bad salon experience. She probably had a bad prom or updo experience. Ask her about it. Or she may be very nervous and it comes out in impatience and anger. You have to win her trust first and get her to communicate her wishes.

Arnold Zegarelli gives this advice. It is taken from *The Zegarelli Credo,* which he and his late brother published in 1977. It still works today. "Respond, don't react. If someone tries to put you on the defensive, try to stay calm. Look for the real reason for the behavior so you can diffuse it."[3]

Give her permission to complain and share. She will feel you care and that you wish to understand her. As

> *The nonvisual client is the one who cannot visualize her wedding-day hairstyle.*

hard as it is, all she needs is a little love and tenderness. The ones that need the most love are the hardest to love because they won't let you.

If the defensive bride is nonverbal she will show a lot of body language. Watching you, rolling her eyes, and touching her hair all the while she is letting out big long sighs. I know sometimes you just want to ignore all these signs and get her out of the salon as quickly as possible. Nevertheless, these clients do make very loyal customers and are usually willing to spend any amount for a little bit of happiness. Watch those hands. Sometimes I even ask this type of client to show me what she wants done with her hair. She will grab her hair and pouf it just right and say "like this." It's not that I need her help, but it allows her to feel in control. She may pull it up high and loose, or she may pull it to the back tight and low. Then I have something to go on. There is no room for a stylist with an ego for this client type.

If this defensive bride is verbal I listen, again maintaining eye contact.

"By looking people in the eye, you project a positive, credible image. Otherwise, you risk appearing nervous or unsure of yourself," says Connie Glaser a communications expert in Atlanta, Georgia. Glaser is the coauthor of *Swim with the Dolphins: How Women Can Succeed in Corporate America on Their Own Terms.*[4]

If you appear unsure of yourself with this client she will sense her power over you and exert it. Try adding some of your own body language. A gentle touch on the shoulder shows her you are not afraid of her. The defensive client needs to know that you are willing to understand her. With this client, once I have communicated about her style, I get her involved in conversation, offer her a magazine or get her a beverage. I try to keep the focus off what I am doing to her hair and on her as a person. Make her experience pleasant.

HOW TO HANDLE BRIDESMAIDS

Bridesmaids also fall into any of the above personality types. Usually you do not have the liberty of a trial-run appointment with bridesmaids, as many are from out of town. Others are not able to afford a trial run. Personally I do not encourage them. Trial runs are not to practice a style; practicing on your down time is for that purpose. A trial run is to find the style the person wants to have. If you find you need a trial run to see if you can do the hair then you have not practiced enough. Your wedding department will not become profitable if you take too long to perform a service.

With bridesmaids, be on the watch for personalities and image styles and handle accordingly. Follow the same way of handling them as with the bride. You will have to assess their personality type and communication style much quicker because there will not be a separate trial run. More than likely you have many girls to work on. I prefer working on two to three girls at a time. Working on two or more at a time takes your full atten-

The defensive client needs to know that you are willing to understand her.

Bride Type	Personality	Service Tips
Verbal	assured, possibly demanding, wants to feel understood and respected	have good eye contact, listen well, don't interrupt, repeat back requests and concerns
Nonverbal	does not offer much information, keeps opinions to self	make client comfortable, ask pointed questions or use a written questionnaire; show encouragement and reassurance
Nonvisual	cannot visualize abstracts, may buy whole ensembles	be open to a few trial runs and variations, have others in salon offer input, reassurance
Defensive	generally a pessimist and unhappy, has predetermined not to like what you do	maintain eye contact, be patient and calm, ask about possible past experiences that may have been bad, give permission to complain/share

tion off just one person. Finish the most difficult person last, even if it is the bride. Once they pay, they leave. If the fussy client is done first, she will spend her waiting time looking in the mirror and ask you to fix things no one else would even notice. Trust me, I have learned the hard way.

You do not have to match the hairstyle to the dress in the case of the bridesmaid, because every woman is in the same dress. Instead match their features and textures to the hairstyle. Someone is sure to be in a dress style not complimentary to her body type, so at least give her a hairstyle that will make her feel pretty.

However, the bride may want the bridesmaids to match perfectly. I have had brides insist that whoever is in the wedding had to grow their hair out for an updo. If this is the case you will be sure to have some angered brides-

maids. Also, if the bride insists that everyone in the party has to have the same updo, you are sure to run into some trouble. There is usually someone who does not want an updo at all. This is my main reason for working quickly with the party.

I had one bride who talked me through each bridesmaid's style; this was to ensure that the bridesmaids would not have the same hairstyle as her, or each other.

Most of the bridesmaids I have worked on want a style to reflect who they are personally. Because they are all in the same dress they want their hair to make them stand out as individuals. Brides who recognize this have a happier wedding party.

If you are free to create a style for the individual take into account her personality. The outgoing bridesmaid wants a great hairstyle to stand out. The city girl may want the latest retro look. The one with the longest hair wants everyone to know it, so leave out a tendril. The quiet wallflower does not even want to be in the wedding much less have an updo making her feel conspicuous, so do something simple without height.

If you have gotten into a trouble spot with a client, take a walk for a breather. Reassess the situation and think about where the problem may have started. Ask yourself these questions:

- Is it communication?

- Is it a lack of skill?

- Is the bride demanding of how her party looks?

- Is it a lack of trust on the brides-maid's part?

- Is it just a person you do not click with?

- Is she just unhappy about being in the wedding and she won't like anything?

I have had more problems with bridesmaids than with brides. Some-times the worst clients are the bride's sisters! I have had a bride in tears over her mother and sister arguing. I had a sister storm out of the salon with the bride chasing her back in. They may be having some of these feelings:

- They are nervous because they have to do a reading at the ceremony.

- They feel the dress is unflattering.

- An "ex" is going to be there.

- They hate the color of the dress.

- Even before the updo, they are taller than their partner.

- They never wear makeup.

- They are angry because they really can't afford the updo the bride wants them to have.

The out-of-town bridesmaids may be the most difficult. You are not their regular hairdresser, their dress does not fit right, and they did not sleep well at Aunt Susan's last night. A lot of times bridesmaids are more nervous than the bride. You, on the other hand, are more concerned with the bride and may become resentful of a demanding bridesmaid. At this point many brides are happy to get the whole wedding thing over with while the maid of honor is a mess, and you are glad she lives five states over.

I had one bridesmaid whom I could not please. It was a matter of trust in this case. She was from out of town and would not let me do anything creative. But the simple look she wanted did not work with the decorative comb that needed to be put in. I had to stop working on her because I had other bridesmaids to do. I kindly told her, with a smile, that I was not able to please her and suggested she try another stylist. She looked at me funny but couldn't say anything to such a polite, smiling request. I sent her to the stylist who was doing the bride, so I could start the other girls from the party. When she saw my creative work on the other updos she had the nerve to ask if I could take out what the other stylist did and give her a creative updo!

A lot of times bridesmaids are more nervous than the bride.

With all the professionalism I could muster I was happy to tell her there wasn't enough time.

Sometimes you just have to get through a situation as best you can.

Marcy Blum, who publishes *The Bridal Business Report* and owns and operates The Bridal Group Inc. in New York City has gone as far as to say "this is still a frivolous business—we're not curing leukemia. If the shoe dye isn't exactly the perfect shade, no one is going to die, most people won't notice."[5]

Sometimes you need to have this attitude when working with the bridal party. You can't win them all.

If a salon truly wishes to cater to the bride, if their research has been completed, if their image is in place, if their stylists are trained, their packages are spelled out, and the system is in place, "most" brides will be easy to handle. However, when a bride is difficult from the first phone call and the consultation does not go well, end the relationship there or try another stylist. I only run into problems when a mature client gets a younger stylist who cannot relate to her needs. *Doing brides is not just doing hair.* The hair almost becomes secondary to making her feel comfortable and special.

> **D**oing brides is not just doing hair.

HOW TO HANDLE CHILDREN IN THE WEDDING PARTY

If children are involved there may also be problems, especially if the bride wants the child's hair a certain way. Sometimes the child is too young and won't cooperate. Or she is just too tired from all the excitement and sleeping in a strange bed.

I had a six-year-old who seemed hyperactive. She was related to the bride through a family member on the groom's side. Her parents were divorced and the child was with her father for the wedding. The child had to sleep at the home of the bride whom she did not know well. It was left to the bride to bathe her in the morning and get her to the salon for her hair. The bride was a little late getting to the salon and, needless to say, stressed out. The bride wanted the child's hair all up on her head in curls. This child had enough hair for six people. It was very thick, naturally wavy, and down to her backside. Did I mention she was "active?"

It is important to get a child's hair up with as few bobby pins and as quickly as possible. Their heads are more sensitive than an adult and they are not quite ready to "suffer" for the sake of beauty.

Many times this is what I do when the bride requests curls on top of the head:

1. I stand behind the child and take 1/3 of the hair from ear to ear and put it in a ponytail on top of her head.

2. I set that ponytail in small, hot rollers.

3. I gather up all the rest of her hair and put it in another ponytail up close behind the first one.

4. This second larger ponytail I braid.

5. I wrapped this braided ponytail around the base of the first ponytail and the base of itself.

6. Bobby pin the braid in place. This technique pulls the two ponytails closer together, hides the elastics, and gives a solid braided base for the curls to be later pinned into.

7. Let the child get down and run around a bit while her curlers are cooling.

8. Take out the hot rollers. Loosen and fluff the curls with your fingers and spray them.

9. Pin the curls along the braid and let some "nest" in the

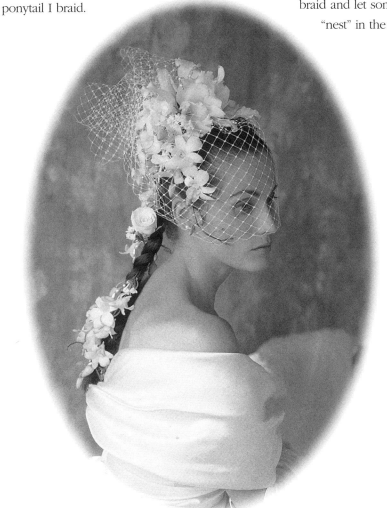

Photo Courtesy of Salon Pereau

middle, pinning them into the ponytail holders and not the scalp.

10. Let the child down again and while standing behind her spray the updo well. Let her walk away from the cloud of spray.

This method allows the curls to be pinned into the braid and not the scalp. Only three or four bobby pins touch the scalp which secured the braid. Also, by having most of the hair braided and 1/3 in curls the style is not top heavy.

The stylist who handles this situation needs to have patience and understanding for the small child. Their routine is disturbed. If you can keep these things in perspective when working with children it can be an enjoyable experience. If the child is crying and very fussy you may be able to explain to the bride that a simple braid or ponytail bun will be best for all concerned. Patience is definitely more important than skill when it comes to kids. Lollipops help, too!

Working on older children and junior bridesmaids also calls for understanding. The child is in an uncomfortable situation. A child can't say "no" to being in a wedding if cousin Mary and her mother insist.

The stylist who handles this situation needs to have patience and understanding for the small client.

During a trial-run appointment with an older bride I had asked about the rest of the bridal party. She said it was just her and a flower girl. She choose a ten-year-old niece to be a "flower girl." The bride said her niece was calling herself a junior bridesmaid. She did not want to be a "flower girl." Since I have daughters around this age I knew there would be trouble. I sided with the kid on this one and told the bride ten was too old to be considered a flower girl. "Just call her a junior bridesmaid and she will be fine," I told the bride. The bride had wanted her to wear a floral wreath and drop petals from a basket. The kid was not crazy about the idea of a wreath on her head. One fussy, sad, and miserable kid standing up at the altar with the bride can ruin a wedding. I told the bride I would work fresh flowers into the hairstyle. I kept the style low and around the back of the head. I surrounded the design with beautiful fresh greens and flowers. Everyone was happy!

One note here about kids and teens. Keep their bangs the way they are used to seeing them. Save the curls for the back. Curly bangs seem to bring tears.

TIPS

❧ Study image types and personality types. The whole salon will benefit from this knowledge.

❧ Make a list stating the qualities in communication styles.

❧ Make a heading of each client type on a piece of paper. Write in some of your clients to form these groups stronger in your mind.

❧ Try to take one people-oriented seminar a year.

❧ Use these skills with your everyday clients and not just brides.

❧ Take a breather and step away for a moment.

❧ Smile.

❧ Tell yourself you'll get through it.

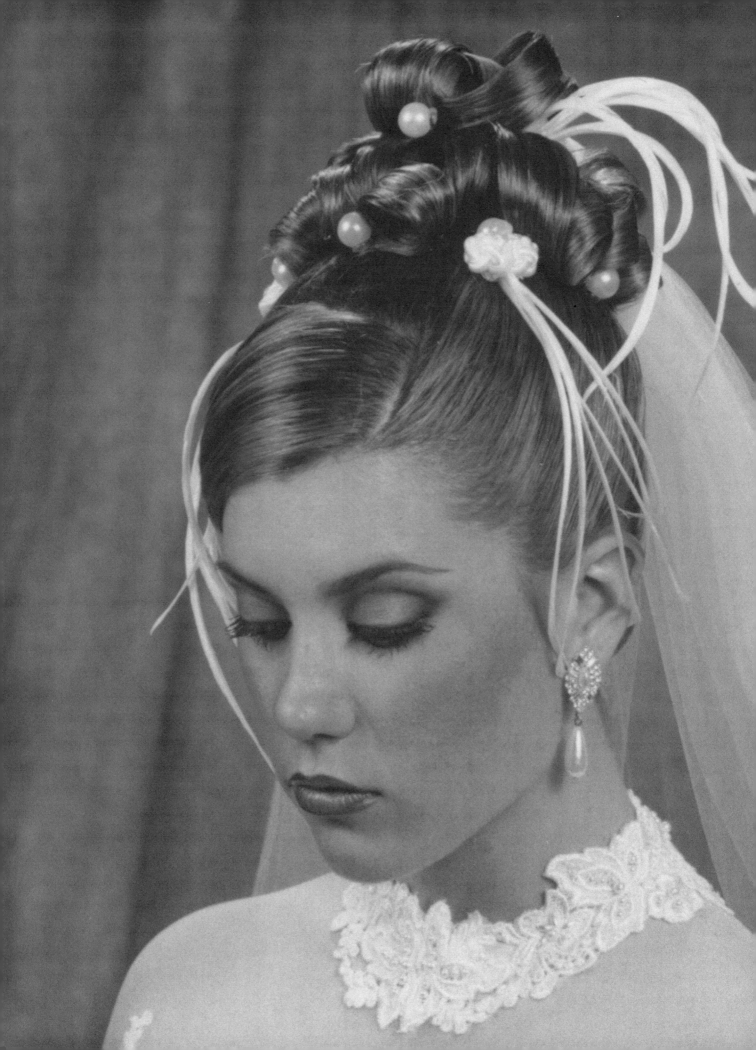

CHAPTER 7

Makeup

A bridal department would not be complete without offering makeup services. Any of us who have witnessed the transforming power that properly applied makeup has on a person could not send a bride home with a bare face. To fully meet the needs of the bride and to have a plan for her from head to toe, a salon needs to have a makeup person on the bridal team. I would have to say 95% of the bridal parties I see coming into the salon want the services of a makeup specialist for their wedding party.

WHEN YOUR SALON *DOES NOT* HAVE A MAKEUP SPECIALIST

What should a salon do that does not currently have a makeup department yet wants to create a bridal department? Becoming a well-known bridal salon does not mean it has to be big, fancy, and have a lot of employees. Bigger is not always better. Having a plan, setting goals, being committed, and following through are the important elements that foster success. Many salons do not have a makeup department or offer makeup retail and services. The need to have a makeup person on the bridal team does not necessarily mean the salon should invest in a full line of makeup and hire a specialist just for the bridal department. If doing so is not in your salon's budget don't despair—there are some other options. Many times not having a large budget forces you to become

more creative and resourceful. What you do need is someone to commit to being on the bridal team, someone who specializes in makeup.

- That person could be available on an on-call, part-time basis since weddings are booked so far in advance.

- That person could sell her own makeup and be hired as an independent contractor and work part-time so there is no initial investment for the salon.

- There may be a stylist already on staff who would like to get makeup training.

Considering makeup services for the bride is something to discuss in the beginning stages of creating the bridal department. A commitment to education is very important whether it is a current staff member or someone independent. Product companies offer a variety of makeup education and videos. Also available are many great books from the Milady/SalonOvations' catalog. Nothing is better than practicing, plus it's fun! It is also important to study the fashion magazines very closely and try some of the looks you see, even if they are outlandish. You will learn by doing.

When you are ready to look for a makeup person here are some ideas to get you started:

- Run an ad in the newspaper and interview respondents.

- This is a time to ask questions and listen to them.

- Explain in detail the demands of being on the bridal team as well as have everything in writing to give to them after the interview.

❧ If you feel they made a good impression have them come for a second interview.

❧ Make sure they bring a model to the second interview.

❧ Plan on having a second model that you pick out for them to do as well.

❧ Watch how they relate to the model they do not know.

❧ It is a good idea to have a model who is middle-aged. More than likely they will bring someone young who will make their work look good.

Here are some questions to ask yourself about this potential employee:

❧ Did they arrive on time?

❧ Did they come neatly dressed?

❧ Did they come prepared?

❧ Did they have an organized makeup kit?

❧ Were they hygienic in their application methods?

❧ Did they clean up when they were done?

This person may be hired independently or on a part-time basis. In the beginning of creating your bridal department you do not have to sell makeup to offer wedding-day services to the bride. However, the eventual purchase of a makeup line for retail and hiring a makeup artist could be a goal tied to the growth of the bridal department.

When contemplating the purchase of a makeup line here are some things

to consider:

❧ Try to **work with** a makeup distributor who will allow you to purchase in small quantities.

❧ **Look into** a makeup line that is offered by the same product company you are already dealing with. They will be more apt to offer you a payment plan.

❧ If you **have built** a strong name and reputation for your salon consider a no-name product line you can put your name on.

❧ Always try to **negotiate** the huge price that comes with the purchase of an entire line. Be aggressive.

❧ **Shop** a few lines for the best deal and use the information as a bargaining tool.

❧ When purchasing an entire line **make use** of the education that is offered.

❧ **Keep** your eye **open** for a less-expensive display case. You pay a lot of money for a lot of plastic. Consider a small antique dresser, or a unique vanity table. Barter with a client who has a husband who is a cabinetmaker.

❧ **Make your own** makeup palette by gluing small pots of shadow onto a mirror or a Lucite frame for display and use. (An artist uses a palette when painting. This enables her to see all of the color choices at once, allowing the eye to mix and create before the paint hits the canvas.)

❧ **Group** the colors in complementary shades and textures. Seeing two or three colors displayed together, you

Considering makeup services for the bride is something to discuss in the beginning stages of creating the bridal department.

and the clients will be more apt to use a variety, paving the way for better retail sales. (I even do this for my traveling makeup when I am doing hair shows. The small containers always slip out of my hands.) I also do this for the makeup I use at home.

🖋 **Display** makeup brushes and use them when doing services. You will have more sales of makeup brushes.

🖋 **Encourage** clients to try the testers. Have plenty of disposable applicators on hand.

🖋 Each day someone should **be responsible** for keeping the makeup station and brushes clean as well as stocked with Q-tips, tissues, and sponges.

WHEN YOUR SALON *DOES* HAVE A MAKEUP ARTIST ON STAFF

Ideally, having a full-time makeup person is a great benefit to the entire salon. Many times clients are in the salon for other appointments and want to talk to me regarding their upcoming wedding. It is an asset to the image of the bridal department to be able to introduce this bride to our makeup specialist. This future bride is greeted by an entire department set up just for weddings including a department head stylist, and a makeup specialist. Some of the larger salons, like Adam Broderick Image Group, are able to employ a full-time Bridal Coordinator.

If your makeup display is collecting dust and your stock is not turning over, then that department is in need of

a makeover itself. Creating a bridal department in the salon may be just what a tired old makeup area needs to boost retail sales. The person you have currently doing makeup may need some additional training. So much time and energy is spent educating the cutting and coloring staff that the makeup artist may not feel part of the team. Continuing education for the makeup artist keeps that department fresh and exciting.

I spoke with national educator Lori Neapolitan who travels the country teaching makeup seminars for Your Name Cosmetics as well as being a makeup artist for Pivot Point International. Lori has been in the makeup business for twenty years. She has worked in research and development of products along with having editorial credit in *Skin Inc., Elle, Vogue,* and the Oprah Winfrey show. Lori stresses the importance of educating the salon in makeup as well as the significance of having a profitable makeup department. "I help the salon with every aspect of promoting and educating the makeup staff. I consult on where the makeup area should be set up, what cabinets work best, ...how the lighting should be. Also covered is pricing, marketing and especially retail," says Lori. Lori and I played telephone tag for a week till I caught up with her in California. The class I particularly was interested in is her bridal makeup class. Lori not only teaches about camera-ready wedding-day makeup application but she also stresses the importance of marketing the bride with promotions. "I teach the makeup artist how to stress to the bride the importance of having a professional makeup application for her wedding day."[1] Lori's classes teach the makeup artist how to create a personal portfolio, tips for photo shoots, pricing, contracts for services, in addition to putting together a traveling makeup kit. If you are interested in a class contact Your Name Cosmetics, Long Island City, New York or Lori personally at (630) 871-0520.

Some other ideas are:

- Talk to your distributor about creating promotions and displays.

- Give the makeup artist a budget to use for retail purchases and help them set some goals for improving the department.

- Have the entire salon educated in the basics of makeup so they can talk about it to their clients.

Most important, have the makeup area displayed where clients can see it. If the makeup department is given a sense of importance it will become an important department. If it is treated as an afterthought it won't be thought of. Tobi Britton, owner of The Makeup Shop, a New York makeup boutique, adds, "too often, makeup is an afterthought in many salons and the counter reflects that."[2]

As you are considering the layout of the bridal department make sure your makeup is visible and available for clients to experiment. It is important for the bride and clients that the area set aside for application be somewhat private, or screened off.

Even as a bridal hair specialist it is a good idea to become trained in makeup application and product knowledge yourself. I find it very helpful in many ways to be able to apply makeup. As the wedding department grows it is important to have a few people in the salon who can apply makeup. Many times part of the bridal team may be called to offer services out of the salon on a busy Saturday. There should be someone back at the salon who can sell makeup and apply it while the team is away. Five out of the thirteen stylists in the salon where I work can do makeup applications. There are times when I go to the home of a bride and do her makeup as well as her hair. Another time our makeup artist was called to do makeup for a wedding party on the same day I had to do a wedding that needed hair and makeup services. Many times I have had to do makeup at photo shoots and hair shows. If you can do it, you can sell it.

STATISTICS FROM *MODERN BRIDE* HEALTH AND BEAUTY SURVEY

Modern Bride was kind enough to send me their survey to use for this book. Let me tell you who responded to the survey:

- 94% of respondents are first-time brides

- Average age of respondent: 26, Average age of fiancé: 27

- 92% are college educated; 89% are employed, 73% full-time, and 16% part-time

- Average annual pretax income of respondents and fiancé: $48,400[3]

As you are considering the layout of the bridal department make sure your makeup is visible and available for clients to experiment.

The brides are ready and willing to spend. Are you marketing your makeup and skin care products to them?

When *Modern Bride* did a survey of a percentage of their readers one of the many questions was:

Where do you normally shop for each of the following products?

Listed were fragrance, cosmetics, hair care products, skin care products, nail care products, and sun care products as well as three areas that do not apply to the salon—feminine hygiene products, eye care products, and birth control. They were asked to choose from:

🖎 department store

🖎 discount store

🖎 drug store

🖎 grocery store

🖎 beauty salon

Let me list only those that concern us. Listed are the most popular compared to the beauty salon:

🖎 Cosmetics: Department store 54%, Beauty salon 4%

🖎 Hair care products: Discount store 33%, Beauty salon 34%

🖎 Skin care products: Department store 37%, Beauty salon 10%

As a whole we have done well with the selling of hair care products. There is no reason why we can't compete in the areas of skin care and makeup.

Then the brides were asked:

If you will purchase any of the above products specifically for your wedding day and/or honeymoon, where will you purchase them? Watch the changes!

🖎 Cosmetics: Department store 64%, Beauty salon jumps to 12%

🖎 Hair care products: Discount store drops to 24%, Beauty salon jumps to 50%

🖎 Skin care products: Department store 48%, Beauty salon jumps to 14%[4]

According to *Modern Bride*'s survey, 7 in 10 engaged women will spend more than usual on skin care, hair care, and makeup for their wedding day and/or honeymoon. Department stores see increased activity, as do *beauty salons,* when engaged women shop for products for their wedding day and/or honeymoon; and discount stores and grocery stores experience a drop in activity. Significant proportions of brides-to-be will try different brands of various products when planning for their wedding day.

What does this information say to the beauty salons out there? The brides are ready and willing to spend. Are you marketing your makeup and skin care products to them? Most brides who know you have a wedding department will come to you at least four to ten months ahead of their wedding day. This is ample time to get them interested in some new products for their wedding and honeymoon.

We know most brides purchase a bridal magazine to look at wedding dresses. *Modern Bride* also wanted to know how interested brides would be in reading about certain subjects. Guess what the top areas of interest were? Hair and makeup. The brides-to-be in this survey felt that articles about these topics were important or extremely important:

- Wedding-day hairstyles (88%)
- Tips for keeping your hairstyle looking great all day (88%)
- Choosing the right hairstyle for your headpiece (84%)
- How to keep makeup fresh all day (82%) [5]

These were the top four answers. If one thing about this survey leaves any impression, it has to be that brides and beauty salons are meant for each other. They are a marriage made in heaven. It is high time salons wake up to the beauty needs of the bride. If the services are offered and packaged properly, the bride will purchase her beauty products from the salon over the department store.

Here are some other interesting facts:

- 78% will hire a professional to do their wedding-day hair
- 45% will have their makeup applied by a professional on their wedding day
- 59% indicated the professional will use the bride's own makeup
- 68% will spend more on products for their wedding day
- 32% will spend about the same [6]

Hopefully it will be makeup and products that they purchase from your salon.

I had a bride who NEVER wore makeup on a regular basis. So, when it came to her wedding day, I assumed she would just need us to use our makeup for that day. I neglected to even mention makeup needs to her. When she came in for her trial-run appointment, I was shocked to see her bring a bag full of new makeup she had purchased at the department store. I made the wrong assumption. Too bad I had not read the makeup study sooner! Sometimes we may get too personal with our clients and feel that we know them too well. We assume they would not want to purchase products they don't use on a regular basis. Yet when these products are offered to them they will make a purchase, especially when it is their wedding day. It was obvious that the client did not need some of the products she was sold and she knew it.

Use this as an angle when showing the bride makeup from the salon. You may choose to say something like, "Let me show you what you need for your wedding day to keep your makeup fresh. If you wait and go to the department store they will be sure to push you into purchasing products that you really don't need."

Susan Bergeron McKenna, a makeup artist with whom I have worked for six years, was trained by a big company and did work in a department store for some time. She is quite familiar with their tactics. Some might say this is fine and good for sales, but if department stores have earned a negative reputation for this, why should a salon want to as well? It is because we do establish a relationship with our clients that we should meet their beauty needs with respect. They will feel much more comfortable to come back to us than to go back to a department store. They know we want to keep them as a salon client.

Anticipate the bride's needs. The Bride Line Network has this to add:

If the services are offered and packaged properly, the bride will purchase her beauty products from the salon over the department store.

> *"Although it is not wise to monopolize the conversation, it's extremely valuable that the bride is aware that you are mindful of all possible concerns on her part. The fact that you know your business well enough, and would make obvious to her all the intricacies, and all their solutions, so that they will never occur during her celebration, is an endearing part of genuinely caring for the bride's needs."* [7]

Whether it is salon services or makeup for the big day, a salon should be fully ready to anticipate any needs that may arise.

Whether it is salon services or makeup for the big day, a salon should be fully ready to anticipate any needs that may arise.

I ran into a situation with a bride concerning her wedding makeup. I thought I was meeting this bride's needs by anticipating any problems that could possibly arise. This particular bride was getting married at 10 A.M. She and her party were due to come in at 6:30 A.M. and were to be out of the salon by 8:30 A.M. The bride's request to me was, she had a friend who wanted to do the makeup for the wedding party. It was to be this friend's gift to the bride. Since the party was coming in so early and there would not be time for makeup after their hair appointments, the bride asked if her friend could bring her makeup to the salon and do the party while they were getting their hair done.

I know you are all thinking NO! NO! You didn't let her did you? I did. I didn't want to do it; I knew it was totally unprofessional. However, this bride was special for two reasons. One, she had me make her a very expensive floor-length headpiece. Two, she was allowing our local news TV station to

come to her wedding and videotape it. Portions of the video were going to be used for a segment showcasing my custom headpiece work and would air just before the evening news. I rationalized that our salon's regular hours start at 9 A.M. on a Saturday and the party should be out by then. Here is where I was anticipating a problem. I explained to the bride it would be OK for her friend to do the makeup at the salon but I stressed to the bride that she needed to make sure her friend understood that she had a very important job that morning. I told her many times "friends" do not understand the importance of the wedding morning remaining on schedule. I told her to have her friend come in at the same time as the party and for her not to be late.

You guessed it! The "friend" came late and ran the whole party behind. Plus, she was still doing makeup after 9 A.M. When the makeup artist came in for work she had a fit! Beside all this, I knew the photographer who was doing the wedding and was upset that he was going to think it was the salon's fault for a late-starting photo session. I took all the blame on this one, cooled down the makeup artist, and vowed never to let this happen again!

I am sure each and every one of us has a wedding-day horror story to share. Speaking of sharing, I want to thank *Modern Bride* for letting me share this enlightening information with you. The percentages provided by *Modern Bride* in this section are very informative and convincing. Brides want special services. They want a special atmosphere. They want special products and are willing to spend more. Now use these statistics wisely and get ready for the brides!

MAKEUP FOR PHOTOGRAPHY

There are many seminars and schools concerning this subject and if you are interested in doing makeup for print work I encourage you to do some research and attend a class or two. For our purposes I want to give you a few tips concerning makeup for wedding photography. It is important for the bride to understand that she needs a little more makeup on her wedding day than she would normally wear. This is especially the case for the bride who normally wears very little makeup and will feel uncomfortable with too much.

Two things to think about when consulting a bride regarding her makeup:

1. Most brides will be in a white dress. All that white can be overpowering and void of color.

2. She will want her features to show up in the photos.

National makeup artist and consultant Lori Neapolitan says, "Film, and especially video, flattens out the face. This needs to be explained to the bride. The bride's makeup needs to be defined and given dimension. Special attention should be taken to defining her features such as her brows and eyes because her image will look washed out on film."

Susan Bergeron McKenna also stresses, "Paying attention to brows is important because they tend to fade in photographs."[8]

B. J. Gillian, Cover Girl's makeup pro says, "The camera sees more than your friends do." Gillian also suggests that you apply a bit of earth-colored or brown eye shadow under your bottom lashes, and smudge. "This gives the illusion in photos of long, thick lashes."[9]

I spoke with Laura Geller of Laura Geller Makeup Studio in New York City. Laura suggests, "to avoid shimmery colors, which often look too shiny in photographs, especially in the eye area. However, don't be afraid of using a gloss with shine on the lips. Adding shimmer to the lips makes the mouth more voluptuous, more kissable."[10]

Darac, a Prescriptives national makeup artist, warns against applying cool colors heavily, because they tend to "jump off your face" in photos.[11]

The flash from the camera will actually bounce off any shiny surface and cause a white-looking spot. Also, too much cover-up under the eyes will cause a raccoon look in the photos. If you need to use cover-up make sure to apply a powder finish over it to blend. This will help to avoid white areas caused by the flash showing up in the photo. Studio lighting will eliminate this from happening but that is not the lighting used during a wedding ceremony.

I worked with one bride who had a distinctive image in mind for her total bridal look. She worked in Manhattan and wanted a modern hairstyle which looked great. She had light blonde hair, she was wearing white, and her bouquet was all shades of cream and light beige. She seemed to have an angelic soft vision for herself because

It is important for the bride to understand that she needs a little more makeup on her wedding day.

she insisted on very pale makeup as well. The makeup artist and I tried to explain how she would look lost in the photos, but it was to no avail. She did not like the makeup done at the trial run even though it was done in neutrals. She would not trust the makeup artist to make changes and decided she would do her own makeup on her wedding day. Sometimes with certain strong personality types you have to let the bridal client have what she wants, even if it is not going to complement her. Her happiness is what matters most.

When doing the bride's makeup for her black-and-white engagement picture the emphasis should remain on the eyes and lips. Avoid using blush. It will show up as a shadow instead of a highlight. Any shade of red or pink will become black or a tone of gray in black-and-white photos. Do not neglect the bride's brows, especially if she is blonde. Line the lips well and go for a darker shade than normal.

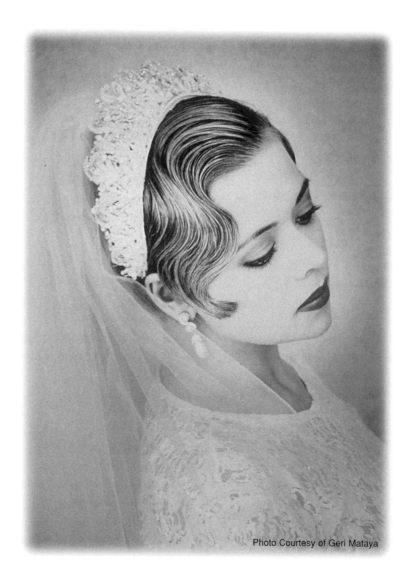

Photo Courtesy of Geri Mataya

TIPS FROM THE EXPERTS

Who are the experts? As far as your bride is concerned, if she is happy with the results of what you do for her, then *you* are the expert! "Expert" comes from the word *experience*. It is experience that will allow you to call yourself an expert. Experience comes from practicing and making decisions. *Don't* experiment on a paying client. *Do* practice on your free time. When the salon has a night set aside for practicing updos make sure the makeup artist is included.

Susan Bergeron McKenna, who did most of the makeup for this book, was a joy to work with. I love having Susan on the bridal team with me because she is an expert at calming the bride. Her patience and soft-spoken manner is as just as important as her skill with makeup. One trick I always see Susan do with the bride is having the bride walk across the room. She then asks the bride to look down as if she were holding her bouquet of flowers and instructs the bride to slowly walk toward her. Susan uses this method to check the bride's eye makeup as well as her overall palette. Susan stresses, "This special bouquet trick just for the bride leaves them with a further impression that our salon is bridal friendly. Look and make sure she is well-blended. Double-check, and recheck. Also, take her hairstyle into account. If the bride has short hair or an updo make sure there are no visible lines in her neck area or leading into her ears, match the shade to her neck and blend it well below the jaw line.

Finish with pressed or loose powder and you'll have the the perfect canvas for the rest of your makeup."[12]

At Diane Young Skin Care Center, New York City, the bride gets a minimum of three makeup lessons if she'll be applying her own makeup. If the salon will be doing the makeup, the artist does the application in advance to experiment with colors and perfect the look.[13]

Louis Salvati, Artistic Director of Education for Graham Webb, feels a bride should have a more natural look for her wedding day. "Accent the cheeks and lips more, do not overdo the eyes."[14]

Laura Geller also has this information for the eyes: "Draw attention to your eyes by adding extra eyeliner in the outer corners. Don't use extreme shades; natural colors tend to look better when you're wearing white."[15]

Lorraine Altamura, of Seven Arts NYC, says, "The lips are the most important feature, with all that kissing going on. For color that won't bleed or smear, use a creamy lip pencil to outline the lips, then fill them in with the same pencil."[16]

The makeup artist, esthetician, or stylist doing makeup has the power to transform the bride into her most beautiful self. The bride's moment will be captured in photos that she will look at for years to come. The sentiment coupled with the responsibility of taking care of the bride's needs is an ever-present incentive to do my best. I welcome the responsibility accompanied with the occasional challenge.

> *Experience comes from practicing and making decisions. Don't experiment on a paying client. Do practice on your free time.*

As I have stressed many times in this book, reading the personalities and clueing in on the wishes of the bride will make you a success. You need to hear where she is coming from and avoid defining any stereotypes where makeup is concerned.

Dee Alicia, the makeup artist for Noelle Spa for Beauty & Wellness, in Stamford, Connecticut, was so kind as to offer her makeup services for the last photo shoot for this book. She gladly would have done more but the timing for my project fell in the middle of her pregnancy. I waited till Dee was back on her feet and was so fortunate to have her input. As I worked with Dee she would ask what was the "look" I was trying to achieve with each model. She would look at the model's gown and ask what kind of hairstyle I was going to do. Based on listening to me and reading what I was trying to achieve with each model, she produced beautiful results.[17]

As a makeup artist there will be someone you need to please. It may be the photographer at a photo shoot, a set director, or, in our case, the bride.

"The bottom line is how the bride feels about herself; she needs to feel beautiful and it is my job to help create that for her," says Susan Bergeron McKenna.[18]

COLOR UNDERTONES

Education, practice, and becoming visually aware of slight differences in skin tones will make you an effective and sought-after makeup artist.

With the makeup service you have to be able to see color. You need to be able to see the color of undertones in the skin. A person's undertones will influence the color you put on the skin. The same foundation color applied on two blue-eyed blondes will look different if one has warm undertones and the other has cool undertones.

It can be difficult to pinpoint someone's coloring exactly. Dee Alicia has this further advice to share when trying to determine a client's skin tone.

First I look at the client's eye color, her eyes may be a blue-gray, a bright clear blue, or a golden blue. This will help me to determine what colors will complement her. Then I look at her hair color if it is natural, or I ask what her natural hair color was. Thirdly I check her skin tones. Studying these three areas is the best assurance to find out if the bride or client has a cool or warm skin tone."[19]

Someone who is cool, meaning blue undertones in the skin, next to someone who is even cooler may throw off your judgment. Dee's method of having three checkpoints is a great idea.

Diane Young, owner of Diane Young Skin Care Center NYC, also has a three-point system that works every time to determine whether someone is cool or warm. First, she asks the bride or client to list her three favorite clothing colors, then she asks her to list her three worst clothing color choices. "Then I ask her what family of colors her favorite lipstick comes from. These three questions always tell me if she is warm or cool." Most people are attracted to colors that complement them.[20]

Be careful not to have your ideas set in stone. A bride who looks best in a certain color may resist wearing it. Trying different colors combined with the bride's input is your best source of information. I witnessed a conversation between the makeup artist and a bride who was cool, and considered by the makeup artist a "true winter." The makeup artist asked this bride if she was wearing a white gown because white would be best. The bride got a little worried because she was not wearing "pure" white. Certain fabric, mainly silk shantung, does not look pure white, but when placed next to a cream or an ivory gown, does look white. When the bride explained what fabric her gown was made of the makeup artist assured her it was perfect for her skin tone. When you look at white satin it is considered a cool white because it gives off almost an iridescent purple glow.

Another trick from Susan Bergeron McKenna is to ask the bride what colors she has chosen for her bridesmaids. This always tells you where the bride's favorite colors lie. Also ask her what colors are in her flowers. Use these colors as a guide in choosing her makeup colors.

There will be some brides who purchase one shade of lipstick based on the color of the bridesmaids' dresses and bring it in for the entire party to use. Here is how Susan handles that dilemma:

Explain to the bride one color will not be correct for every person. Assure the bride you will keep the color tones in the same family but adjust the base tone to complement the individual. If everyone is to be in pink someone may need a slight bit of coral added, where someone will be able to wear a cool pink. On film everyone will look like they are in pink. This will avoid having unhappy bridesmaids or allowing someone in red, someone in burgundy, and someone in fuchsia which will not produce a coherent image for the party, or look good in the photos." [21]

The *correct* colors will do just that, correct or diminish flaws. Properly matched colors will smooth and clarify the complexion. A healthy glow to the face, created by using the correct makeup colors, will minimize lines and circles, while shadows will disappear into the background. By applying inappropriate colors to the skin the complexion will look sallow, pale, or muddy. Shadows, fine lines, blotches, and dark circles will then tend to pop out. Use the trial run to make appropriate adjustments. Educate your bride, have her bring in all of her makeup so you can see what she needs to replace or add to her assortment.

THE TRIAL RUN

How many times have you heard someone complain about a makeup artist who used the same colors the makeup artist herself was wearing— colors appropriate for her but not the client? Or she didn't seem to listen when the client said, "I'm not used to too much makeup," and came away looking like a clown. I had a friend

> *Properly matched colors will smooth and clarify the complexion.*

who actually walked away mid-sentence from a makeup person in a department store because the woman kept offering colors and products she did not want. Listen to your clients. Even if the bride has the perfect palette and is beautiful, yet wants to look simple for her wedding day, you need to listen to her.

The wedding day is not the time for a makeover. However, good use of the time you have at the trial run will allow you the chance to establish a rapport with a bride who may become a makeup client for life.

Laura Geller feels the trial run is an important time for the bride to visualize what kind of look she wants. "I talk with her, listen to her, and together we create a little magic." Geller knows the secret to wonderful bridal makeup: communication paired with the absence of attitude. "I never force colors or new looks on a bride; if she has a favorite lipstick that makes her feel great, I'll use it instead of my own makeup. The key is for the bride to look and feel comfortable and confident, and she must be able to recognize herself when she looks in the mirror!" [22]

Follow these steps to ensure a happy client:

1. Listen and ask questions.

2. Show her a wedding-day look complimentary to her.

3. Write down everything you did and every color you used.

4. Purchase face charts and actually apply the makeup itself to the chart for further reference.

5. File it the same way the stylist files the bride's hairstyles and information.

6. At the end of her trial run use this time to show her an evening look, something she may like to try on her honeymoon.

7. Encourage her to ask makeup questions that may not pertain to her wedding.

8. This is the perfect opportunity to sell her some products.

9. Also encourage the bride to schedule a season-change makeup lesson.

The bride is all ears at her trial run. It gives her a chance to feel pampered. She will feel more comfortable in a familiar atmosphere. She will look to you more as an artist than as a salesperson.

BASIC WEDDING-DAY MAKEUP APPLICATION

Concealer

Work on a clean, well-moisturized face. Look for any areas where the skin pigment is darker. The corners of the nose, mouth area, and under the eyes are the most common. The dark circles are caused by blood vessels showing through thin skin in the eye area. Remember not to use white or to conceal in a complete semi-circle under the eye. This will cause raccoon eyes and any light from the photographer's flash will reflect from this area. If the bride has allover ruddy pink areas, conceal with a green base concealer. If

The wedding day is not the time for a makeover.

the bride has bluish undertones near her eyes, use a yellow base concealer (yellow is also great for broken capillaries). A lavender base concealer is also good for dark circles under the eye. Refer to the laws of color. In the color spectrum, colors opposite one another will cancel each other out, leaving a more neutral base to work on. Apply concealer in a stippling, dotting manner with a makeup sponge, and blend.

Foundation

Choose a foundation color closest to the bride's own skin tone. Apply over the concealer with gentle strokes. Apply over the entire face including the eye area and lips. Go into the neck area and near the ears. Since the foundation should match the bride's own natural coloring, you do not need to cover all of her neck or shoulder area. A powdering of these areas afterwards will be enough to merge the finishes. Blend the foundation and finish with downward strokes. This allows the little facial hairs to lie smooth.

I asked Dee Alicia to offer some wedding-day makeup tricks. Here's what she does to make the foundation last all day. "Start with an oil-free toner or a colored concealer to correct any flaws. Over this apply a fine layer of foundation. Then mist the face with a water-base face spray. Let it dry for a few seconds and apply a loose powder. Repeat with a thin layer of foundation and end with powder again, this time skipping the water mist." [23] Dee also suggests asking someone from the wedding party to be responsible to check the bride's makeup just before any important photos.

Eye Colors

After choosing the eye colors, apply the lightest or medium shade over entire eye area. The foundation in conjunction with this shadow over the eye will create a smooth, nonmoisturized area and help keep the colors from creeping and creasing throughout the day. Contour a deeper shade in the crease of the lid just under the brow bone. If there is not a distinct brow bone ask the bride to open her eyes and look straight at you. As her eyes remain open put a small amount of color where her brow bone should be as if to mark the spot. Have her close her eyes again and blend in this deeper color at the brow bone area.

There is no application method set in stone. Some artists line the eye first, some apply the shadow first. One thing I have learned over my many years of experience is, if something works for you, have confidence in your decisions because they will prove reliable.

Lining the Eye

Lining the eye can be done with a pencil or eye shadow and a fine brush. I prefer working with an angled brush and shadow for a more pronounced look. However you choose to apply liner, never leave a harsh line, always blend.

Look at the eye shape. Is it almond shape, large and oval, or small? Think of designing the liner in a way to create the opposite effect and make the eye do what you want it to do. Large eyes can handle eyeliner applied all around the eyes. Smaller eyes look best

In the color spectrum, colors opposite one another will cancel each other out, leaving a more neutral base to work on.

with a concentration of tone more toward the outer corner of the eye. The idea is to widen the eyes a bit.

The Brow

Make sure at the trial run you introduce the bride to waxing her brow. Nothing transforms the eye and the entire look of the face more than beautifully shaped eyebrows. When filling in the brow, brush the brow hairs down and give the top of the brow a smoother line. Brush gently up and fill in empty spaces lightly. Finish by combing up and following the natural arch. You can work with pencils or compact powders. Think "light touch" and step back to look from a distance. You can always add more of anything. A trick I like to do is to cup my hands around one eye like I am looking through a camera. It helps my eye to focus solely on the face.

Blush

For the blush, choose a shade complementary to the bride's coloring. Start at the apple of the cheek, the area directly below the eye. Stroke up toward the hairline along the edge of the cheekbone. This is not the time to contour under the cheekbone. Contouring in conjunction with a photographer's studio lighting is the best time to create cheekbones; done incorrectly it can look like a bruise or a dirty smudge. Keep blush natural looking. You may also choose a pressed powder a shade or two darker than the skin tone. This gives a change in tone without color. If the bride has a high forehead I like to apply pressed powder in a slightly

deeper tone along the hairline. Blend, blend, blend!

Lips

Line the lips in a color as close as possible to the lip color you will be using. Line the natural lip line. The bride will feel foolish if you go outside the natural line. She wants to feel beautifully enhanced on her wedding day, not made-up. Fill in the entire lip with the lip liner; this helps the color to last. Using a lip brush, stroke on the lipstick over the lip liner. Remember, any shine or frost will reflect light of any kind, emphasizing fine lines around the mouth. Depending on your height and the height of the chair you are applying makeup at, it is always a good idea to have the bride stand up to check her lips. Look at them at your eye level and make sure they are even and match. Don't neglect applying color in the corners of her mouth. Have the bride say a few words to see if her lips are perfect. Check her teeth for lipstick stains and have her blot excess lipstick with a tissue.

Powder

Nothing finishes off the look better than a dusting of face powder. If she is dry skinned her makeup will set in about twenty minutes and last all day. If she is oily have her use rice papers or an oil-blotting paper to remove the excess oil throughout the day. This is better than adding more powder. By applying more powder to cover the shine the skin will get coated and blotchy. Color over color always turns darker. A dusting of loose powder one shade lighter than the foundation even lightly over the eyes creates a beautiful finish. Or you may choose to use a translucent powder so you don't discolor the foundation. If you feel the need to powder before you begin the eyes, go ahead and do so. Sometimes when applying eye shadow it spills onto the under eye area. By applying some loose powder there first, spilled eye shadow is easily wiped away.

Mascara

"Waterproof mascara is a must for the bride," says Dee Alicia.

"Another trick I do with the bride is, after curling her lashes, I put on one coat of regular mascara. Then I use the waterproof mascara as my second coat. This seals in the color and makes it easier to remove the mascara later." [24]

When selecting makeup colors make sure to choose those combinations from the same tone, warm or cool, for a balanced natural look.

🦢 Cool tones consist of: Soft blues or vibrant clear blues, forest greens, aqua greens, grays and gray/taupe, mauves, pink/roses, blue/purples, blue/reds, wine, burgundy, purple/plum, and silver.

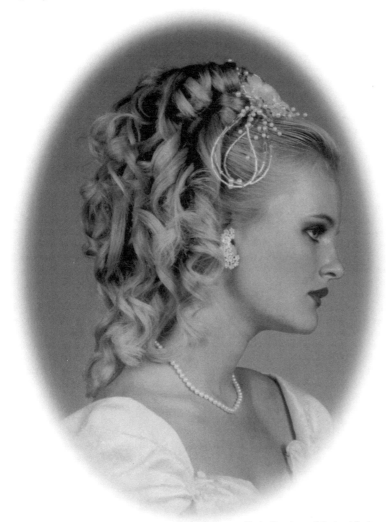

Photo Courtesy of Garland Drake

❧ Warm tones consist of: Terra-cotta russets, red browns, tan, sierras, dark brown, golden beige, yellow gold, yellow greens, earth greens, coral, peach, salmon, orange/pinks, red/plums, and gold.

CHOOSING COLORS

Lois Pearce, president of Beautiful Occasions, an event planning service in Hamden, Connecticut, as well as the Association of Bridal Consultants Connecticut State Coordinator and Director of Ethnic Diversity, recently shared the following information in an ABC newsletter:

" *By the year 2056, an 'average' U.S. resident defined by census statistics will be able to trace his or her descent to Africa, Asia, the Hispanic world, the Pacific Islands, or Arabia; almost anywhere but White Europe. Statistically, there are five major minority populations in the United States: African American, Asian American, Native American, Hispanic, and Pacific Islander. Although identified as 'Hispanic,' the truth is there are no Hispanics; they are Mexicans, Puerto Ricans, Dominicans, Colombians, Cubans, etc. Depending on where your service is located determines the percentage of these minority populations you may serve. However, it does not mean you should not make yourselves aware of these cultures and how they can add to your bottom line."* [25]

In the area of makeup it is important to become educated in how to address the needs of the multicultural population. You don't need to have a foundation on hand for every person on earth but you do need to know what to look for in the skin tones and how to mix your colors accordingly. Seek out as much education as you possibly can.

I am fortunate enough to work with three very experienced hair colorists in the salon. They understand color—hair color, chemical color, underlying tones, cool and warm skin tones—no matter what color line comes into the salon they can work with it. I have interviewed colorists who can only work with one hair color line. How limited! If you understand the laws of color, some chemistry about the colors you work with, and take the education that comes with carrying a line, you will understand color. Period. You will be able to use your knowledge and work with any color line. You will become more creative and have more options to offer your color clients. You will be better able to do color correction correctly without waste. The same goes for makeup. When a bride or client trusts your instincts about their makeup needs they will seek you out again and again, for services in addition to retail.

Once you have decided the bride's skin undertones and you have inquired as to the colors of her wedding party, what colors will look best on her? Of course this is the reason for a trial run. With the bridesmaids, however, there is no trial run so a knowledge of color is important. In this next section I take a general look at colors and choices. You can use the chart below for a quick reference.

Brunettes

To enhance the brown eye color of a brunette look to see if she has golden highlights or copper specks in her eyes. Bring out those colors by using them on her eyes. If her eyes are a very dark brown leave the lid light and define with eye liner. Smudge black or use a dark brown eye liner. Avoid the overall brown look. Having no color will make her look tired. Remember she will be in white. The only color will come from her makeup. Purples, plums, and greens as well as bits of gold or silver are beautiful on a brunette. Lips should be as vibrant as the bride will allow.

Blondes

Deep-toned pastels work beautifully on the blonde bride. Light golden browns with a hint of peach or pink are also nice. Do not overdo the undereye area with too much liner or mascara. Light corals are best as long as they complement the skin tones. Avoid blues and greens. Lips should not be too dark or rich. A matte berry is nice, so is a shade of mauve. A blonde bride can easily look washed out in photos. Don't neglect her brows.

Redheads

If freckles are present, they should be allowed to show through a sheer foundation, if the bride allows. Usually the pores are very small on a freckled face so there is no need for heavy founda-

Features	Eye Colors	Face Colors	Lip Colors
Brunette	purples, plums, greens, bits of gold or silver (bring out colors within eyes: gold, copper specks)	bisque, medium beige foundation	as vibrant as bride will allow
Blonde	light corals, deep-toned pastels; avoid blues, greens	ivory, fair to medium color foundation	berry, mauve, not too dark or rich
Redhead	corals, earth-tones, neutral shades	blush—soft pink or peach	corals, soft pink, deep berry
Latin	burgundy, plums, deep blues, jewel tones	avoid pink-based foundation	berry, soft fuchsia, red, plum
African American	wines, fuchsia, purples with cool undertones	blush—orange or peach with warm skin	orange, peach, burgundy or deep pinks
Asian	neutral shades	medium to dark foundation	reds

tion. Blush can be a soft pink or peach. Remember, a beautiful head of red hair takes center stage. This bride can wear the natural and neutral shades on the eyes. Blend these with shrimp, corals, or apricot. Greens in the earth tones are best. A little gold on the center of the eye lid or under the brow bone opens up the eye. Soft brown eye pencil on the outer edge and brown mascara frame the eyes nicely. Don't let the red hair fool you into thinking she is always warm. A cool redhead has a bluer shade of red and very sheer skin with blue undertones. Her eyes are usually a clear blue with white flecks and to use products with a gold tone will not complement a cool redhead.

Latin

If you do not have the colors to work on Latin skin, have the bride bring in her own foundation. You cannot use a pink-base foundation on an olive or yellow-green skin tone. For eyes and lips, choose beautiful rich shades. For an evening wedding and formal affair rich burgundy, plums, and deep blues are a good choice. For a day or morning wedding, jewel tones such as emerald green, amethyst, or sapphire are striking. These bright or dark colors can be blended with a neutral to tone them down. On the lips, a bright berry or soft fuchsia is lovely for daytime. Save plums, deep berries, and red for evening receptions. Never do a brown natural look on a Latin bride; she will look tired and drained.

African American

Here you can run into red or gold undertones in the skin as well as olive. Then you need to determine if the skin is dark, medium, or light. Take special care to the areas of the eyes, nose, and mouth and blend in concealer well. To complement gold undertones you can use orange or peach for lips and blush. Red undertones in the skin are best complemented with wines, fuchsia, and purples.

Asian

An Asian face has a flatter-surfaced bone structure. Depth needs to be created in a subtle way. Avoid too much depth around the eyes; allow her natural features to take center stage. Keep any eye liner soft and smudged. Playing up a beautiful mouth with a true red to set off her lovely dark hair is ideal. Crystal clean brows are a must. Add a white dress and not much else is needed for the Asian bride. This classic look is lovely.

If you do not have the colors to work on Latin skin, have the bride bring in her own foundation.

TIPS

- Plan on adding makeup to your salon if you do not already carry it.

- Research different product lines.

- Be sure your makeup area is visible and spotless.

- Seek additional makeup education to advance your skills.

- Now is the time for brides. Reread the statistics.

- Educate your bride as to her makeup needs.

- Remember to consider what the lighting from the photographer's flash may do.

- Establish whether the bride's coloring is cool or warm.

- Make use of the trial run to establish a makeup relationship with the bride.

- Consider skin tone, the bridesmaids' dress color, flower colors, the bride's eye and hair color when choosing makeup colors.

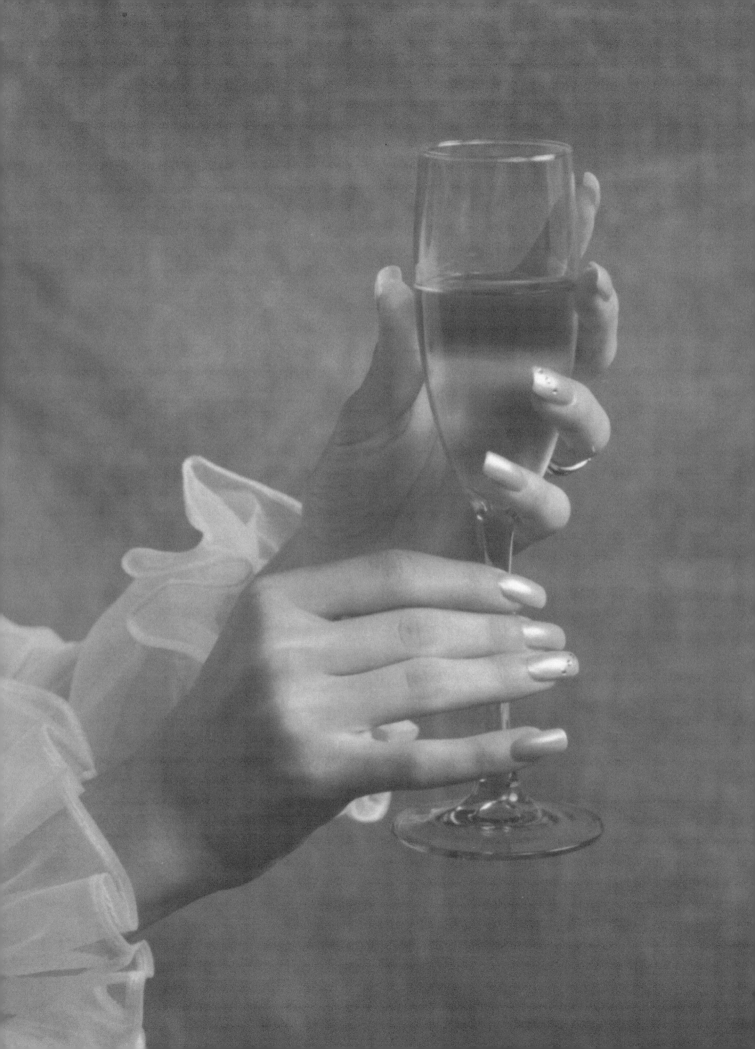

CHAPTER 8

Nails, Waxing, and Skin Care

Three more areas to consider in the total bridal look and meeting all the beauty needs of the bride are the areas of nails, waxing, and skin care. Again, please do not give up on the bridal market if your salon does not offer all of these services.

Go back to Chapter 2, Getting Your Salon Bridal Ready, and study the ideas listed to help your salon work with businesses who offer services you do not. If you believe the bridal statistics and want your share of the bridal market, nothing will stop you.

For those of you who do offer all or some of these services, this chapter will help you to fine tune them for the bride.

NAILS

Apart from her hair, the bride's second main concern is her nails. She wants her nails to be beautiful. Let's face it, the first thing a bride receives is the ring. That alone sends many soon-to-be brides into the salon for manicures. Your job is to try to keep her there.

I ran across an article in the May 1996 issue of *Modern Salon*. It featured a special section on bridal nails. Interviewed was Terri Schmidt of Palos Heights, Illinois. I contacted Terri and asked her to give me some information for this section.

She said, "Nails are a very important part of the bride's total esthetic presentation. She needs perfectly beautiful nails especially when there will be photos of the rings and the cutting of the cake."[1] I sent Terri a list of questions to answer regarding her bridal nail business and advice she has to offer. Throughout this nail section I will be referring to Terri and others who market the bridal client nail services.

Merchandising

Don't forget merchandising and marketing bridal services in the nail department as well as getting out in front of the bride. One of the questions I asked Terri was, "What do you do to specifically market the bridal client?" She replied, "I like to participate in bridal fairs. They are a great way to get in front of the bride and a lot of fun. I set up a beautiful booth including photos of nails I have done for other brides. I also raffle off free full sets. This allows me a list of names of brides who are interested in my services."

In Chapter 2 I talked about making up bridal gift baskets. Separate nail gift baskets are also a great idea for the bride to give her bridesmaids as gifts. These can be priced lower than a hair product-filled basket, giving the bride a variety of choices. Small baskets filled with a file, a bottle of polish, and a gift certificate make adorable gifts. Avoid putting in too many products that promote do-it-yourself nails. Do an all-white theme for weddings and other colors other times of the year. These are a sure seller.

American Salon magazine interviewed Suzi Weiss-Fischmann, executive vice president of OPI Products, North Hollywood, California. "The key is to

> Apart from her hair, the bride's second main concern is her nails.

set up a retail center that has ample lighting, is well-stocked with plenty of product choices and is neat and clean."[2] These three elements make all the difference in the world when it comes to selling retail in the nail department.

Start collecting photos of brides' hands which you have done. These can be framed and placed in a bridal nail display. It takes a little effort but ask any of your brides if they will be having a photo taken of their rings or a close-up of cutting the cake. Offer to pay for a copy and keep on her. Everyone will be trying to get photos from her so you will need a little persistence. There is no reason why a nail technician cannot have a portfolio of her best work.

Besides using photos of the brides you have already done, why not look for a model and plan a photo shoot? When looking for a model to use to photograph your nail talents look for an overall lovely hand and nail bed. Too many times when we try to think of someone to use for a model we only think of that person's long, strong nails. When I was on the lookout for a hand model for this book someone would say, "I know so and so; she has great nails," and I would ask how old the woman was and she would be in her forties. Touchup work on photos can run hundreds of dollars an hour. Look for great hands and long nail beds— "great nails" can always be added. Look at nail photos in the magazines and you will see great nails and too many ugly hands. Look for smooth skin as well as slender hands.

I had a twelve-year-old classmate of my daughter in my appointment book for a haircut. As Jessica started to describe what she wanted for her hair by using her hands to show me, all I saw were lovely hands in the mirror. I interrupted her, grabbed her hands, told her how beautiful they were, and asked her if she would be a hand model. She looked at me like I had twelve heads until I explained a little bit more of why I wanted to use her hands. Hats off to Susan Trischitti who managed to give a lovely full set to an active adolescent! We had a great time and Jessica had to wear her full set for a week for two photo shoots. Susan Trischitti who works with me on the bridal team did the nails for the photos in this book. Susan has been a nail technician for thirteen years, eight of which she owned her own nail salon. The hard work produced beautiful results.

NAIL SHAPES TO COMPLEMENT THE NATURAL NAIL PLATE

When deciding on what shape and length to give to the nails of the bride you must look at her hands, fingers, and shape and length of the nail plate. The same laws of balance and design used for the hair and jewelry to complement the shape of the face are used for the balance of the nails to the hands. Owner of Diane Young Skin Care Center NYC says, today a shorter, functional nail length is best, but many times the younger brides still desire length.

Short hands and a short nail plate are horizontal in shape compared to long slender hands and nail plates which are vertical. We are talking here about the nail *plates* and not the nail *tip* or free edge. The nail plate is the visible part of the nail attached to the nail bed. This may seem as general information to some of you. Nevertheless, the laws allowing nail professionals to work vary from state to state. In my state there are no laws governing who may perform nail services. There are those who have no idea about nails, their disorders, diseases, or the structure of hands, arms, and nails. Look into further education if you happen to be performing nail services in a state without requirements; you owe it to yourself and your clients.

"What are the specific shapes you like to give the tips in regard to the shape of the natural nail plate and the size of brides' hands?" I asked Terri Schmidt.

Longer nails are best to take away from the width of a shorter nail plate. If the nail plate is long, then the bride can wear a more natural length and still look like she has longer nails. I advise tip application approximately three days before the wedding so the bride has a chance to adjust to the new length. If the bride has large hands, longer nails are best to take away from their size. Most importantly I recommend a full color and not a French manicure for large hands. The French cuts larger nails in half, emphasizing the size of the bride's hands."

I also asked Terri what shape she finds most popular for the bride. "Oval is requested more often; it keeps the nails looking natural."[3]

If the bride is used to wearing a square nail soften the edges a bit for the wedding. Your key to what she wants and what you as the professional feel is best can be discussed during the consultation. Stay away from too much nail art when doing the bride's nails. I have seen wedding designs in some of the nail magazines where the model has a lace design on her nails with pearls. You may perform great airbrushing designs and wish to show off your creative work, but try to keep the designs understated and simple. I have also seen where the bride has just her ring finger designed with some nail art.

CONSULTATION QUESTIONNAIRE

What color is your gown?

White _____

Off-White _____

Cream _____

Ivory _____

Other: _____

What type of wedding are you having?

Formal, evening wedding _____

Morning wedding _____

Afternoon wedding _____

Casual wedding _____

Themed wedding _____

If so, what is the theme (Renaissance, Medieval, Black-and-White, etc.)? _____

Is the entire wedding party receiving nail services with us?

Yes ❑

No ❑

If not everyone, who is?

Bride	_____	Mother-of-the-Bride	_____
Maid of Honor	_____	Mother-of-the-Groom	_____
Bridesmaids	_____	Groom	_____
How many?	_____	Groomsmen	_____
Flowergirl	_____		

Other: _____

Do you prefer everyone's nails to match?

Yes ❑

No ❑

What color are the bridesmaids wearing? _____

What color are your flowers? _____

Where is your reception? _____

Where will you honeymoon? _____

Do you wish to wear:

Tips	_____	An Airbrush Design	_____
Acrylic Nails	_____	Pearl/Rhinestone Appliqués	_____
French Manicure	_____	Single-Color Polish	_____

Which nail shape do you prefer:

Square/Rectangle _____

Oval _____

Round _____

Pointed _____

Would you be interested in a pedicure?

Yes ❑

No ❑

Bride's Name _____

Date of Wedding _____

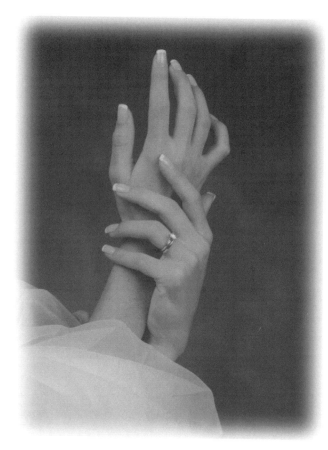

your client's preferences (feel free to add your own):

- What color is your gown?

- Is it a formal evening wedding or a day wedding?

- Is the entire wedding party receiving nail services with us?

- Do you prefer everyone's nails match?

- What color are the bridesmaids wearing?

- What color are your flowers?

- Do you wish to wear tips?

Look at her hands, skin, nail beds, and overall shape of her hands in proportion to her body type during the consultation.

"If the bride does choose to have tips or artificial nails for her wedding, I ask her if they are to be just for the day or does she wish to attend to them on a regular basis. Tell the bride she can wear her tips a little longer for the wedding and then can have them cut down for everyday,"[4] suggests Susan Trischitti.

Terri Schmidt says, "I ask the bride about her wedding gown, its' style, what shade of white it is, as well as what color the bridesmaids' dresses are. I also ask her where the reception is being held."[5]

Don't pass over the bridal nail consultation. Make it a separate, important part of the bridal department.

CONSULTATION: LONG OR SHORT, COLOR OR NATURAL

Your salon offers a consultation for the bridal hairstyle. Make sure the bride also receives one before you begin her nails. A benefit of having a bridal department set up is that the receptionist is able to show the bride all the services your salon offers upon her first contacting the salon. Hopefully, contact is made a few months before the wedding and proper arrangements can be made concerning the care of her nails.

Consultation Questions

You may use these questions on the attached questionnaire to get a feel for

Long or Short. Don't forget to ask the bride about her honeymoon. Today's bride is very active and she may want her nails to be a shorter length because of activities planned on the honeymoon. Again, refer to the overall size and shape of her nail beds and hands to determine the best length for her wedding nails.

Color or Natural. When consulting a bride as to her nail choices for her wedding there are endless options. Most prefer and end up with the French manicure.

> *I do prefer a French manicure as opposed to the California French or the addition of rhinestones or pearls. The focus of the hands should be on the ring. Healthy skin and beautiful nails should complement each other. With the bride there are so many choices available today. You can offer your advice and experience but ultimately you need to please the bride,"[6] says Susan Trischitti.*

For the French manicure shown in this book Sue chose colors by Essie Cosmetics. Blanc was the tip color and the overlay was Coconut Grove, a nice ivory beige.

Terri Schmidt's personal favorite in a French manicure is a pinky-lavender. It gives the nails a healthy glow and is pretty against the white dress. Moreover, consider the color of white of the gown. A cream or off-white dress may look best with a soft, natural beige overlay. Remember to consider the bride's skin tone when choosing the color of the French overlay.

Diane Young, owner of Diane Young Skin Care Center NYC, says, "The French manicure is, hands down, the Number One choice of brides-to-be. For the client who has yellow or gold undertones to her skin, use transparent peach polish; if her undertones are pink, use soft pink."[7]

Solid, clean nails in a subtle overall color are a nice choice as well. A day or garden wedding and lovely spring colors call for an overall soft pink nail. A more elegant evening wedding allows more choices, like the new metallics. The color Susan chose for the solid nail is a beige metallic. Today's metallics are very different from yesterday's frosted colors. New technology has added to this advancement. The metallics produce a lovely soft glow without the garish iridescence that takes away from the ring, plus bounces back the photographer's flash, much the same way as it does in makeup. Offer the bride options of colors during the consultation. Try a few against her skin tone.

A good suggestion for the bride is to have her nails done the same day she has a fitting for her gown. This way she can see the color choices against her gown. For that skittish, sensitive, otherwise nervous bride, offer to do each hand in a different color. *Make sure you write down what you used.*

WHEN TO HAVE SERVICES

I spoke with Stacy Bollen, manager of the Gene Juarez Salon & Spa in Seattle-Tacoma, Washington. In June of 1996 Gene Juarez moved his 1,400-square-foot salon to the other end of the mall and opened a 9,300-square-foot day spa which earned him *Modern Salon's*

> A *good suggestion for the bride is to have her nails done the same day she has a fitting for the gown.*

Your Beautiful Wedding

It's the biggest day of your life...and Gene Juarez Salons want to make sure everything comes together as beautiful as your dreams. Proper planning of your hair and beauty needs today will ensure a wedding day you'll always remember.

Bridal Parties

For bridal parties of four or more, we request a **$25.00 deposit per person** at the time the appointments are made. Deposits are refundable if appointments are cancelled 48 hours in advance.

We strongly suggest brides schedule a trial appointment for makeup and hair, with veil and/or hair accessories, at least three weeks before the wedding. These appointments assure you'll have no surprises on your special day.

Wedding Day Planning

The following are suggestions for achieving the perfect look for your wedding day.

❑ Three Months Before

❖ Begin a facial treatment program (every 4–6 Weeks).

❖ Think of a style change? Now is the time to try something new before the big day. You'll have plenty of time to get adjusted to your new style or redesign if necessary.

❑ Two Months Before

❖ Enhance your nails with a manicure every other week.

❖ Make bridal-day appointments for you and your bridesmaids and relatives.

❑ One Month Before

❖ Technical services—perm, color, and/or conditioning.

❑ Three to Four Weeks Before

❖ Haircut.

❖ Trial airwave or updo with veil and/or hair accessories.

❖ Makeup lesson.

❑ Two Weeks Before

❖ Full-set of nails (acrylic, linen, silk).

❖ Facial.

❖ Waxing (lip and/or brow).

❖ Haircuts for men in the wedding party.

❑ One Week Before

❖ Pedicure (bring a pair of thongs).

❖ Waxing (underarm, legs, bikini, and/or arms).

For Your Comfort:

❖ *We recommend that waxing services be performed after 3–4 weeks of hair growth.*

❖ *Please allow 24 hours before sunbathing or using a tanning bed after waxing. Newly waxed skin is more sensitive to sun and will burn easily.*

❖ *We regret that we cannot perform waxing services on clients who are taking Accutane, Retin-A, or antibiotics, due to the sensitivity these products cause to the skin.*

❑ One to Two Days Before

❖ Nail fill or manicure.

❑ Wedding Day

❖ Makeup application.

❖ Polish change or manicure.

❖ Bridal airwave or updo.

❖ Bridal party hair styling, manicures, and makeup applications.

We Recommend

❖ Identify yourself as a member of the bridal party when scheduling your appointments.

❖ To alleviate last-minute problems, please schedule your appointments 6 weeks in advance.

❖ Please provide day and night phone numbers with all wedding party appointments.

❖ Please ask each member of the wedding party to confirm or cancel their own appointment 48 hours in advance.

❖ Wear a button-down shirt for your wedding day appointment.

❖ For chemically treated hair, avoid chlorinated water in hot tubs, swimming pools, and jacuzzis.

Your Appointment Schedule

Date/Day   Time   Service   Salon/Artist

_____

_____

_____

_____

_____

_____

_____

_____

_____

_____

_____

_____

_____

GENE JUAREZ SALONS

FOUR SEASONS OLYMPIC HOTEL 528-0011 • DOWNTOWN SEATTLE NORDSTROM 628-1405
BELLEVUE SQUARE 455-5511 • NORTHGATE MALL 365-8000
SOUTHCENTER MALL 432-8695 • TACOMA SALON & SPA 472-9999

"Salon of the Year" for 1997. Stacy told me about their bridal prep card and directed me to Linda Rackner, in the corporate offices, who faxed me a copy. Out of all the research I did for this book I personally love what Gene Juarez provides for the bride. I must share the entire program. Please note where the nail, skin, and waxing services are scheduled. I plan to implement much of this information in my own bridal department immediately! I hope you do as well. Simply titled "Your Beautiful Wedding," this two-sided card can easily be slipped into a standard salon brochure. "It is also designed so the bride can check off her progress as she gets closer to her wedding day,"[8] adds Stacy. Great idea!

There are ample lines available for many appointments and listed at the bottom are the six Gene Juarez Salon locations. They were wonderful to deal with over the phone and I thank them for sharing this information.

I posed a few more questions to bridal nail specialist Terri Schmidt.

How many weeks before the wedding do you suggest the bride come in for weekly manicures to get her nails in shape for the wedding? "About four weeks, depending on what kind of shape her nails are in."

Do you encourage entire parties to come in together to get their nails done? "It's great when the bride and bridesmaids all have their nails done at the same booking. Preplanning means the nail colors can be coordinated to the dresses and all the hands will be professionally finished. The girls love it, too. They can take time to kick back and make a party of it. It's easy to achieve a uniform look when they're all together. Later they'll be happy to see in the wedding pictures that everyone's hands look beautiful."

For the bride who wishes to grow her natural nails she should receive weekly manicures with paraffin treatments for eight weeks prior to the wedding day. This will give her natural nail time to grow out. This time also allows her to see the benefit of regular manicures, a routine she will hopefully keep up after the wedding.

Diane Young offers an even more assertive time period for getting bridal nails in shape. "If the bride makes the commitment to getting her own nails in great shape, start weekly treatments four months before the wedding. For the woman who doesn't have the time or money for this, apply tips one week before the wedding. At T-minus three days and counting, redo the manicure."[9]

Don't forget the groom! Remind the bride it would be a good idea for the groom to receive a manicure as well. Offer groomsmen wedding packages that include a manicure.

When thinking of nails don't forget the needs of the bride's feet. When you begin working on her hands for the big day remind the bride of pedicure services. Most brides take a tropical honeymoon and will need to have her toes in shape for the beach. I have seen brides laugh in a sweet, scandalous tone as they are sporting red toenails inside their white wedding shoe waiting to come out of hiding on the honeymoon!

Don't forget the groom! Remind the bride it would be a good idea for the groom to receive a manicure as well.

While you are preparing the bride's toes ask her if she will be needing the services of waxing.

WAXING

One of the areas I decided to look into when researching this chapter was *The Standard Textbook of Cosmetology* published in 1995 by Milady Publishing. It was interesting to read again some history behind the removal of unwanted hair.

In 1875 Dr. Charles E. Michel, an ophthalmologist, used an electric current directed through a thin wire to remove ingrown eyelashes. Thus, the beginning of electrolysis. Early Egyptians used to pumice and literally sand their bodies smooth to render them hairless. Women, mostly in the upper class of society since the beginning of time, have been removing their hair. Today, the service of hair removal is available and affordable for most everyone. The bride is no exception.[10]

As the bridal statistics prove, brides are willing to spend more and try new services in preparing for their wedding. What better time to introduce her to waxing services?

Kristin Wall, spa director of the Adam Broderick Image Group in Ridgefield, Connecticut, suggests that the bride begin seeing the esthetician a couple of months ahead of time. "This way the esthetician can see and access the growth rate of the bride's hair as well as check for any reactions. Then we suggest hair removal be done 4 to 5 days before the wedding. We also remind the bride to take special care in the sun."[11]

Diane Young recommends a leg and bikini wax no later than one week before the wedding. She also stresses the importance of using a loofah sponge to prevent ingrown hairs. This advice leads us into discussing the bride's skin care needs surrounding her wedding.[12]

SKIN CARE

A bridal department that encourages and promotes all bridal-specific salon services will have the most success with the bride. This is true across the country. Paula Fierson, consultant for Noelle Spa for Beauty & Wellness, in Stamford, Connecticut, spent some time working in Japan introducing them to the "Noelle Spa concept." I asked her if they were interested in the bridal services. "Yes, the Japanese women are very interested in having all the services available to them, especially if they have a important event such as a wedding."[13]

A perfect time to introduce a young bride to a lifelong relationship with skin care is during her engagement. The fine lines of time are beginning to appear. The stress related to juggling all the worries of planning a wedding has taken its toll on the weary bride. Skin care services directed her way will be a welcome relief.

Skin care has ridden a tidal wave of aging baby boomers the last two decades. The oldest baby boomers turned fifty years old in 1996, leaving many more skin care converts in their wake, mainly their children—your new brides. Product companies have turned much of their research and advertising dollars toward skin care product development and exposure. Makeup advertisements used to fill the pages of the magazines; now skin care ads have taken precedence. Proper skin care, its requirements and retail, should only be offered by a well-trained salon professional. Not a person trained in selling, but *a person trained in skin care.*

This is why you and your salon should include the skin care department when planning a bridal department. How does an unqualified client or bride know what her skin care needs are? Does the average person know and understand skin? A product does not "not work." It has been improperly prescribed or the bride has misdiagnosed her own skin and purchased the wrong thing. You, the esthetician, who can touch and study the skin, are the one person who can meet the needs of the bride. The bride is looking for what to do, where to go, and is willing to spend more on skin care for her wedding day!

According to *Modern Bride's* Health & Beauty Survey, 1996:

- 93% of brides-to-be will make a personal care change during their engagement

- 58% will make more of an effort on skin care

- 33% will try different products, brands, and formulas when planning for their wedding day and are willing to spend a little more than usual[14]

I picked up a wedding magazine that offered skin and body care tips for

You and your salon should include the skin care department when planning a bridal department.

> *It is so important for the bride to be using skin care products prescribed for her skin type.*

the bride. I thought I could learn something to share with you in this chapter. The information only cemented what I have been trying to say so far. Essentially, it was a list of seventeen different retail and professional products a bride may wish to "try." How does a bride know what to try if she is not educated in what her needs are? She can only guess and waste her money. That is where you, as a salon professional, must be prepared with the answers. The bride may be reluctant to purchase more products if she can hardly close the cabinets in her bathroom as it is. Educating her is the key. Talk about what she has and how she is using it. Prescribe a program for her. Help her to use up some of what she may have at home that is perfectly fine for her. Be sincere, uplifting, and honest.

Kristin Wall, spa director of the Adam Broderick Image Group in Ridgefield, Connecticut, shared with me a special service they created especially for the stressed-out bride, The Bridal Facial. This facial is a non-aggressive facial designed to hydrate the skin and relax the bride. Kristin also mentioned this procedure is done with a water-soluble oil that will not interfere with the bride's hairstyle. Let me share just how this service is worded in their salon brochure.

> *This is an Adam Broderick Image Group exclusive, designed to help the bride look her absolute best on the most photographed day of her life. Because makeup lasts the longest on well-hydrated skin, this facial is very simply a gentle cleansing and hydration treatment. We also offer a mask designed to calm most stress-*

> *induced skin irritations. It's a relaxing way to begin the day."*[15]

This service is offered on a page in their salon brochure booklet entitled "All Eyes on the Bride." It is target-market specific. Did they have to invest in new products? No. Did they have to hire a bridal skin specialist? No. They just took what they already were offering and changed the wording to specifically target the bride. The brides are already coming to see you. Just changing the way you already do business to target the bride specifically will increase the revenue this "new" client market will generate.

For the bride who wants more of a treatment plan prior to her big day let me share what skin care veteran Diane Young suggests. She has plenty of advice to offer the estheticians who will be working on the bride.

> *Always ask the bride if the wedding gown has an open or sheer back, or a deep neckline. If your client has clogged pores or breakouts on her back or chest, treat the problem areas well in advance. My rule of thumb is, never perform a facial closer than two weeks prior to the wedding. Even if the woman is a regular client whose skin you are very familiar with, she's so nervous that the chances she'll have some sort of reaction are too great. If she needs corrective care and will invest the time and money, start a facial series four to six months before the wedding. During the last facial before the wedding, avoid any facial massage. Book the full time, but instead of the facial massage, concentrate on the back of the neck,*

upper shoulders, and upper back. This is where the client carries tension. A massage releases it and increases blood circulation to the face, giving her a warm glow."[16]

Diane also suggests that the bride use products that she is familiar with to avoid unexpected reactions. Any exfoliating should be done no closer than three days before the wedding. The night before, the bride can use a hydrating or clay mask to tighten and refine pores.

This is why it is so important for the bride to be using skin care products prescribed for her skin type. You must go beyond selling and prescribing. To assure success with your clients you need to be concerned about their skin, much the same as a doctor or dentist is concerned about preventive care. Keep records on your clients. With regular usage, products last only so long. Chart when they should be running low and give your client a call. You want them to experience success. You need to know if a product is not performing properly. If you don't show you care they will think you don't and not take their skin care seriously.

This is what I call going the extra mile for your clients and your career. Chapter 9 gives you some other tips and motivation to go the extra mile.

Honeymoon Reminders

Remember to ask your bride where she will be taking her honeymoon. This information not only allows the bride to become more comfortable with you but is a good tool for knowing what ser-

vices she will need in the days leading up to her wedding. Of course, tropical honeymoons call for sun protection. Diane Young advises, "Don't let the bride forget to bring skin care protection and a hat on her honeymoon. Also eyelash tinting is a great idea."[17]

Rock climbing, hiking, and biking honeymoons will call for shorter nails. Why not offer a small nail travel kit for the bride so she can remove her wedding polish and have a color appropriate for dancing the night away?

Honeymoon travels call for travel sizes of all your salon products. Add combinations of these and display them along with your bridal displays. The bride looks forward to the honeymoon as a release from a year or two of intense planning. Don't forget to be there for her with reminders of services and products she will need to have a great and safe time to remember for the rest of her life.

TIPS

- Market bridal nail services.
- Collect photos of nails you have done.
- Make sure the bride has a nail consultation.
- Have a list made up of when she should begin nail and skin services.
- Educate your client regarding waxing precautions.
- Get the bride on a skin care routine.
- Remind her of what she needs for the honeymoon.

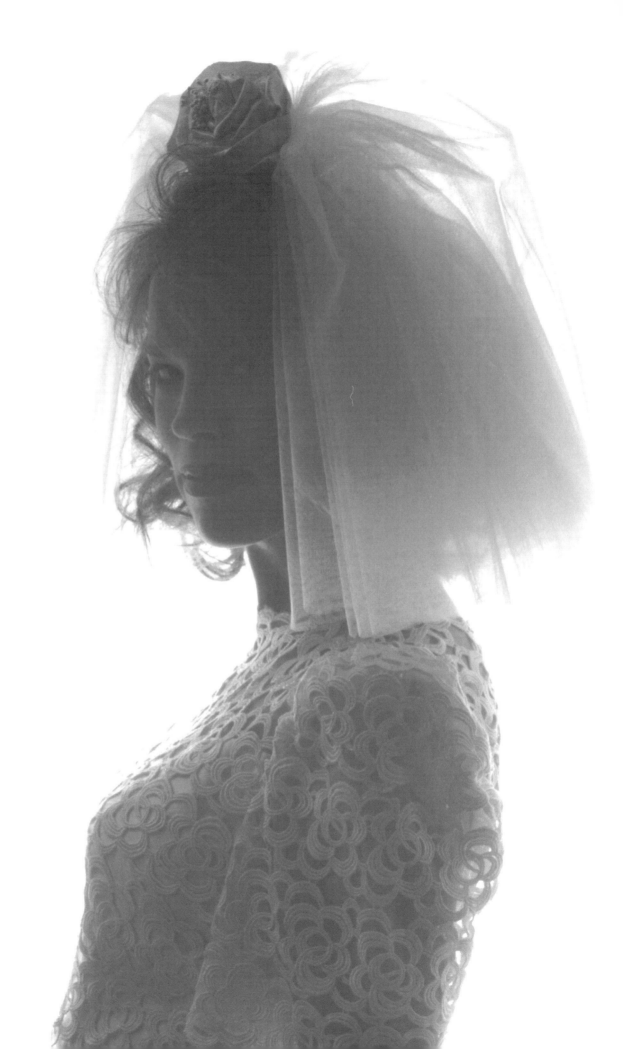

CHAPTER 9

Going the Extra Mile

*W*hen a builder puts up a structure what is the first thing he makes sure of? That the foundation is solid and secure enough to hold the structure. Paul DiGrigoli says, "I believe in mastery. A strong foundation of basic skills will support one's continuous upward growth. However, a weak foundation is impossible to build upon successfully."[1] The building of a bridal department needs to rest on the solid foundation of the entire salon. You can't build your house on the sinking sand. Jumping in and developing a bridal department when the salon is not solid is asking for trouble.

> "*A strong foundation of basic skills will support one's continuous upward growth.*"

It is not easy to move or change, is it? You hate to have to clean house and throw some things out, don't you? But it is sometimes necessary. New beginnings need to have a clean start. Good materials, just as good people, will make for a good structure that lasts.

I want to end this book with a chapter that ties together many of the factors I have already shared with you, yet takes them one step further. I wish to leave you with the encouragement to go the extra mile.

- Going the Extra Mile is written to motivate you above and beyond the call of duty.

- Going the Extra Mile is not necessarily geared to the bridal department per se, but to you as an individual.

I hope you feel that I have given you the tools you need to become very successful with the bridal market.

Please review this entire book. Please make sure no step is overlooked or neglected. Each section, each chapter, is a piece of a puzzle. Just as each piece of a puzzle interlocks with, and depends on, another to make a beautiful picture, the same is true of each chapter in this book. I have shared everything I know, everything I have experienced, researched, and developed. I have enjoyed every minute of putting it all down for you to read and learn from.

Going the Extra Mile is a whole chapter of "Tips." It's about all the little extras I do that I feel are important and have given me the success I enjoy.

In order to be able to give of yourself, there must be extra to give. If you are personally burned out and creatively spent, you have nothing left over to give. If your vessel, yourself, is void, you cannot possibly give. You may get by, but you will not be able to go the extra mile. If your personal goals are "just get me through this day," then that is all you will achieve. If you say you have dreams and visions of success but do not actively take steps toward them, then they will remain only dreams.

DRESSING HAIR ON ANYONE YOU HAVE TIME FOR

I went into this business because I love making people feel better about themselves. As a child I was always drawing pictures of princesses in beautiful gowns. They all had beautiful hairstyles with pointed hats and long flowing veils. I always loved the story of Cinderella. Remember the powerful transforming effect that feeling beautiful had on Cinderella? With her new dress and beautiful hairstyle her face brightened, she floated about, and giggled happily. She was beautiful inside first. Her stepsisters were ugly inside and no amount of clothes and jewels could help them.

Reach your bridal clients on the inside first. Put into practice the information on relating to the bride. Once you relate to them on the inside, you will be able to transform them on the outside. You will have a lot of happy Cinderella brides floating about. And a lot of referrals.

Go the extra mile for all of your clients. If you can, give extra time and attention to your finish work. You may not have any control over the salon that you work in, but you do have control over the work you do and the attitude you project. Nothing influences your clients more. If they love what you do for them, then they will overlook many other things.

Get started!

1. Look at your appointment book every morning.

2. Pick out a few people with whom you would like to spend a little extra time.

3. Think about what it is you want to do for them ahead of time.

4. Pick out some pictures with them in mind and have them ready to show.

5. They will be blown away by this gesture.

6. Tell them you were thinking about them.

7. Give them a blow-dry lesson.

8. Put the brush in their hand.

9. Offer to blow-dry straight someone who is naturally curly.

10. Give a quick updo or braid for no charge.

11. Make sure your finish work is precise and tell your clients you enjoy finish work.

12. Remind them you are available for their holiday office parties, weddings they may be attending, or nights on the town.

Women have gotten out of the habit of thinking of the salon as a place to go for styling. They only come in for their regular haircuts and chemical services. This is our fault. The last thirty years of wash-and-go haircuts have replaced the need for a special-occasion service. They get a new outfit, shoes, and maybe a manicure but wear the same old hairstyle. Speak up and get them in your chair! I always remind my clients that I am available to give them a beautiful blow-dry or a Velcro roller lift anytime in between their haircut appointments. I mention that any reason they may desire to look special is a reason to come see me. An important meeting, an interview, a night out, or a pick-me-up. Weddings, reunions, and proms needn't be the only reason for a pretty style. If you go the extra mile on a regular basis they will see that you have more to offer them.

You may not have any control over the salon that you work in, but you do have control over the work you do and the attitude you project.

Don't forget the younger generation. They are very loyal. I make sure my teens—male and female—feel very important. I make a point of finding something to compliment them about and read their magazines to keep up with the trends.

I had one young boy recently who was referred to me by a former employee who had to quit the industry because of medical reasons. This twelve year old had hair to his shoulders and had been wearing it this way for a couple of years. When he walked in, I thought he was a girl. His mother's eyes told the whole story. She wanted him to feel good about himself and he needed a change but he was unsure of what to get. We looked at pictures together but he could not settle on a style.

Having had this hairstyle for so long he could not picture anything else. He and his mom came to me because it was left up to me to gently push him into a change. I asked him what music he listened to. "Hard core alternative." OK I said, "seems to me I need to leave some hair for head banging then," he smiled and was pleased that I knew his music. I decided to use my razor instead of scissors because I knew he would think it was "cool." He did. As I took my razor out, he said "Hey, what's that?" I said, "A razor." As I expected, he responded, "Cool." I started to slice off his hair and his mom started to cry for joy. I shook his hand when I was done and I made two new clients.

Small children also love extra attention. Make sure at some point in the haircut you squat down to their level and speak to them eye to eye. By their second or third appointment they will feel comfortable enough to let you hug them. They will kick and scream to make their mom bring them to you. Every kid with long hair should walk out with a little updo or a French braid. Even if it is a complimentary bang trim, the little girl gets a braid.

PAY ATTENTION TO REGIONAL HAIRSTYLE TRENDS

Bridal parties bring in bridesmaids from all over the country and the world. In one party I had an American woman who had been living in Paris, France. Another party combined women from rural Vermont and Southern Connecticut. In another party there were bridesmaids from California, Texas, and the

Carolinas. Why is this important to think about? Because every area has its own regional hairstyle and clothing trends. Every once in awhile the fashion magazines cover what trends are being seen where and why. Different regions of the country are influenced by what is happening there and what is acceptable. The Southern women usually go for more feminine looks. They like their hair longer and bigger. They are usually not makeup shy, either. The women from Europe and the larger cities in the United States are willing to wear some of the more trendy styles. Bridesmaids coming from the rural areas will need your suggestions and may be wearing a dated haircut. I had one bridesmaid from Ohio who said to me, "Well, when we get bored we go get a perm." Be careful not to put a trendy look on the wrong person. Others, on the other hand, may want to fit in with the rest of the fashion-forward party.

Also be aware of climate differences. Natural curls will flop in a dry area. Curly hair will frizz and expand in the humidity, causing frustration for the bridesmaid in Arizona. Hard and soft water may cause problems for a bridesmaid. Her hair may not be "working right" since she arrived here for the wedding. Also, borrowed shampoo may be leaving a buildup on someone who shouldn't be using it. We are used to dealing with our own climates and water. The next time an out-of-town bridesmaid is frustrated over the way her hair is behaving ask her what may be different for her here.

Cultural differences may also come into play. Even though a particular bridesmaid came in with her hair

Every kid with long hair should walk out with a little updo or a French braid.

dry, as she was told, she was used to keeping it "oiled" because of her ethnic background. Another bride was new to America. Her hair was poorly cut and overprocessed from an inadequately executed perm.

VOLUNTEERING AND ITS BENEFITS

If you need to do something for yourself, *don't* go on a shopping spree. Volunteer instead! Giving of yourself, your time, and your knowledge will give you much more in return. Look for ways to get yourself and your salon involved with your community. It does not even have to be related to hair, or it can be directly related to hair. Read your local paper and see what groups are running fund-raisers. Contact the chairperson or organization. Buy a ticket and attend the fund-raiser. Plan on helping with it the next year. Many months of planning go into a large dinner dance, fashion show, or wine-tasting reception. Some of the things you can help with are:

- Marathons
- Road races
- Theater productions
- Cocktail receptions
- Auctions
- Talent shows
- Soup kitchens
- Shelters
- Food banks
- Fund-raisers
- Telethons

Always challenge yourself and take risks.

- Grand openings
- Galas or balls
- Recitals
- Fashion shows

Some of the things I have been involved in over my career personally or with my coworkers have been haircuts at our local shelter, a bicycle marathon, cut-a-thons for children's camps, walk-a-thons, Earth Day, beer- and wine-tasting evenings and casino nights, hair shows to raise money for domestic violence, a rape crisis center, and AIDS. We have purchased Christmas presents for children of incarcerated parents, our local shelter residents, and Toys for Tots. Also, makeovers for Girl Scout troops, Newcomers club and Junior Women's group. Some are fun and some tug at your heart strings. But they are all worth it. Once your salon is known for getting involved, the groups and organizers will start calling you.

Many of your clients are also a rich source of information. Volunteer to do makeovers for your client's local church group or synagogue. This is a great way to start talking in front of people. When I first had my salon, one of the things I wanted to do was to hold evening seminars for our clients. I had a mature, experienced esthetician/makeup woman at the time and I wanted her to give a small evening presentation for our clients and their friends. We had about forty people in attendance. All I had to do that evening was introduce her. My heart was racing, I was sweating, and my face was beet-red. But I did it and it was a start! All you have to do is get the first one under your belt whether it is speaking in public or organizing your first fund-raiser.

Everyone starts out unsure and nervous when it comes to planning a big event or speaking in public. Always challenge yourself and take risks. Miette Levine, a financial services manager told *McCall's* magazine her way of gaining confidence is to take risks.

Nine years ago I became involved in a local women's organization. I started off as its secretary, then became program chairperson, and now I'm the president. I've learned that when I stretch myself, I feel more secure in all areas of my life.[12]

This is so true. When you have a feeling of power and confidence you have more success.

FASHION SHOWS BEYOND JUST DOING HAIR

Don't just show up to a fashion show, get everyone's hair done, and leave. *Get involved.* Every show I have done I have made some form of contact that benefited my career at a later date. Remember networking? This is where it happens. Whether I have made a new client, learned a new skill, or just had fun, every experience has been worth it. I have met great makeup artists, new photographers, and seen professional models in action.

Volunteer to do the hair for the country club's fashion shows, bridal fashion shows, or any that you hear about. When doing the hair for these fashion shows and bridal shows stay throughout the show and help in the back. The organizers will find something for you to do. The models need help dressing—tags get left out that need fixing, hair gets messed up, clothes need to be hung up. Your involvement will always be appreciated and remembered. Any shows that my salon participated in always asked us to come back the following year.

College sororities are another source for fashion shows. As are Newcomers clubs, women's groups, country clubs, senior centers, boutiques, department stores, and yacht clubs. Before doing a fashion show find out who the audience is going to be. If the audience represents your client base or one your salon is trying to reach, then do the show. Eventually, when your salon becomes busy doing these shows, you will need to choose to work only those beneficial to your salon.

School plays and theater groups are another source to use your hair-dressing skills. I have done hair for numerous schools plays even when my children were not participants. It is great fun to do exaggerated looks on the kids. Fifties' flips, beehives, Victorian updos, finger waves, braids, and buns. I also have a couple of clients who are opera singers and need period looks for the characters they are playing. If the person does not have a picture to show you, then it is a good idea to research the period of history in which the story takes place.

Try what you haven't done or do what you like. If your personal goals lean more toward the salon industry call your local distributor and see how you can get involved with a salon prod-

> When you have a feeling of power and confidence you have more success.

ucts company. Volunteer backstage in the prep room. After a show speak to one of the educators and see how they got started.

Cold Calls

Make cold calls. Call organizations you want to get involved with. Call product companies you would like to work for. A photographer friend I work with made a cold call to a large marketing company with which he wanted to get involved. He called to ask if he could make an appointment to bring in his portfolio. The woman on the phone said to him, "Sure, no problem, now wasn't that easy?" and she laughed with him and gave him an appointment. When making cold calls it is important to learn some facts about the company you are calling. Who their top educators are, what products they represent, etc. When this photographer is interested in approaching a beauty-related company to do photography for them, I research what that company is presently doing. I send him ads from magazines and photos from their product boxes. We plan a shoot and he takes the photos into that company. He has sold some of his photos with my hairstyles this way.

When you are starting out don't always look for the almighty buck; experience is worth more than money. You never know who might see the photos and want to know who did the hair or makeup. Go the extra mile. Eventually you will be able to set your fees. Go beyond just doing hair in the salon. Networking gets you involved. Involvement prevents burnout and fuels your creativity.

> **W**hen you are starting out don't always look for the almighty buck; experience is worth more than money.

SUBMITTING TO THE PAPERS

Nothing gives your business a shot in the arm like a little press! The best place to get your feet wet for seeing your salon's name published is to start with your local papers. Anything your salon does, the local papers should know about it. Get to know your salesperson for your local paper. A friendly relationship with that person helps move things through back at the office. Especially if your salon regularly advertises with them they should be willing to give you a mention.

How about a weekly beauty column? If there is someone on staff who enjoys writing they can contact the beauty editor and see if the paper is interested in receiving a small beauty-related feature each month.

Another plus of press is the writers of the larger paper in your area may read something of interest about you in the local paper. That was how my salon got featured with a large color photo in the Living section of the Sunday paper. In our smaller and less-expensive paper I ran an ad in the children's section featuring our special "Babies First Haircut." The larger paper saw this ad and thought it would make for a great story.

"You never know who might be reading those little papers," says Tamara Friedman, owner of Tamara Institute de Beaute, in Farmington Hills, Minnesota. "Every reporter looks for something new and exciting,"[3] says Friedman.

What I have found to work best at getting results with the local press, is you have to word your information to focus on what you are doing, and not who you are. If the press release reads like the salon is the main focus, the paper will not print anything that sounds too much like free advertising.

If you are doing a show to raise funds for a national organization call your local chapter. They should help your salon get press coverage as well. Remember their main focus is to raise funds for the organization, not to get you press. Keep that in mind. They also may have specific requests regarding how their name is to be represented in print. It is very important to comply and respect their guidelines.

Press Releases

"The press release is key to opening the doors to the media," proclaimed Tana Fletcher, in *American Salon* magazine. "You can't demand of the media. You have to make your presentation as pleasant as possible."[4]

The major theme I kept hearing over and over, as I researched for this section, is that editors are very busy and receive a lot of material. If it is not simple, direct, and eye-catching it will be tossed in the wastebasket.

Kim Lord, of Kim Lord Public Relations, in New York, says, "The senior editors are very busy. The press release must be unique and creative. Anything boring gets overlooked." Lord goes the extra mile for her clients and ensures that the press kits she puts together get a second look. How does she do this? She takes the time to get to know her clients.

It is so important to establish a relationship with the salon owner. I like to know the salon's strengths, and weaknesses." Kim helps the salon owner define their image. *"I need to find something unique about the business or person and help create a concept. That way I have a better understanding of how they want to be represented. Then I can put together a great press kit and find the best avenue for that person or salon. Because the senior editors are very busy I like to deal with the associate editors and establish an ongoing relationship with them. They call me directly and I can give them information about a salon immediately."[5]*

Whether you hire a public relation person or start by doing the work yourself the press release must include some specific information. Jayne Morehouse of Morehouse Communications, Brunswick, Ohio, says,

Include background information on you and your salon in your initial presskit folder. Incorporate a brief page on your salon and what makes it unique, a straightforward list of important facts about your business, a salon menu, a business card, copies of any press clippings, your newsletter if you do one, and a personalized cover letter to the editor."[6]

To learn more important facts from Jayne get a copy of her book. Jayne has written an information packed book entitled *Salon Public Relations*. It is published by Milady/SalonOvations. Jayne's book is a must have for every salon's library.

Ginger Boyle, who ownes Planet Salon in Beverly Hills, California, also

> I f it is not simple, direct, and eye-catching it will be tossed in the wastebasket.

co-owns Elantis Productions with her photographer-husband. Elantis Productions is a visual marketing company. I was very excited to be able to take their seminar at the International Beauty Show in New York City one year. I sat for three and a half hours to make sure I got to hear both of their seminars and not lose my front row seat. It was worth going the extra mile. The first seminar was entitled "Get Exposed." Here are some of Ginger's tips for getting exposure in our industry:

1. Press Release (who, what, where, why, how). This should never be more than one page.

2. Biography (six important features in your biography). List these features and make sure you have a contact name.

3. Cover Letter (what editors look for). Gear your release to what the editors are looking for. Is it real people? Theme projects? Make-overs? Call and ask them.

4. The Overall Package (what to include and what it should look like). Short and sweet. Simple packaging. Professional letterhead.[7]

The more you and your salon go the extra mile the more you will get published. Local press is good for business, but trade press makes you feel great because you are reaching your peers. Trade press is also a great boost for the staff's morale and sometimes leads to consumer press coverage. Remember, just as the larger newspapers' editors read the local papers, the national magazine editors read our trade magazines.

John Hickox of Hickox and Friends of Portland, Oregon, confesses, "I really don't know how we got there," referring to making it into a *Glamour* feature. "It was a real gift. I do know that doors are opened for us as Intercoiffure members. But we also have a strong local reputation and dominate the Portland market."[8]

Whether it is local press you are after or the bigger press from the top magazines, repetition is the key to seeing your name in print.

Andrew DiSimone, who owns DiSimone Studio, in New York City, knows what it takes to get press coverage. Andrew relies on the services of Kim Lord Public Relations. Andrew knows being committed to ongoing press coverage is crucial to his success in the Big Apple. Andrew has been mentioned and quoted in national magazines such as *Glamour, American Health, Allure, Star Magazine, Marie Claire,* and *Ladies' Home Journal,* as well as on television shows including *Montel, Maury Povich,* and *Rolonda* to name a few.

"I send out press kits every three months," Andrew told me. "You need to first ask yourself, who am I and what hair do I do? Do you want to do fashion? Editorial? Makeovers? Catalogue work? Photo sessions? Or just reach more clients? It is also important that the coverage benefits the whole salon. You as the owner need to ask yourself, will the entire staff benefit from the press kit?"[9]

In gearing a press kit about hennas toward a health magazine, Andrew was able to get coverage not only for his salon, but also for the staff member who specializes in henna. This is a win-win team attitude.

The same happened for my salon when our press kit caught the attention of a cable TV show. We were focusing a lot on makeovers at that time. Makeovers are great because everyone loves to see them and they involve the entire salon. The press package included a cover letter, before and after photos, our menu and copies of our referral cards, a business card, newsletter, and our new client card. I sent the package to newspapers, magazines, and our local cable TV show. The cable TV show called back and invited us to do a live makeover segment. They wanted a show about redheads so I was able to plug our chemical director and her services. It was great fun and motivated the entire salon.

Trade press has a trickledown effect right to your clients and your bottom line. And for the same amount of money you may be spending on advertising weekly, you can hire a public relation (PR) person. To make the most of your money and your PR person, Andrew DiSimone says, there are some things you need to know about the person you are going to hire:

Is this person familiar with the fashion world? Who are their friends in the industry? Who are their contacts? Ask for client references. What editors do they know? Ask to see their portfolio. Your PR person needs to be creative and willing to get to know you. PR is PR, anyone can sit at the phone all day trying to reach an editor, so think about what you want to pay for.[10]

Don't jump right in with a PR firm and hope for the best. Just like you need to plan and organize the evolution of your salon's bridal department, you need to lay out the steps to take toward press coverage. Start small, start smart, but take that first step.

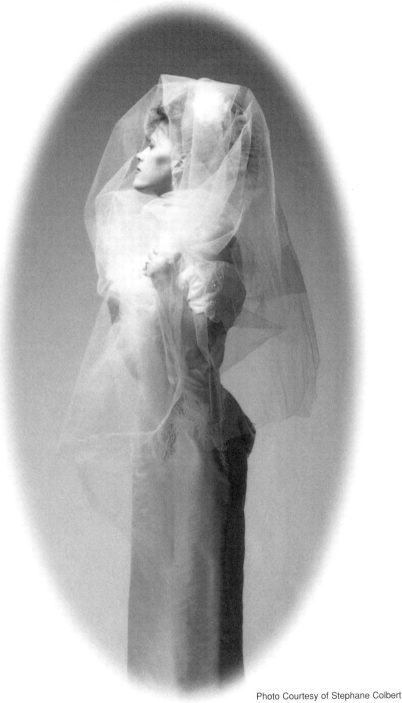

Photo Courtesy of Stephane Colbert

GETTING PUBLISHED

Getting published is more than just doing great work. You need to know what an editor wants. Earlier I talked about finding out who you are and what work you do. Now you need to match your talents to the editor's needs. Do you want to be in *Passion* magazine? You must get to know them and what they want. You can request from them a detailed list of what they look for in a photo and what to avoid. Many times editors are looking for certain looks, such as styles on men, children, and mature models. If your goal is to see your name in print think about doing a photo shoot with these subjects in mind. Most people submit women's styles, but there is less competition in these other areas and a better chance for publication.

Each hair book has an image. It is a waste of time and money to send mature-hair shots to a progressive magazine. I sent a bridal photo into *Passion* and they published it in *Coiffeur Q* magazine because it better matched that book's image. Study the work already published in a book in which you would like to be.

- Look closely at the poses, the models, the makeup, and the lighting.

- Look at the book with a photographer before planning a shoot.

- Look in the back of the book for guidelines to follow.

- Look for an address or a phone number to call and request submissions guidelines. (See example of photographer's guidelines.)

- Follow their guidelines strictly.

If great work is sent in the wrong size or the wrong film format it will be overlooked. Do they want 8 x 10 prints or is 5 x 7 acceptable? Can you send photos or do they want only slides? All photos and slides need to be marked with your name, the photographer's name, the salon's name, and anyone who should get credit. Do they want models' releases? Are the photos and slides of top quality? I had some work sent back with a letter explaining that the pictures were good but the slides were scratched and unusable.

These publishers receive thousands of photos. Just as the press release has to address the editor's needs so do any photos you may send. Some editors like a series of photos that have a theme. Come up with a catchy name for your release. Seasonal shots are also good but need to be planned accordingly. You will need to think holiday looks in the heat of the summer, for example. Send seasonal photos at least six months in advance.

When we look at hairstyles in a book we know we can do just as good a job. Sometimes we have said, "I can do better than that," and toss the book aside. That's an attitude problem, and a poor attitude will stop you dead in your tracks. Paul DiGrigoli has this to add: "Never foolishly believe that you know everything. Once your mind falls prey to your ego, you lose your competitive advantage." [11]

Consumer magazines are another source for getting published. Remember the readers of the consumer magazines are much different than the readers of

> Remember the readers of the consumer magazines are much different than the readers of the trade magazines.

PHOTOGRAPHER'S GUIDELINES

Catherine Frangie, Publisher/Editor-in-Chief
Bonnie Sanford, Managing Editor

SalonOvations Magazine is the industry magazine for all salon professionals and is the Official Publication of the National Cosmetology Association. Editorial content focuses on personal and professional development. Published monthly by Milady Publishing Company, the leader in beauty industry publishing.

All photo submissions should be of the highest quality, and appeal to our reader. We are seeking work that can be used for full-page feature photos and "Your Work" pages. We also consider step-by-step technicals. We also accepts shots of good-looking, contemporary salons for use with features and other articles.

Accept 35mm slides or 2-1/4" x 2-1/4" transparencies only, preferably in color. Slides and transparancies must be clean and of good quality. Will consider high-quality B&W.

All submissions arrive with the following:
    1) A signed model release form allowing us to use this photo in the magazine and/or promotions for the magazine.
    2) Credits for artists involved in the production of the photo, including the photographer, hairstylist, nail technician, makeup artist, photo stylist, and company should accompany the submission.

Payment is in copies or as negotiated.

We also use high-quality illustrations to accompany editorial features as well as to illustrate technicals.

All submissions must be accompanied by the proper-size return envelope with sufficient postage attached, or work cannot be returned.

All queries and submissions should be directed to:
Bonnie Sanford, Managing Editor
SalonOvations Magazine
3 Columbia Circle
Albany, NY 12212

MILADY SalonOvations'

3 Columbia Circle
P.o. Box 12519
Albany, NY 12212-2519
Tel 518-464-3500
1-800-998-7498
Fax 518-464-0358

the trade magazines. They are our clients. Many times magazines want information about how clients can do their own hair at home. They want trade secrets and many salons do not keep these magazines in the salon because of this.

The book *Salon Public Relations* by Jayne Morehouse I mentioned earlier goes into detail about "who wants what." She lists top magazines and what they are seeking. Editors also have editorial calendars that list what they plan to put in the magazine months ahead. You can call any magazine and request a copy of their calendar. (See example.)

Have you seen all those makeovers they feature in the women's magazines? Well, I wanted to know how I could get my salon to do some. I looked in the table of contents and called the beauty editor. She was very nice and said that their regular makeovers are done in house by a stylist who works with the magazine, but she did say that they like to do one big beauty story a year. If I had anything to send her she would love to see it. My point is, make the calls. It is as easy as picking up the phone. Anyone can do it!

INNOVATIONS IN
SALON EDUCATION

MILADY
SalonOvations'

1997 EDITORIAL CALENDAR

MONTH	THEME
January	Exploring Your Sale Chemical Crazy
February	The Power of Promotion Multicultural Clients
March	The Art of Being the Boss Fresh Heads: Cuts for Spring
April	Consistent Customer Service Beauty Is Skin Deep
May	Safety in the Salon Color, Color, and More Color!
June	Beauty Is Big (and Small) Business Pedicures
July	Techno-Talk A Nail Extravaganza
August	Fall Fabu! Hair and Clothes Classic and Carried Away
September	In Pursuit of Profits Making Faces
October	Partnerships: How to Make Them Work Men, Glorious Men
November	Untapped Salon Services After Eight—Party Hair
December	Achieving Your Goals The Wave of the Future

3 Columbia Circle
P.o. Box 12519
Albany, NY 12212-2519
Tel 518-464-3500
1-800-998-7498
Fax 518-464-0358

THE PHOTO SESSION

Nothing sends the message of success to your clients better than for them to see your work in print, whether you are an individual stylist or the owner of a salon. Photos of your work are a powerful tool in establishing a positive image in the mind of the client. Go the extra mile! We as individuals and salon owners have to wake up! We have to think like the "big boys." If we want success and recognition for our talents we have to make it happen. A good place to start is having a photo session. If you are a salon owner it is a good idea that the entire salon is included. To create a team effort each team member needs to feel their significance.

The first thing that needs to take place is a meeting to discuss the importance of a photo shoot. Then you must ask yourself and your salon what are the goals of this photo session. They may include:

⚘ The colorist wants to do color makeovers.

⚘ The nail technician wants to submit her designs into a magazine.

⚘ The updo specialist wants a portfolio for his clients' to choose from.

⚘ The owner wants posters for the walls.

There may be many reasons and each reason has a different purpose that needs to be drawn out of the photos. If you do some planning you may be able to cover a few agendas with one photo shoot.

Ginger Boyle of Elantis Productions, in Beverly Hills, California, offers a seminar entitled "Preparing for a Photo Shoot." She lays out a road map to get you started. Following is some information from that seminar. (For further information please call Elantis Productions at (310) 550-1766.)

Preparing for a Photo Shoot

1. The Creative Process

   A. Why do it?

      1. editorial

      2. local advertising

      3. business cards

      4. personal portfolios

      5. salon posters

      6. co-op advertising

2. Details That Count

   A. Selecting the Photographer

      1. select one who specializes in beauty

      2. look for good lighting in their portfolio

      3. look for creativity and good direction

      4. make sure the photographer understands your needs

   B. Model

      1. a marginal model means a marginal photo

      2. good skin, hair, or nails if that is the feature of the photo

   C. Makeup Artist

      1. must have experience doing makeup for photography

      2. understands the photographer's lighting

3. takes direction well

D. The Crew

    1. who is important and when

3. Marketing Yourself

A. Past (how clients and fellow professionals see you)

B. Present

    1. personal and professional features

    2. special talents

    3. how much is your time worth

    4. how to become included, quoted, or mentioned in journals

C. Future

    1. setting up your educational calendar [12]

Learning from the experts is always best. Thank goodness there are successful professionals in our field who are willing to share. The Milady/SalonOvations catalog is rich with information to guide and motivate you. The trade magazines are for us. Frankly, there is no excuse for any of us to sit back and be bored!

So maybe you don't have the money for a "good" professional photographer or professional models, or know a makeup artist with experience. Do it anyway! Experience and knowledge is a process that grows with time. No one gets it right the first time. I started out by taking Polaroids of some of my hairstyles. From there I used my auto-focus 35mm camera.

Then I picked up my Dad's old Minolta that had a close-up lens. I worked with black-and-white film because I liked it. From there I took photo classes at our local camera shop. Then I took a full day portrait session class.

Then I bought a new camera. Then I bought lights. Whenever I was involved with a photo shoot I always asked questions. I read books. I subscribed to a photography magazine. I set up shoots and learned by doing. I still have more to learn about the technical aspect of photography.

I began to see the power and influence photos of our salon's work had on the clients and staff. So I decided to plan a big staff photo session with a professional photographer. Then we did another one.

Here are some quick tips for getting your photos published:

🖎 Use the best models possible.

🖎 Look for good skin and great bone structure.

🖎 Avoid deep set eyes or too-strong features.

🖎 Make sure the makeup is flawless.

🖎 Keep accessories simple and timeless.

🖎 Don't use overly trendy clothes or anything that takes away from the hair.

🖎 Don't let your background compete with the model.

Use color well. Make it strong and bold or go for a monochromatic look.

A boring background of cream or gray is average and may not catch the attention of the editor. A vibrant orange-red behind a blonde model will. Or shoot in black and white. Think about the entire photo as a whole. Just as the total bridal look must balance and complement, so must the whole photo shoot process.

Putting out the money for our photo shoots was worth it. We used the photos for our ads in the paper and were the first salon in our area to do so. We blew up copies of our makeovers and hung them in the salon. We submitted some work that was published. We used our makeover slides in talks to women's groups. We showed them at hair show fundraisers. We used them for press kits.

Even if your salon does not want to get involved, do it for yourself, or approach the owner about a shoot. Try to get everyone excited and interested. Maybe everyone can chip in to cover expenses.

The Photographer

After you have established your purpose for your shoot you have to choose a photographer. Doing an interview and having a consultation is very important and prevents wasted time and money. I wish someone had told me this years ago. I had to learn from many mistakes.

When you are consulting with the photographer, it would be a good idea to have some pictures from books ready to show. Pick out poses you like. Ask about the lighting. Talk about backgrounds. Before planning a trend

release or a show I like to make a large collage of "looks" (cut out from magazines) to hang up for inspiration and direction. This is also something you can show the photographer at the consultation.

Ask to see their portfolio. You want to make sure they have an eye for beauty and are not just a portrait photographer. Just as there are technical hairdressers who are good but don't have a feel for the hair, there are technical photographers who are good but don't have a feel for capturing mood or beauty in a picture.

For example, with this book I needed the artistic control because I had an agenda in mind. My agenda is to teach and share. My goal is to have you, the reader, try some of the styles on your clients who are real brides. I didn't feel it was the time for me to push my creative avant-garde limits, so I needed a photographer who would look to me as the client and meet my needs. I thank Steve at S.M. Cooper Photography for being artistic, technical, and willing to listen to me.

Some photographers are very artistic and into their own interpretation of how the model should look. During your consultation see how they are acting and what they are saying. Are they listening to you and your wishes? If not, don't try to work with someone like this if you want control. However, do try to work with someone like this when there is no set agenda and you both are free to create. If you are always working within limits you may not experience the freedom to become creative.

Just as the total bridal look must balance and complement, so must the whole photo shoot process.

A talented artistic photographer I like to work with is Stephane Colbert. I met Stephane while networking at an ABC meeting. He is published in many books, has national ads to his credit, and has produced many beautiful images. When I work with Stephane he leads me. I allow him to push me to cross over any artistic boundaries I may have subconsciously set in myself. Stephane will say, "I don't want anything average. Here, I have these little birds. Do something with them." Or he may give me a great pair of earrings that inspire an updo. These sessions are great fun and get creative juices flowing. They only cost time. Beautiful work results.

One photographer I used never came back for a second shoot. I did not interview him prior to the session, so when I first met him and saw all the equipment he had, I knew he was a hobby/gadget technical photographer. He got so nervous by all the models and stylists, I could not get him to come back. For straightforward make-overs, his work was fine.

Another photographer made me use a model for whom he was granting a favor.

Another rushed us and was expensive.

Another photographer fell off the face of the earth. We even got our work published. I tried to contact him and let him know, but I couldn't track him down.

Another one set up at an educational show and was taking pictures for everyone. But he never followed through and got the pictures back to us.

At another session a stylist brought too many models and did not stick to our agenda. This caused negative feelings and wasted time and money.

I thought I would find the "right" photographer for me. What I have found is that different photographers bring out different things in me. If you look, you will always learn something from an experience. Go the extra mile!

YOUR PORTFOLIO

A portfolio needs to show a variety of your work and talents. Brides love to look at other brides. They also like to see what you as the stylist are capable of. Going the extra mile by having a portfolio is taking the time to invest in yourself. No one else is going to do it for you!

Before starting, ask yourself, who is going to be looking at your portfolio?

❧ Editors?

Your portfolio must be professional by their industry standards. Call someone who you read about that gets published frequently and ask how they got started. Most people are flattered that you call and are willing to share. All you need is a name, and a town, then call long distance information. Make sure you tailor your portfolio and press releases to the editors with whom you want to work.

❧ Clients?

Clients love looking at photos of hairstyles. They will build a great deal more trust in you if they can see some of the work you have

A portfolio needs to show a variety of your work and talents.

done in the past. A portfolio also shows you how your work is evolving and should be updated yearly.

🖎 Photographers?

What images are their specialty? It may be a variety of looks and you will be asked to meet a specific agenda. I had a stylist in one of my classes whose portfolio was full of undergarment ads. If they specialize in wedding sittings and wedding photography you may be able to get some bridal clients from the photographer. Most important, when working for a photographer keep in mind you are working for them. You have to be able to take direction well.

🖎 New color clients?

If you are a specialist in a specific area tailor your portfolio to that specialty. If you are a colorist, share the expense and photos with a haircutter who would like to show their work as well.

🖎 Brides?

Ask every bride you do to get a picture to you after the wedding. Offer to pay for it. Also have a camera with film in it at the salon when you have a wedding party coming in. Set up a bridal photo session and get creative. Put these creative bridal shots in your portfolio. Tell the client this is being done for fun. Sometime when they see you can be creative they may let you do something a little over the top for their wedding. If they see it they will ask for it.

Whatever photos you put in your portfolio make it neat, organized, and easy to look at. Celebrity makeup artist Roxanna Floyd says, "Make sure everything in your book is uniform. You don't want to have to turn it around to look at the pages, and all photos should be the same size."[13]

Show only your best work; too many pictures can be distracting and take away from the best ones.

ON THE ROAD

Many times you may be called to go on the road to do services. Large wedding parties may want you and your wedding team to come to their home. Photo shoots, fashion shows, bridal fairs, and hair shows require you to pack up and come to them. It is very important to be prepared.

Remember I talked about your skill being only 15% of why someone wants your services? When traveling, your image, whether you arrive on time, and being prepared all adds up to make the other 85%. You will be asked to come back or referred for your services if you can keep in mind the importance of the 85%.

Busy organizers and fund-raiser chairpersons don't have time for an unprofessional stylist. We all have to take a part in raising the level of professionalism for our industry.

What to Pack

Here is a checklist of everything I put in my bags when traveling. Whether it is for a bride, a hair show, or a fashion show, you can use it to make sure you

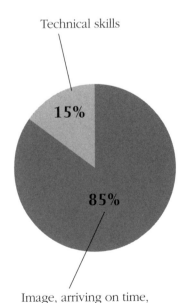

Technical skills

15%

85%

Image, arriving on time, and preparedness

Client Satisfasction

Travel Checklist

TOOL	PACKED	NEED	DON'T NEED
multiple outlet bar			
3-pronged extension cord			
converter plug (for 3-pronged tools)			
cloth hand towel			
sewing kit			
bobby pins/hairpins			
curling irons—all sizes			
portable hood dryer			
craft scissors			
products			
masking tape			
large, black marker			
tissues			
safety pins			
brushes/combs			
hot rollers			
Velcro rollers			
blow-dryer			
hair scissors/razor			
makeup			
Blistex/Vaseline			
face cream/makeup remover			
extra pantyhose (black, cream, nude)			
hair accessories/coated elastics			
Other:			

have everything at hand. You can make check marks in the column to see at a glance what you still need to pack.

Even if I am not planning on doing the makeup I bring my own. Blistex and face cream are a must for nonprofessional models. So is extra panty hose. Professional models are usually well prepared. Old inns and homes may not have updated electrical outlets. A converter with two prongs that goes into the wall and has space for your three-prong power bar is a *must*. In every show I do someone needs to use my large craft scissors, tape, and marker to make a sign.

One time I did a bride at an old inn and we blew a fuse. I needed an extension cord to reach one of the outlets that was still working. When working at a bride's home I always need my power outlet bar, because there are never enough empty outlets in a kitchen. If I have a lot of tools to plug in I spread them out to other rooms to heat up to avoid blowing a fuse. When doing fashion shows there is always a need for a safety pin or a sewing kit. I even had to sew a button on a shirt while there was still a handsome man in it!

Another time I had a bride with short hair that I had cut two weeks before the wedding. When I styled her hair at the inn where she was getting married, I noticed her dark neck hairs had grown in. I had to use her leg razor and shaving cream to remove it. After that I put my close clipper razor in my travel bag. I do have doubles of some of my tools because repacking the bag is a hassle. Use the packing list. Laminate it. Keep it in your bag and check against it each time you pack to travel.

Being Prepared

I am the type of person who likes to learn from others who have "been there." Someone who has "been there" is Ken Reeder of the Ken Reeder Experience. Ken is a DJ entertainer who has performed at many hair shows. Ken is a one-man show. He is extremely talented in what he does. He listen to his clients and delivers what they want. He is always fun, easy-going, and very helpful.

At one of my first hair shows I brought some of my camera equipment and I needed an extension cord. Ken found one for me through the hotel staff but as he gave it to me he explained the importance of always being prepared. His manner was friendly and sincere. He said it is important to be professional, ready, and have what you need. It leaves a good impression and will get you a chance to be rehired or referred. He also said it would be a good idea for me to get an outlet bar as well for all of my curling irons and hot rollers. So what did I do when I got home? I put an extension cord in my trunk and bought an outlet bar to keep in my travel bag.

Another time I was doing the hair for a school play, teasing up a perfect French twist, when a mother asked if I was a "real hairdresser." Ten minutes later she brought over her twelve-year-old daughter. She told me her daughter was good with hair and would be able to help us if we needed her. Not wanting to discourage a budding

U*se the packing list. Laminate it. Keep it in your bag and check against it each time you pack to travel.*

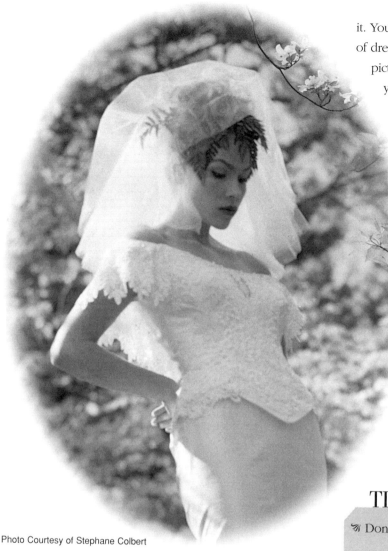

Photo Courtesy of Stephane Colbert

it. You have the talent. You have a lot of dreams and goals. Take the big picture and go backwards planning your steps. When we all learned to walk it was one step at a time. Don't start off running. My friend, Paul DiGrigoli, says, "You have to crawl before you walk and walk before you run. Don't start off running, it may be in the wrong direction."

The Business of Bridal Beauty is a great tool. Just as you need to use a hammer over and over again throughout a project, the same goes for this book. Look to it as a tool, pick it up again and again. YOU CAN DO IT!! BEST WISHES!

TIPS

❦ Don't wallow in negativity.

❦ Go the extra mile for your regular clients.

❦ Get involved! Look to help in the community, salon industry, fund-raising.

❦ Get your name in print.

❦ Never give up!

❦ Plan a photo session.

❦ Prepare a portfolio.

❦ Be available to travel.

❦ Be professional at all times.

❦ Be prepared.

❦ Use the packing list as a reminder.

stylist I told the mother that would be great. I also told her it was important for her daughter to do well in high school and what was the best beauty school in the area to send her daughter. I did not have extra tools for the young girl to use, plus all my irons are marcel. Looking at the kid standing there empty handed I encouraged her to pursue our field and explained to her the importance of always being prepared. I hope someday she will be.

You have a great information-packed book in your hand. You have the desire, or you would not be reading

PART 2

T O O L S

I n this section I explain how I use certain styling products and tools. This is what works for me. Feel free to use something else or use them in a different way.

TEASING PICK

I like to tease or backcomb (which is a better word to use with the client) with a comb such as this. I can get close to the scalp and the varied-length teeth allow me to get through all the hair. The pick end lets me smooth loose hairs. It also lets me check to see if my backcombing is strong enough by inserting it into the tease and pulling outward.

TEASING BRUSH

This brush is called a teasing brush but I do not tease with it. It was made for the days when teasing was overly done, in the 1950s and 1960s. I use it for controlled smoothing. The dense teeth prevent the brush from pulling out all of the backcombing. It is great for detailed work. I use the tail end for sectioning.

How to Backcomb

While there are many styles today that do not require backcombing, a true artist in the field of dressing hair will always look to backcombing for control. Todays styles do not require as much backcombing because we have a larger variety of products available.

Root Tease or Lift

The biggest mistake I see in my classes regarding backcombing is it is started too far away from the scalp. Hold up a section to be backcombed. It should be no longer or wider than the comb you are using to backcomb with. Insert the teasing comb a half inch from the scalp and push down toward the scalp in short little "pulses." It may seem like not much is happening but keep doing it. You are only looking for a *little* matting to be forming near the scalp. This section of hair, when left alone, should not fall over but stand firm at the base. If it falls over the section may have been too thick to begin with or you have started too far away from the scalp.

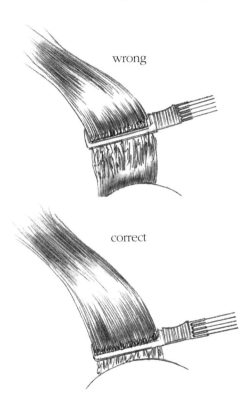

wrong

correct

Backcombing in an Updo to Form Curls

When backcombing a section of hair to form a barrel curl first determine which side will be the inside of the curl. Spray that side with hair spray. Take your teasing comb and lightly backcomb up the strand, make each swipe like you are climbing a step. You only need enough backcombing to keep the curl

from separating and flopping over. Spray as needed with a dry working spray and gently smooth the outer side of the curl before forming it. Pin the curl and repeat.

Backcombing for Sculpting

Section away the hair that is not to be backcombed. Spray thoroughly the hair that is to be heavily backcombed for sculpting. Do not rush by taking too large a section. With regular sections start backcombing at the root, stepping up the hair and pushing down toward the scalp. Spray and re-tease if necessary. Taking the teasing brush, smooth and sculpt the outer layer into shape. Be careful not to brush too deeply and remove the backcombing.

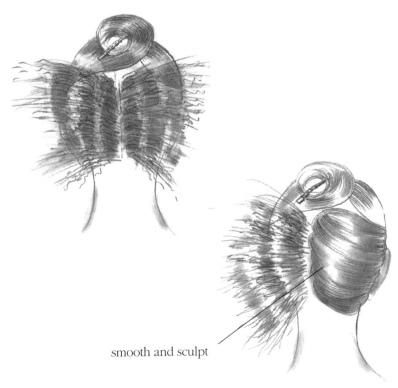

inside

Outerside to be smoothed

smooth and sculpt

ELASTICS

When I mention elastics I am referring to the coated ones, not the rubber kind. The only time I use rubber elastics is when I am braiding small sections and use them for the ends. Rubber elastics can get stuck and pull at the hair, causing breakage.

HAIRPINS

A hairpin is a *finishing* pin, used when finishing the style. It is *not* designed to hold weight or secure the hair like a bobby pin. A hairpin is placed at the edge of a curl, roll, or French twist to keep it in place. One side of the hairpin is to grip the curl or roll while the other side goes close to the scalp.

Place the hairpin at a 90° angle first (a), then at the same time as you are leaning the pin (b) toward the scalp you are pushing it under the curl or roll (c). I never bend my hairpins. They were not designed to be bent. Plus they are impossible to get out if you need to make a change.

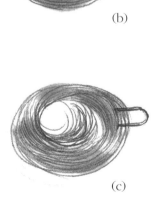

(a)

(b)

(c)

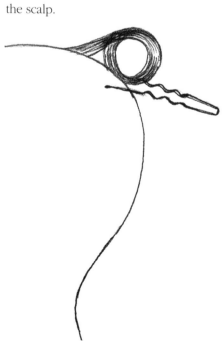

BOBBY PINS

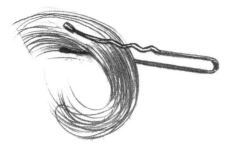

Bobby pins are designed to hold the bulk and weight of the hair. They are for securing the hair to the scalp. When you put your finger in the bobby pin to use it you are leaving a small space for the hair to go in it.

If you shove too much hair in the bobby pin it slides back out. Take it out and put less hair in it. Otherwise you will keep using too many bobby pins to secure the one sliding, when you should be just securing hair. When crossing bobby pins for a strong hold, make sure you feel one bobby pin going over the other. That is why they have the ridges, to keep them from slipping when crossed. Cross as is shown in pictures below.

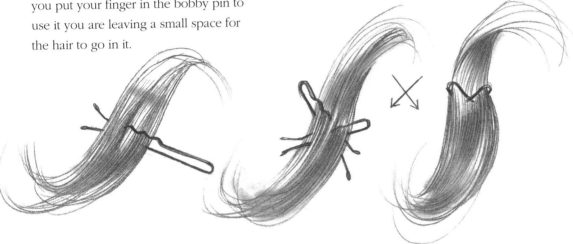

FLAT IRON

I like to use a small flat iron to create smooth curls or loops. Take thin sections and spray with spray gel and smooth down the strand.

CRIMPING IRON

Everything comes back again. Crimping the hair or pieces of it is a fun way to add a mix of texture to an updo. Bring it out again and give it a try.

ROLLERS

Today's brides and clients do not have the time for a conventional wet set. However, the mechanics used in the days of wet setting can be applied to other sets, such as hot roller sets.

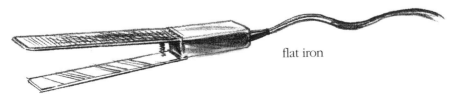

flat iron

HOT ROLLERS

Most of the time I use hot rollers for my updos. They give the hair body, volume, and control. When doing updos you need the hair to have texture to be able to work with it. If you are looking for body put more hair into the roller and use less rollers. When more curl is desired use less hair and put in a lot of rollers. Let them cool completely. I do not roll the hair from the end up to the scalp. I start in the middle of the strand, wrap the ends onto the roller, and then wrap it up to the scalp.

Seecuring Hot Rollers

When working with hot rollers it is best to use conventional silver clips or duck bill sliver clips to secure them in the set. Throw out the hot roller wires that accompany the rollers, they do not allow for a tight enough set. Do not use claw clamps either they will make a "dent" in the hair much like making a crease in the wrong place when you are ironing pants. These dents in the hair are impossible to get out later when the hair is cooled.

Roll the hot roller tight to the scalp. Slip a silver clip between the hair on the roller and the hair from the scalp. You can also pile the rollers on top of one another pinning them together. The silver clips must have a free center. The kind with the little bar at the top will not work, or use the longer duck bill type. See diagram below.

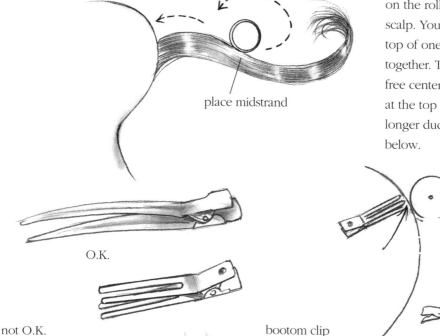

place midstrand

O.K.

not O.K.
bar prevents
sliding into hair

bootom clip
slides along scalp

top of clip slides
into hair from
roller

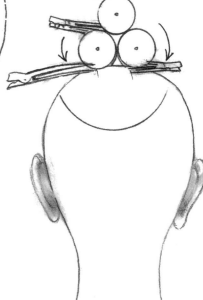

VELCRO ROLLERS

Velcro rollers when rolled with tension, are perfect to help smooth out natural curl. For the bride with curly hair who wants a smooth updo, Velcro rollers are best. Set the hair dry or lightly mist with water. I like to use a spray gel on the section to be rolled up. Take a section, spray it, brush it smooth, and roll it onto a large Velcro roller with tension. Give a final allover spray with spray gel and place the bride under the dryer for about fifteen minutes. Take her out and, while still warm, remove the rollers and brush smooth. Then style the updo.

When you are looking for a firm curl on medium-length hair velcro rollers work better than hot rollers. I have a special trick for a great quick set.

1. Set the hair dry with medium to small Velcro rollers, with tension.

2. Use a styling product if you wish.

3. After the hair has been set, mist it with water. *Do not soak it.*

4. Place a plastic bag over the set and place the client under a hot dryer for ten minutes.

The plastic bag will trap the moisture and create a steam effect much quicker and more evenly than putting in steam rollers. After ten minutes remove the bag and let the client stay under the dryer until dry. Cool completely and remove rollers.

Setting for Direction

Unfortunately many stylists do not learn the mechanics of roller setting. The same principles used for an old-fashioned roller set is used in blow-drying, marcel ironing, and hot-roller setting. Direction is given to the hair and it starts at the roots or base of the hair.

On base: This gives height straight up from the base. The way the hair is lifted from the scalp is similar to giving the hair a haircut at 90°, straight up from the head form. The roller is rolled and rests on the scalp on the base from which it was taken.

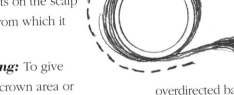

on base

overdirected base

Overdirecting: To give height in the crown area or just for maximum fullness you need to set the roller overdirected.

Underdirecting or dragging: If you need curl at the ends but do not want any height you need to set the hair underdirected. The base has to remain flat and smooth. This is also called dragging the hair or setting off-base.

dragging   underdirecting

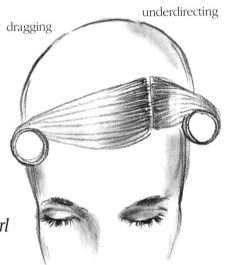

Setting for Spiral Curl

To set for spiral curl, the size of the curl desired and the length of the hair determines what size roller or rod to use.

1. When I set for spiral or use a curling iron to get a spiral curl I take my sections horizontally.

2. I presection the entire head into rows, pinning each row up, starting at the top of the head.

3. Then I take a square section vertically across the rows and curl it.

4. If I am using a curling iron I pin the warm curl to the scalp with a clip or bobby pin.

5. When I am done the entire head is clipped up.

6. I spray it well with a firm-hold spray and let it dry and cool completely.

At the very last minute I take it down or I let the bride leave this way. All she needs to do is remove pins and shake her hair loose. You may set the hair this way with perm rods, rollers, hot rollers, or spiral rollers. Even if I am doing a ponytail updo I will spiral curl the ponytail and clip the curl to hold the set better. Plus, it keeps things neat and allows you to see where you are in the hair.

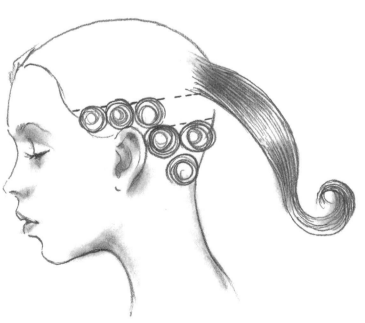

DRY WORKING HAIR SPRAY

A spray that is dry is always in an aerosol can. It usually says it is a dry spray on the label. It is easy to touch the hair right away because it dries fast.

GEL

I prefer to use a gel that is in a bottle and tends to be on the runny side. I pour a puddle of it on the counter and dip my fingers in it as needed. For very wiry, coarse hair I like to use a pomade mixed with a heavier gel.

FINISHING SPRAY

A finishing spray is a final spray to give the bride after you have completed her style. It is very difficult to change anything after you give this final spray so be sure to ask the bride if she is satisfied with her hair before you use the spray. This spray is usually in a pump bottle.

SPRAY GEL

Spray gel stays wet long enough to brush the hair in place before the product dries, yet it gives a softer look than using a heavy gel. I like to use spray gel to tame fly away hairs along the face and at the nape.

SILICONE PRODUCTS

Silicone products help to smooth out the cuticle layer of the hair. I like to use them on naturally curly or thick, wavy hair. I apply it to wet or damp hair, brush it well to disperse it, and then blow-dry the hair.

TECHNIQUES

Debbie

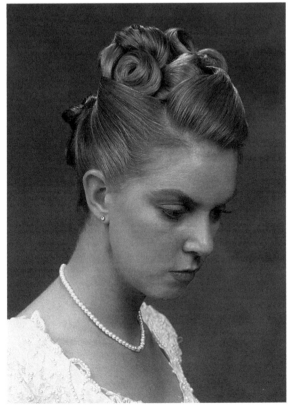 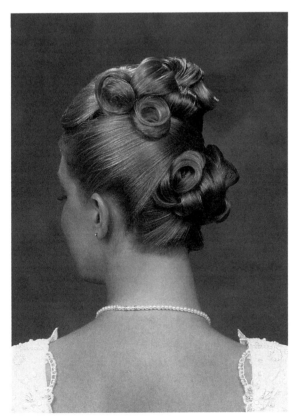

Debbie has long, thick hair with a medium texture. This is a very clean sculpted look. Thicker hair looks nice in a clean, smooth style. Plus this style will hold all day without any drooping.

#1 For texture and volume throughout first set all of the hair on hot rollers. Spray with a spray gel. When the rollers have cooled remove them and do not brush.

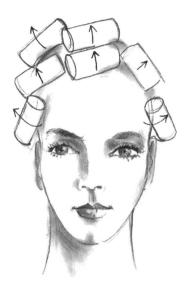

#2 First section a triangle out of the front (1). Standing behind the bride put this front section into a loose ponytail that is not tight to the scalp but has movement. Lay it aside for now. Section out a circle on the crown and draw this section into a tight ponytail (2). Clip it to the side for now. Section behind the ears

and put in another tight ponytail (3). The front sides remain free.

#3 With all the ponytails unclipped and hanging, go to the top, section 1, in front. Holding the elastic between two fingers twist it and push it forward to make a poof for the front.

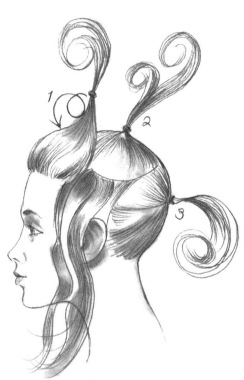

#4 Twist and gently push forward till a nice soft front is achieved. Bobby pin this section securely making sure the pins glide along the scalp. Secure with a criss-cross.

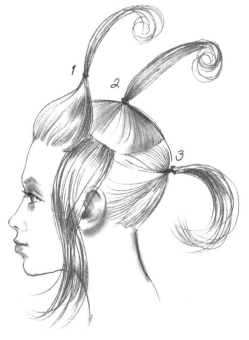

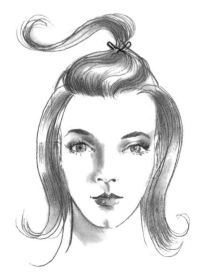

#5 Starting with section 1 separate the hair cleanly down to the ponytail holder and smooth the hair into nice clean curls. Spray each section and smooth it with your fingers before pinning. Pin into the ponytail base. Do this for all the sections. Work from side to side and maintain balance.

#6 Take the right front side and draw it across the back between sections 2 and 3. Bobby pin it close to the elastic in section 2. Do the same for the other side. Shape the ends into curls.

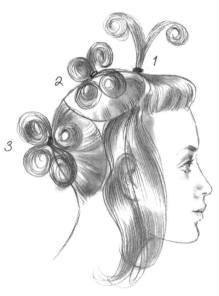

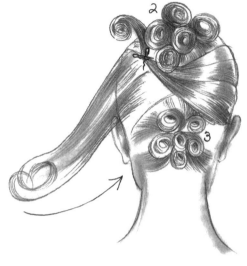

Headpieces suggested for this style:

Backpiece with the veil covering section 3

A **Crown** with curls from sections 1 and 2 coming through

Flowers placed throughout and in back

Pouf style placed in the space in the back

Wreath with a pouf placed in the space in the back

Francia

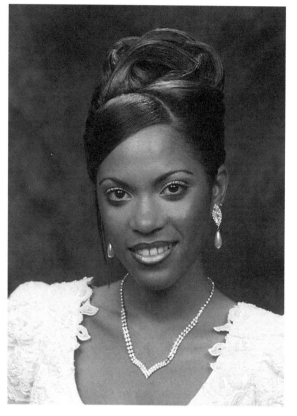

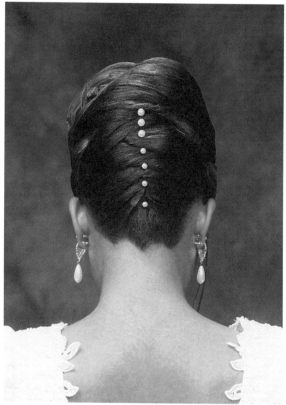

Francia's hair is relaxed with long layers and is a little past her shoulders. Color slicing makes this style interesting.

#1 Section the hair from front to back just above the ears. Section the bottom half into three panels.

#2 Take the middle panel and comb it straight up. Smooth it and pin it to hold. This section will serve as a base for the rest of the hair to be criss-crossed over and pinned.

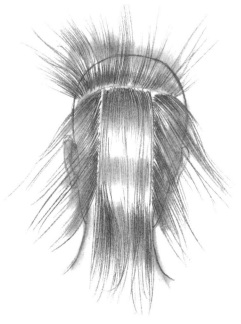

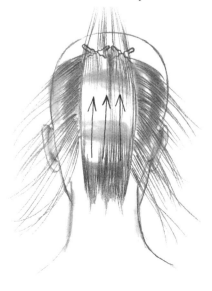

#3 Beginning at the nape on the right side take a small diagonal parting. Smooth and draw that parting over the middle section. Pinch or twist the end for control and pin it along the edge of the parting. Finish with the ends going straight up. Criss-cross in this manner all the way up the section, alternating as you go. Make sure the parting will cover the pins from the previous parting.

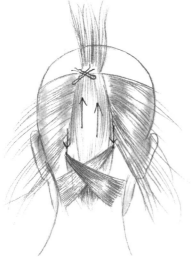

#4 Section the front, top and sides into three sections as shown. There will be only one section 3 which will make the top of the hair design later. The left side and the right side will each have a section 1 and section 2. The section 1 on the right

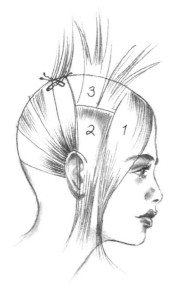

side will be larger because of the side parting.

#5 This is a back view of the sectioning.

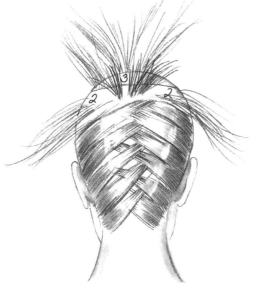

#6 Take section 3 and separate it into four or five smaller sections depending on the thickness of the hair. Make standing up loops or pin curls with these sections. Using diagonal partings work with a flat iron to smooth and shape the sections. Place one behind the other smoothing and pinning them to the scalp. Alternate forming the sections and work the head from side to side. Check for balance and placement as you work.

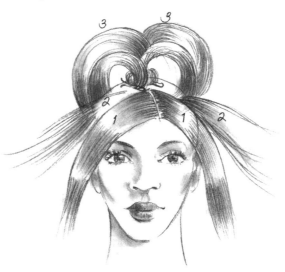

#7 Take section 2 from the left side and draw it up and over the pins from the criss-cross on the top of the head. Pin it down covering the ends and pins.

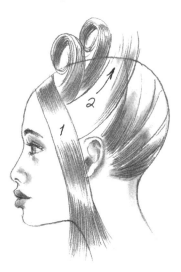

#8 This view shows section 2 from the left covering the pins.

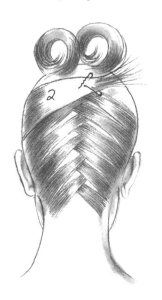

#9 Now take the right side section 2 and comb it into the section from the left side and make it like a small French twist tucking in all of the ends. This will cover all of the pinning in the back. Take section 1 from both sides and blend them over and across the completed hairstyle. An oil spray and flat iron was used to keep this look smooth and clean.

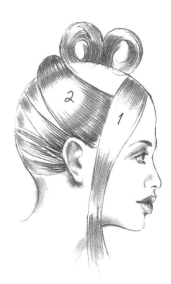

Headpieces suggested for this style:

Backpiece

Crown

Flowers can be placed in the arches

Pearls as shown

Tiara

Paula

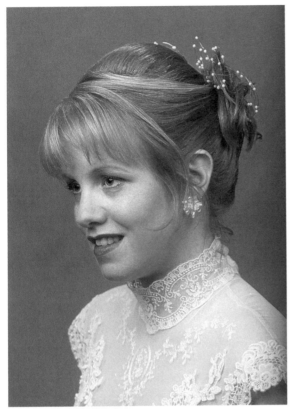 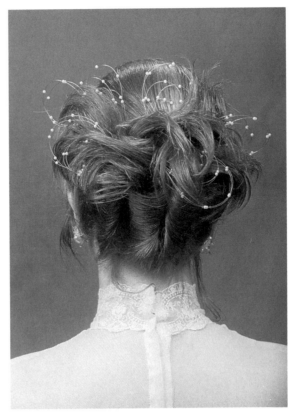

Shoulder length hair with long layers works nice for this style. Longer hair can also work for this style. There is no setting necessary. The idea is to have the ends free and loose.

#1 Section away the front and sides. Draw the crown into a ponytail that rests on the occipital bone. The ponytail should be flat and not sticking out from the head. From the occipital bone down the hair should be loose.

#2 Clip the ponytail end out of the way. Spray the bottom section with a dry spray. Holding out vertical sections, lightly backcomb the hair closest to the scalp. Do not mat up

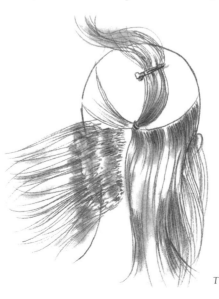

all the hair to the ends. Concentrate the tease close to the scalp.

#3 Separate the back into four vertical sections. Create small twists away from the ear going toward the center on both sides. Smooth the outer section with a brush and pin at the line of the ponytail section. Hairpin the twist if necessary.

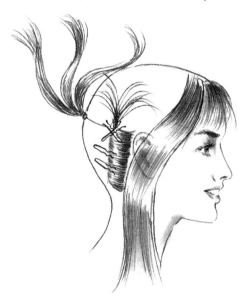

#4 Let the ends hang free for now; they will be sprayed and shaped later. If the hair is longer, twist the section until the hair is used up.

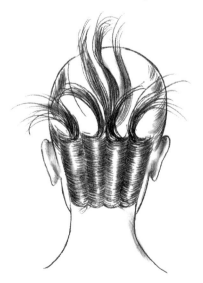

#5 Split the ponytail into two or three sections. Knot or make pin curls. Pin near the ponytail and let the ends hang free.

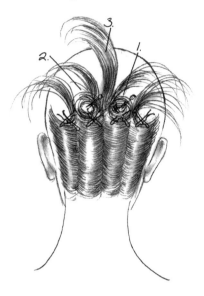

#6 Take the loose ends from the twists and the ponytail and pin up out of the way.

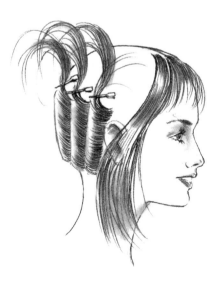

#7 Take the left section and draw it across the back of the head covering the bobby pins. Do the same on the other side.

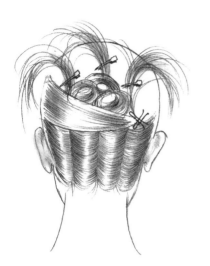

#8 Now release the loose ends from the clips. Shape and spray the loose ends. Fan them out and use hairpins to hold pieces in place. Add the pearl loops.

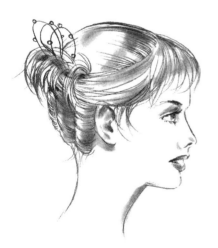

Ornamentation for this design:

Pearl loops can be purchased at a craft shop. They are lightweight and can be stuck into the hair easily. Pin to hold.

Headpieces suggested for this style:

Flowers in the crown area

Hat

Headband

Tiara

Wreath

Kareen

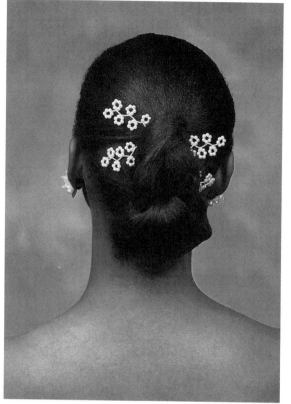

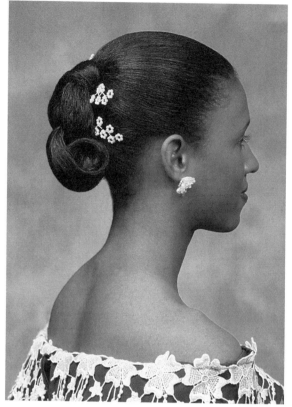

For Kareen's hair type, apply a silicone product for shine and softness to dampened hair. Blow dry hair straight taking special care to control the flyaway hair around the hairline.

#1 Set hair using large hot rollers with tension.

#2 When cool, use spray gel to smooth, and brush hair off face.

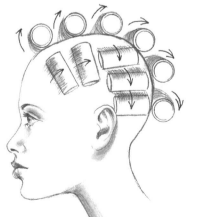

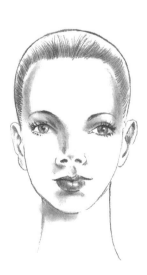

#3 Section off the back of the head behind the ears and draw this section into a smooth tight ponytail at the back of the head. Put in another ponytail under and close to the first one.

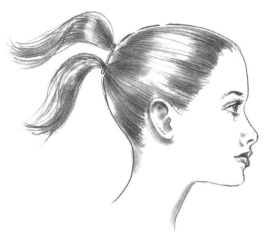

#4 Pick up the first ponytail and spray it while smoothing the hair with *your hands*. (Using a brush to smooth will continually separate the hair and not allow the spray gel to dry the hair smoothly.)

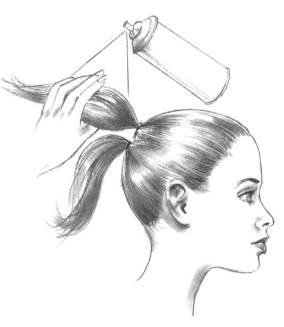

#5 Wrap the first ponytail around the second one and tuck the end under

near the elastic. Bobby pin close to the scalp and elastic.

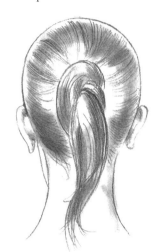

#6 Smooth the second ponytail. Form it into a roll tucking the hair under. Bobby pin it to the scalp on the underside of the roll.

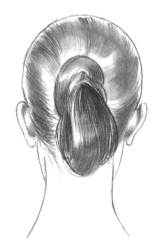

(This style can be done on all one-length shoulder-length hair of any texture.)

Headpieces suggested for this style:

Barrette style backpiece

Crown

Headband

Tiara

Hat

Jennifer

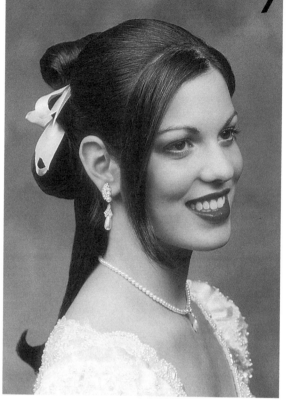

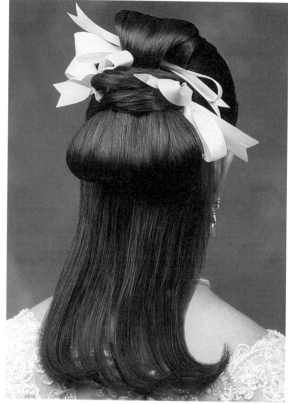

Jennifer has very thick straight hair. This style was done with no setting. This style can be done on long layered hair, longer hair, and any texture. The front of this hairstyle can be done in a variety of ways. Bangs or fringe, a middle part, a zig zag part, or all of the hair can be pulled back into the first ponytail. Ribbon color can be changed or no ribbon used at all.

#1 Draw hair from the temple area and make a smooth ponytail at the back of the crown. Draw hair from the sides to the back and make two additional ponytails below and to the side of the first one. Leave remaining hair along the back out.

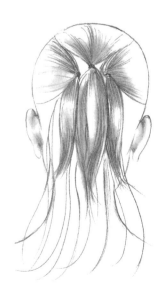

#2 Take three equal pieces of white ribbon and tie bows around the ponytail holders. (Small diameter ribbon to wide ribbon can be used for a different effect. Ribbon size should be decided on at the trial-run appointment.)

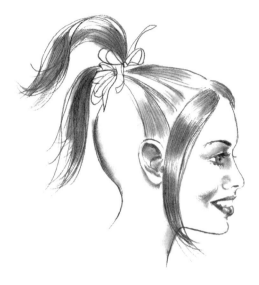

#3 Take the first ponytail and separate out 1/3 of it for the top roll. Backcomb this section, spray with a dry spray and smooth the top side that will be exposed.

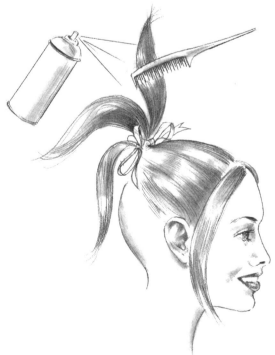

#4 Since this hair type is long and thick, place an additional ponytail at the ends of 1/3 of the ponytail for control. Spray this section and smooth it with your hand. Roll this portion of the top section forward, spreading it out, and pin underneath to the scalp.

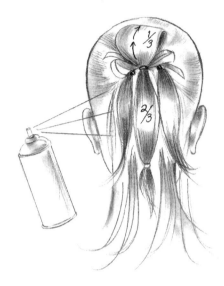

#5 Take the remaining 2/3 ponytail section that is banded at the end and tuck it under in the same manner as the 1/3. Get a portion of the banded end into the bobby pin and pin it up close to the ponytail.

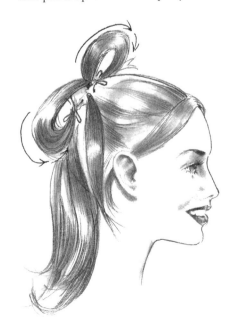

Bobby pin until you feel this heavy piece is secure, pinning underneath and always locking pins. You should still have the two remaining smaller side ponytails left.

#6 Take one of the smaller side ponytails and draw it over and across the middle of the two rolls. Tuck the ends under the top roll and pin. Do the same for the other side ponytail. Adjust the ribbon that is showing for a desired look.

Headpieces suggested for this style:

Fresh **flowers** added near the bows

Ribbons

A simple **veil** on a comb placed in the crown for the ceremony (which can be removed at the reception)

Tiara

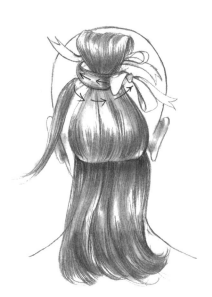

LaKenya

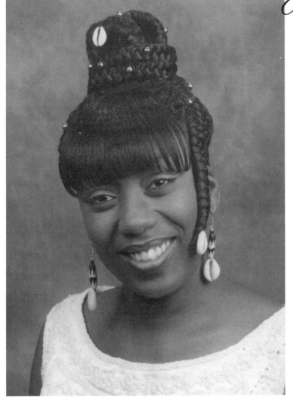

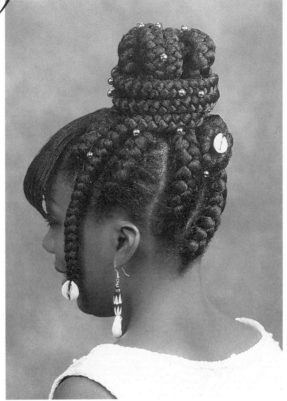

This model has relaxed hair that is about three inches long all around. You must have knowledge and experience of braiding and working with bulk hair to be able to do this style called "Goddess Braids."

#1 Section the bang area out of the way.

#2 Starting at the nape in the middle, braid up into the crown. Add bulk hair. For this style 3-4 packs of 100%

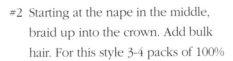

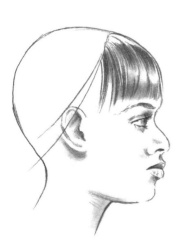

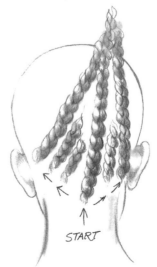

START

Kanekalon fiber was used. Singe the
ends to seal. Braid the remaining
hair working side to side all the way
around the head.

#3 When all of the hair is braided take
out one braid in the back to make
the circle accent as shown in the
picture. Loop up the remaining
braids and pin to secure.

#4 Make one long braid with the
remaining bulk hair and attach it at
the base of the other braids. Wrap it
around the base of the looped
braids and bring the end around to
the front to make a braided tendril.
Add Cowrie shells and gold beads
for accent. Notice the braiding detail
in the bride's dress as well.

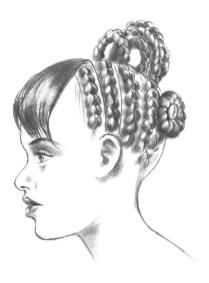

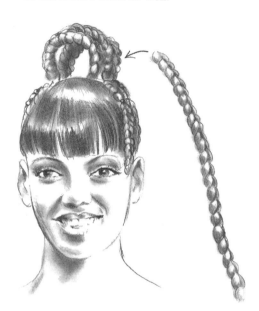

This detailed style should be accented
as shown and not covered up with a
traditional headpiece.

Alexis

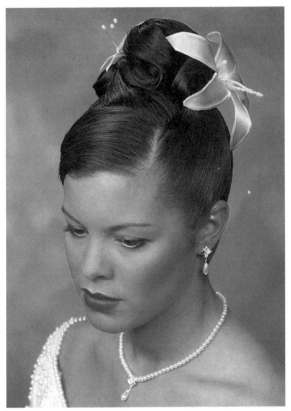 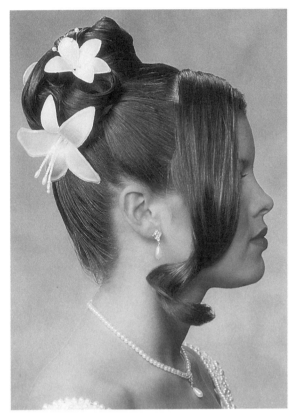

Alexis has silky, straight hair. This hair type does not hold a set well and looks best in a sleek style. The steps to this look can be followed and used for any texture of long hair without layers.

#1 Prepare the hair with a dry working hairspray. For extra hold, each section can be sprayed with a spray gel before going into a hot roller. Set all the hair in the direction it will be going: the sides up and back, the top back, and the bottom up. Everything is going toward the height in the crown.

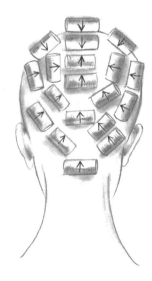

#2 After the hair has set and cooled, section the hair from ear to ear just behind the ears.

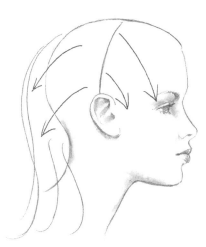

#3 Starting at the section behind the ears, make a circle section taking up the bulk of the hair. Put this into a ponytail at the crown of the head.

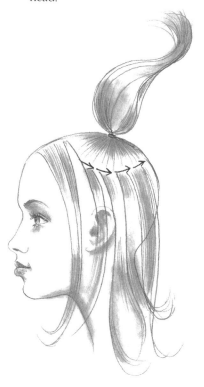

#4 Add three more elastics to the first one. They should be tight and

close together. This helps create a stable base for the updo. All of the pinning from this point forward will be done within the circle section eliminating any need for base tease.

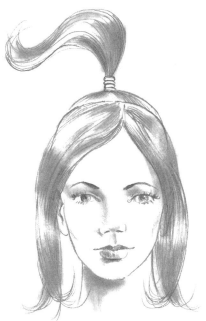

#5 To further stabilize the ponytail, bobby pin the first elastic to the scalp. Two or more pins can be used.

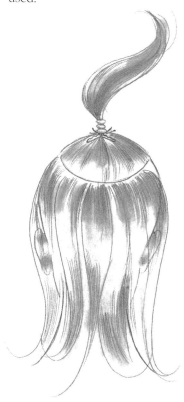

#6 Slightly backcomb the hair that is in the back. Spray it with a dry spray.

#8 Tightly draw one side up smoothing the outer surface. Bobby pin this section to the circle close to the elastics. Do the same for the other side.

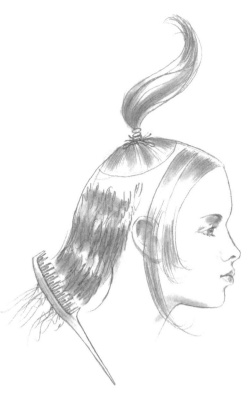

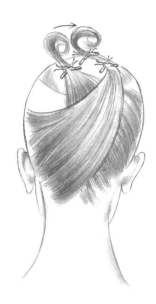

#7 Section this back area into two.

#9 Wrap the loose ends around the elastics covering them. Pin and spray.

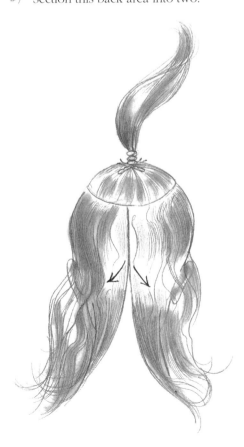

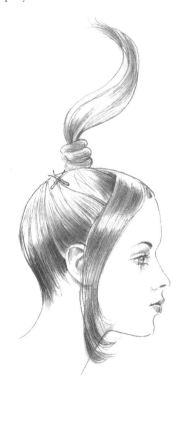

#10 Split the ponytail front to back. Make a clean separation that goes all the way down to the top elastic. Take the front section and backcomb it for control; spray it and smooth out the outer layer all around. This piece should not split and separate; there needs to be enough tease and spray for control.

not pinned will cover the bobby pin. Tuck the ends behind the curl and spray.

#12 Prepare the back section of the ponytail the same as you did the front section. Roll it under but leave a space free to feed hair through later.

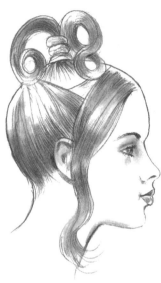

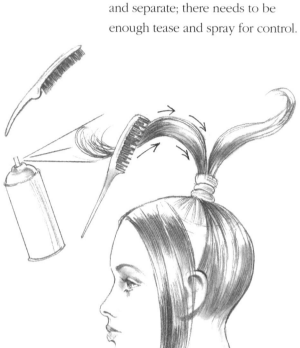

#11 Form this section into a curl shaped like an 8. Bobby pin half the thickness to the scalp. The hair

#13 Take the left front side and hold it up, spray and smooth the outer layer. Bobby pin the hair close to the elastic. Tuck the loose ends through the roll you previously made. For now let those loose ends just hang out the other side. (If

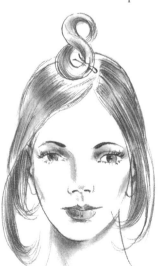

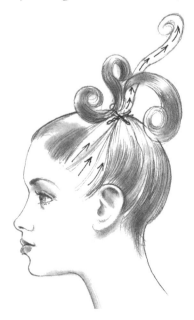

your bride wears her part on the other side or in the middle make adjustments accordingly.)

#14 Now take the right side and do the same but leave out some of the hair around the face as shown.

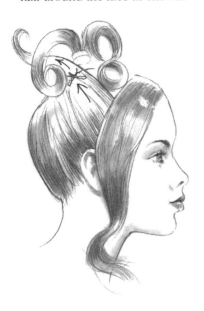

#15 After feeding this section through the roll and bobby pinning it, make a curl with the ends. Also make a curl with the loose ends of the left section you fed through before. Bobby pin the curls in place.

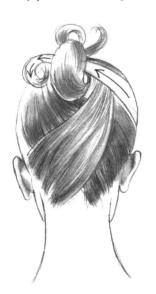

#16 Decorate with flowers. The drawing shows that the piece in front can also be tucked behind the ear. In the photo, the larger flower is opposite the side part creating balance.

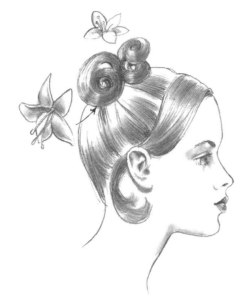

Headpieces suggested for this style:

Barrette with removable veil can be added in front

Headband

Netting on a comb placed in the back under a curl

Melissa

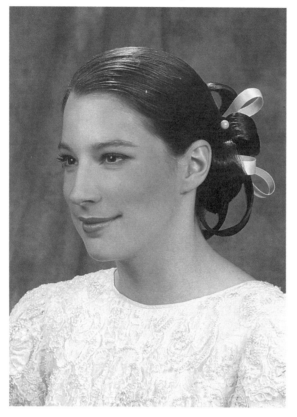 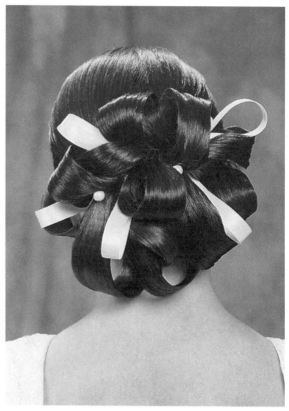

This hairstyle compliments a bridal gown that has back detail. The high neckline of this dress in front works well with the focus of the hairstyle in back.

#1 This model has a slight side swept front. Draw the hair back off the face and behind the ears into two ponytails. Make a third ponytail below and in the center of the first two. Make sure no partings show and that they are tight and smooth.

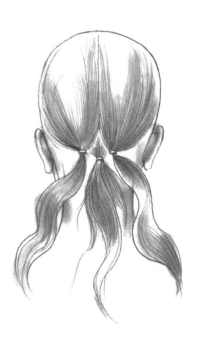

#2 This style is slow going and very detailed. You will need a small flat iron for this design. Each ponytail should make four or more loops depending on the density of the bride's hair. Take the longest sections of hair and use these for the bottom loops.

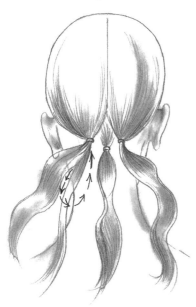

#3 Take a section and spray with spray gel. Run the flat iron over the section and bend it in the direction you want it to loop. It should be crisp and glassy. Bobby pin the end near the ponytail base.

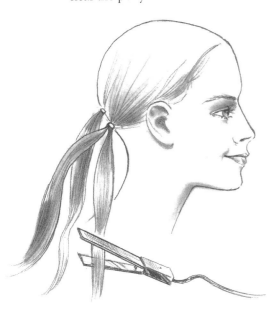

#4 Working side to side doing the outside edges first. Leave sections of hair from each ponytail for the middle. If necessary step back and check your loops for balance. Also turn the bride slowly while she is seated in a salon chair and look into the mirror to study the balance.

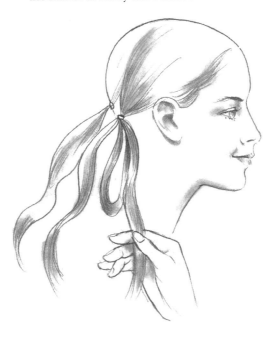

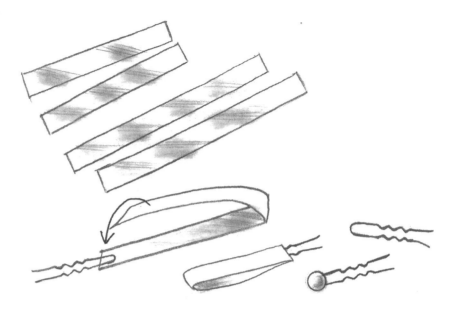

Ornamentation for this design:

You will need:

- ✄ one yard of white ribbon
- ✄ hairpins
- ✄ hot glue gun
- ✄ large pearls

Cut the ribbon into two, four-inch pieces; two, six-inch pieces; and two, eight-inch pieces. Glue a hairpin on one end of the ribbon. Quickly, while the glue is hot, fold over the ribbon and pinch together. Do this for all of the loops.

Glue large pearls onto hairpins.

Add loops and pins into the hairstyle.

Headpieces suggested for this style:

Backpiece worn above design

Bridal hat

Flowers

Headband

Juliet cap

Profile veil

Karie

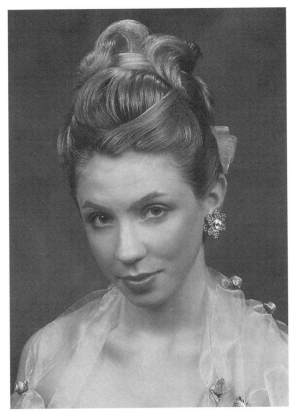

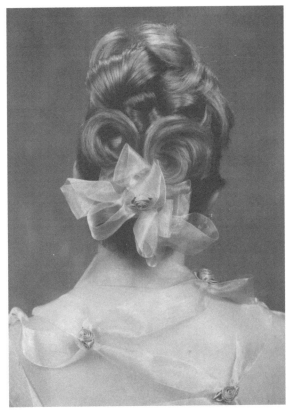

Karie has very thick, all one length, hair. A series of ponytails is necessary for hair such as this. The ponytails help to hold a lot of weight which allows this length of hair to go into an updo without any teasing.

#1 Set all the hair back toward the center with many hot rollers. Spray the set with a spray gel.

#2 Set the bottom hair up. A set should follow the direction the finished updo will take.

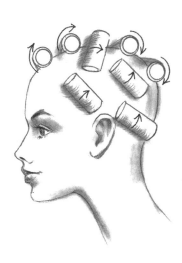

#3 Take out the cooled rollers and do not disturb the curl by brushing. Only finger comb. Section out two small pieces of hair at the front to be criss-crossed later. Take a triangle section at the crown and loosely draw into a ponytail. Place the elastic away from the scalp so the ponytail has room to move.

gently twist and push the ponytail forward. This will create a slight pouf on top. Take a circular section at the top back of the head and put in a tight ponytail.

#5 Split the back remaining hair behind the ears into two sections. Draw up to one side and put in a ponytail close to the scalp. Draw up the other side crossing over the first ponytail and make another ponytail close to the scalp. Pin them to the scalp if necessary, having the bobby pin catch some of the elastic when doing so. Use the criss-cross bobby pin method for hair this heavy.

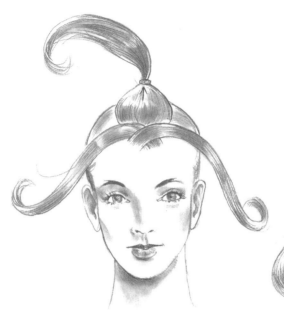

#4 Take that first loose ponytail and with your fingers on the elastic,

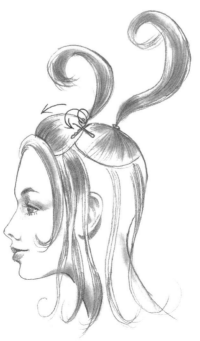

#6 Using the ends of the top two ponytails form some curls at the crown. Make sure your sections are clean all the way down to the elastic. Smooth the hair and spray it with a working spray or spray gel for control. Pin the curls into the ponytail base; be sure the elastics do not show. Your criss-cross sections and sides are still loose.

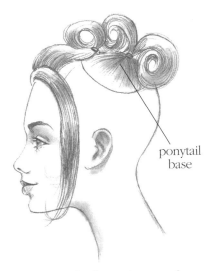

ponytail base

#7 Criss-cross the front pieces and draw softly back into the curls on the crown. Pin them to the scalp in the ponytail base.

curls. Keep checking for balance and work from side to side. Make sure all of your bobby pins that are holding weight get pinned close to the scalp at the ponytail base.

#9 & #10 Loosely draw back the sides of the hair. Pin to the ponytail base and use the ends for filler. Be creative and loop these ends through other curls and let the ends be free.

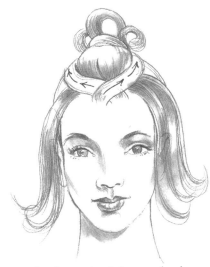

#8 Take the ends of the two back ponytails and form into large pin

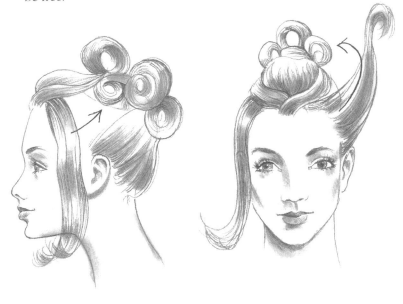

Headpieces suggested for this style:

Backpiece

Crown

Half **headband** with a full veil in front

Random **flowers** throughout

Tiara

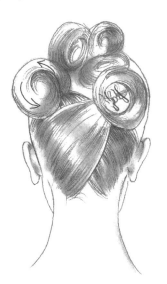

Lauri

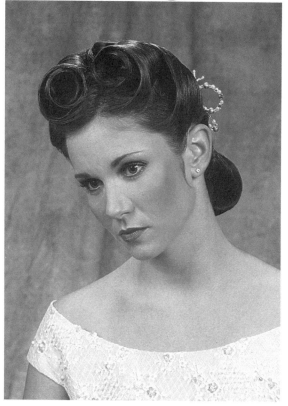 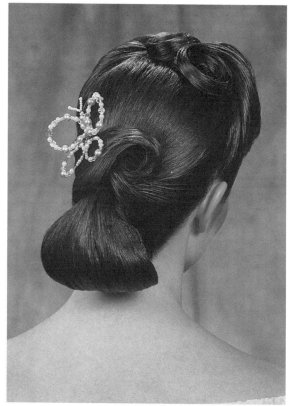

This design is for the more experienced stylist. It takes a steady hand and attention to detail. It is shown here as a bridesmaid style but can be done for a bride as well. The haircut is slightly layered around the face and the length is just past the shoulders.

#1 Section the hair just behind the ear and clip the top out of the way.

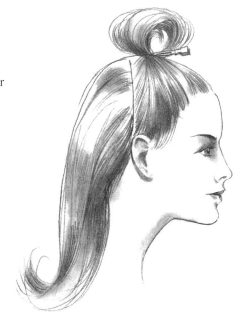

#2 Diagonally slice a section of hair just behind both ears going all the way to the nape. Smooth and spray the remaining hair into a neat, tight ponytail at the nape.

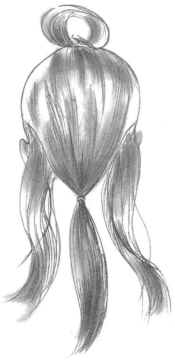

#4 Hot roller placement as well as neatness in setting this design is crucial. The top will be in four sections. Spray smooth and set with tension using one large hot roller for each section. Let cool completely.

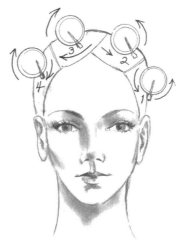

#5 Take down the ponytail first. Brush all the curls smooth into one section. Place an additional ponytail holder near the ends for control. Loop it under and pin near the base elastic.

#3 Roll both side sections up on base with a large hot roller. Spray and smooth with a spray gel before rolling. Make sure these are rolled with tension and clipped with silver roller clips as described at the beginning of the technicals. Set the ponytail in two or three large hot rollers, rolling under.

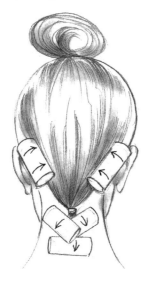

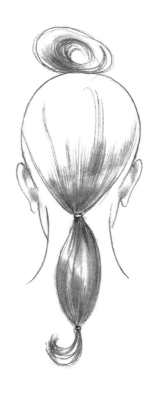

#6 Take out the right hot roller, smooth this section in your hand and bring it across the top of the ponytail. Criss-cross bobby pins as shown.

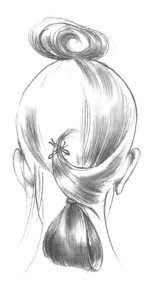

#7 Take down the left side, smooth and draw it over the bobby pins from the right side. Incorporate the ends together into one big pin curl. First pin the pin curl in section 1. You may need to still hold the hair in place at the same time in section 2. Pin some of the underneath from section 2 to the head. You only need a thin veil of hair to cover the bobby pins.

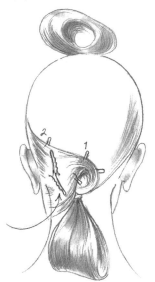

#8 Take out the hot rollers on top. Do not disturb the curl or the partings. Start with section 2. Lightly smooth the hair and roll under. Pin the curl on base in the same place the roller was, minus the roller. Pin inside the curl. Keep the edges of the curl clean and smooth with spray. Now do section 3 in the same manner.

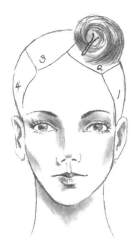

#9 Take section 1, smooth it and draw it up and behind section 2. This curl will lay flatter, more like a pin curl.

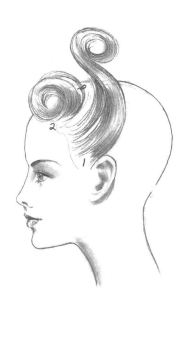

#10 Now draw section 4 up and behind section 3. Pin just behind section 3. These last two curls will cover the ear to ear parting at the top of the head. Use hairpins to hold the edges of any loose curls and spray with a strong finish spray.

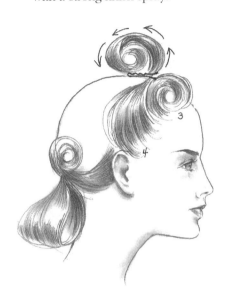

Headpieces suggested for this style:

Crystals or **pearls** glued to hairpins

Fresh **flowers** or randomly placed silk flowers

Juliet cap

Picture hat

Pillbox hat

Katherine

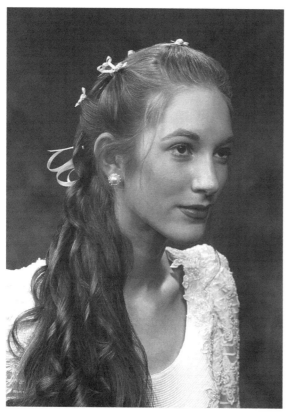
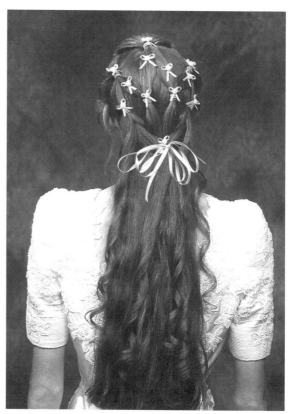

Katherine has very long beautiful red hair. I loved the contrast with the blue ornaments for the "something blue." This is a good look for the young bride. This look can be more dramatic with different decorations.

#1 Take a section in the front from temple to temple. Make sure all of the section partings are clean to the scalp. Put in a ponytail on top of the head. Make two more sections on either side with the rest of the hair along the front. You will have three ponytails: on top is section 1 and the other two are considered section 2.

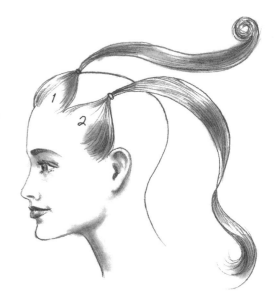

#2 Split section 1 into two parts. Split section 2 into two parts. Add half of section 1 into the two halves of section 2. You will now have five ponytails in the hair.

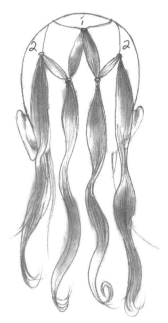

#3 Make a new section collecting the hair behind the ear. This becomes section 3. Before putting in the elastic take the remaining half of section 2 and add it to this new section 3. Do this on both sides.

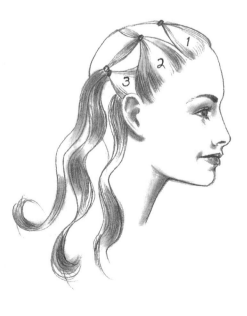

#4 Split this new section in two. The outside half gets curled and hangs free as shown in the photo. Add all the remaining sections together.

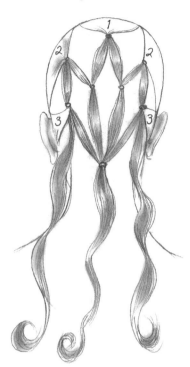

#5 Pin the hanging curl out of the way. At the hairline behind the ear take up a one inch vertical section from the remaining hair. This becomes section 4. Do this on both sides.

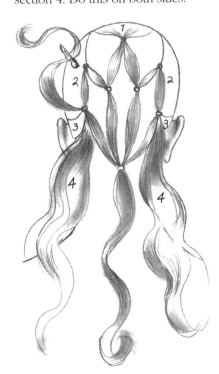

#6 Add the two section 4s together. They will sit over the middle sections. Cover with a ribbon or flowers. Let down the curls that were pinned out of the way from section 3.

#7 Make desired curls with a curling iron using the remaining hair. Decorate with little bows hot glued to hairpins.

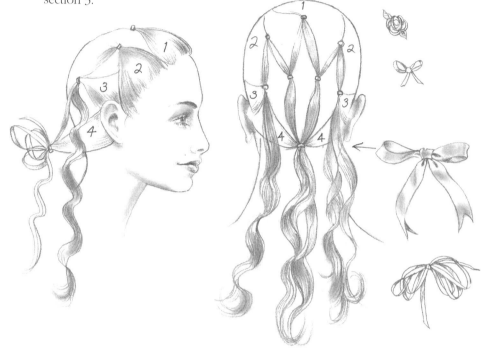

Headpieces suggested for this style:

Blue **bows** and ribbons

Large white **bow**

Long streaming **veil** added to the middle bottom elastic or the top one

Small white **flowers** at the elastics

Tiara

Janice

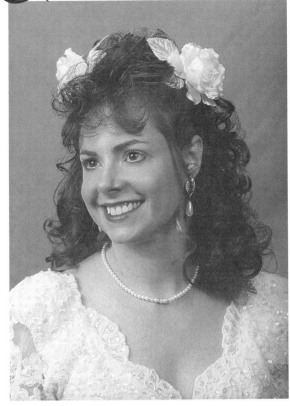

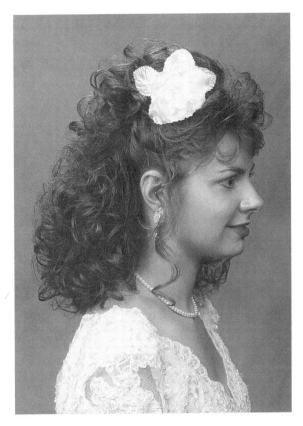

Many brides wish to wear their hair down for various reasons. Don't push the bride into an updo if she prefers it down. A good set and properly prepared hair is the key to this style. If the bride insists on wearing it down and her hair is straight suggest a body wave or perm.

#1 Instruct the bride to put mousse or gel in her hair at home after she washes it. Depending on the bride's natural texture, spray her hair before the set. On coarse hair I like a spray gel or a small dab of gel on each section before rolling. On fine hair I like to use a dry spray. Remember, you will not be brushing this style out after the set. If the products you choose to use make the hair too crunchy and separated it could pose a problem. When setting, take small

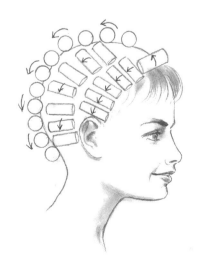

sections and less hair in the rollers than for an updo set. Spray the set when it is complete with a dry spray. Let cool completely.

#2 Remove the rollers and do not disturb the curls. Fluff the hair and rake gently with your fingers. Do not use a pick or brush; it will frizz the curl. Tell the bride the set will relax and settle and that you do not want to disturb the curl too much. To dress up this set draw a small section of hair up on each side and criss-cross pin it in place. Add flowers.

Headpieces suggested for this style:

Backpiece

Crown

Hat

Headband style

Profile

Wreath

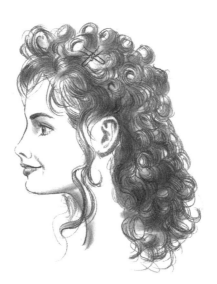

Kate

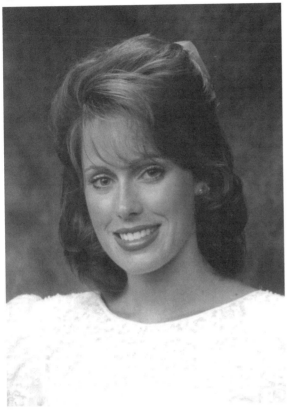

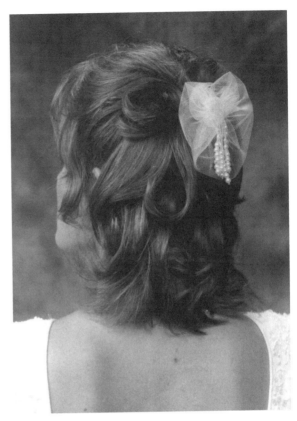

Kate has medium hair that is cut into longer layers. An alternate style for this hair
cut could be a trendy flip.

#1 Leave out some of the fringe bangs
along hairline and set hair on Velcro
rollers for volume. Overdirect the
front curl using a large roller. On
the left side of the first curl set
rollers diagonally going back. Make
sure to overdirect. Set the back all
going down. Spray with spray gel
and a little water and place under a
dryer for ten minutes.

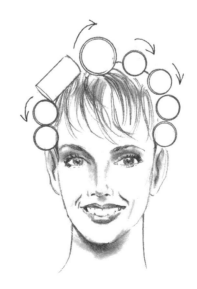

#2 Take out the rollers and finger comb. Spray with a dry working spray. Leave front soft and loose. Draw up the sides toward the back of the head. Bobby pin by crossing the pins. Get the pins close to the scalp. If bride is wearing a heavy headpiece tease the scalp area on the crown before bringing back the sides. Shape the layers in back by pinching them with your fingers while spraying and sculpting.

Headpieces suggested for this style:

Backpiece

Frontpiece with veil

Tiara

Wreath

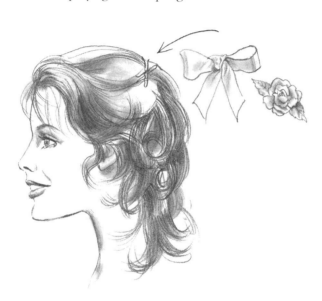

Suzana

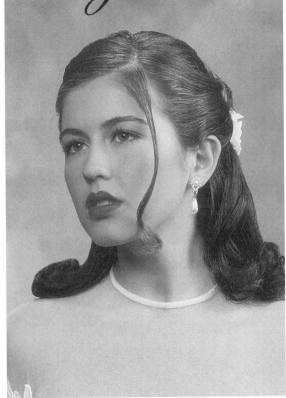

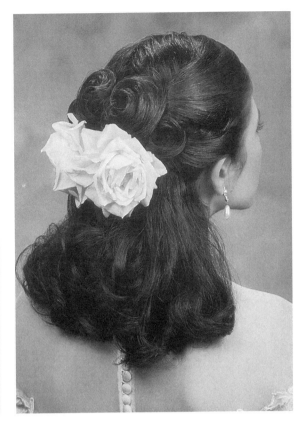

Suzana's hair is thick with long layers. This style is best for medium to thick hair or curly hair. It can also work with a variety of lengths.

#1 Discuss with the bride how she wants to wear the front. This style can be worn with bangs, a middle part, a zig-zag part, or no hair left out. Set the hair on hot rollers all across the back from just above the top of the ear. Set the hair under, even if you choose to flip the bottom afterwards. By not placing rollers on top of the head you will be allowing the front to look more natural.

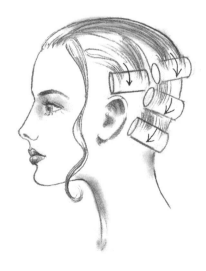

#2 After the rollers have cooled and are removed, make your first parting from ear to ear.

pin the elastic to the scalp. Do the same for the left back ponytail.

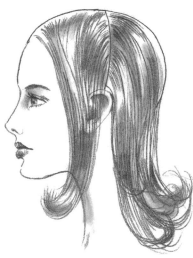

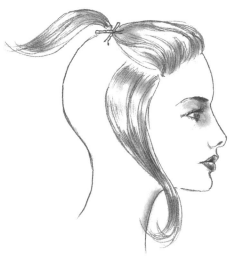

#3 Take the first section at the top of the center front, temple to temple. Draw it back into two loose ponytails. Do not part the section, just split it. The part should not be obvious. Hold the ponytail slightly away from the scalp and put the elastics on. Let the front side sections hang loose for now.

#5 Wrap the end of the right ponytail into a large flat pin curl. Bobby pin the underside of the curl to the scalp making sure the bobby pins do not show in the center of the curl. Do the same for the other pin curl on top. (From the temple down the hair should still be loose.)

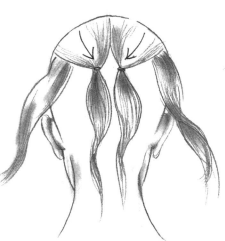

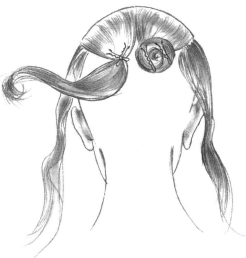

#4 Holding the right ponytail at the elastic, push the whole ponytail up along the scalp. This will create fullness in the top and front. Bobby

#6 Now loosely draw up the right side to just under the first pin curl and pin all the hair with an "X" lock. Wrap the end into a pin curl and

bobby pin. Do the same for the
other side.

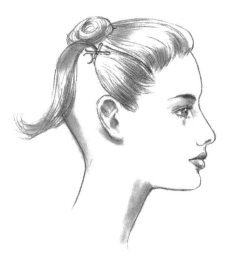

#7 Style the remaining loose hair in the
back. Finger separate the curls and
generously spray the style. First,
spray with a dry working spray
lifting the loose curls and spray from
all sides and underneath. Finish with
a final spray.

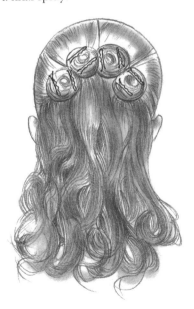

Headpieces suggested for this style:

As shown with **netting** added under
the flowers

Barrette **backpiece** set above the large
pin curls

Headband

Pillbox

Tiara

Wreath

Lori

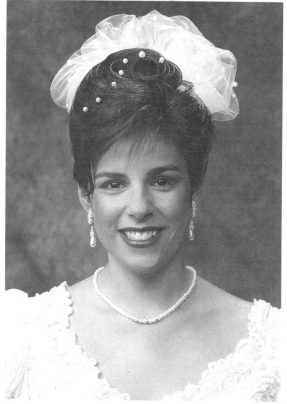 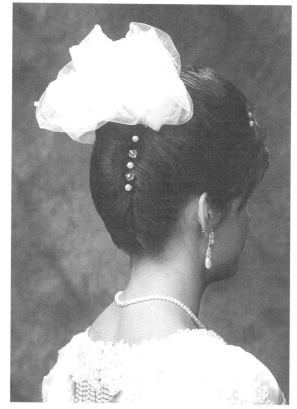

Lori's dark hair lends itself to a smooth style. Her hair has long layers, medium thickness and is fine. This is a traditional French twist yet different. What makes it different is the hair is sectioned in two sections. One twist is in the front and one in the back. The two twists are going in opposite directions. A space is created to place in a headpiece.

#1   Always set the hair in the direction it is going to go. In this case set the sides back with medium hot rollers. Overdirect the front leaving out her bangs and any soft side fringe.

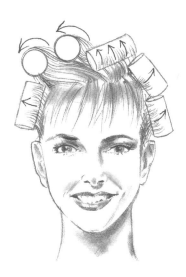

#2 Set the back with the sides and
    bottom all going toward the center.

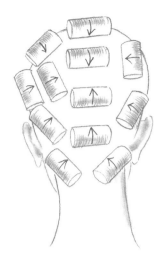

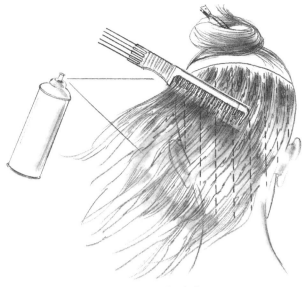

#3 Section the front from the back. Pin
    the front out of the way.

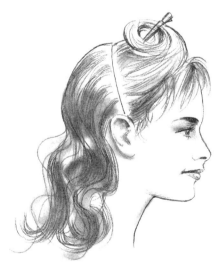

#4 In order to have control and get a
    full twist the hair needs to be
    backcombed. (Fine hair teases
    nicely.) Spray the back with a dry
    working spray. Section the hair
    vertically in about two-inch
    sections. Holding the hair out to
    the left, tease one section at a time.
    Make sure to concentrate the tease
    at the roots. The hair should stand
    out from the scalp and be mostly
    on the left. Spray with the dry
    working spray.

#5 Comb over the hair to the left.
    Make sure not to comb too deeply
    and remove all the backcombing.
    The goal is to smooth out the top
    section. Begin bobby pinning at the
    neck line and pin vertically going
    close to the scalp. Make sure the
    pins interlock and that all the hair
    from the top layer is in the pins.
    Spray with a dry working spray.

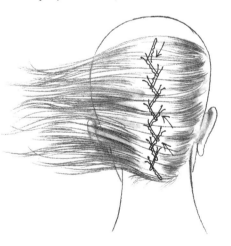

#6 Start to bring the hair over to the
    right side. Now smooth out the top
    layer that is going to show. Tuck
    the hair inside, smoothing and
    rolling. There should be enough
    backcombing so the hair is not
    falling all over the place. You
    should have a cone shape that your

hand is inside of. Bobby pin the *inside* of the top of the cone to the scalp. Use hairpins along the seam.

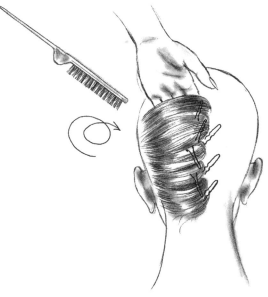

#7 Now backcomb the top section, again having the concentration of tease at the roots. Backcomb in vertical sections and have the hair going toward the right. Spray with a dry working spray.

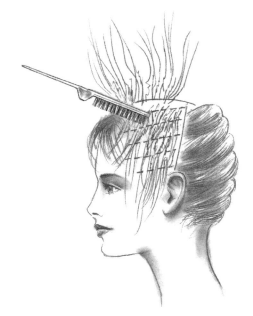

#8 Smooth the top section toward the right. Just behind the bangs pin this section to the scalp interlocking the bobby pins. Spray for control whenever needed with a dry spray. Facing the bride, roll over the top section to your right, smoothing out the top layer. Tuck in the ends and pin inside this roll to the scalp. Use hairpins to tuck the roll close to the scalp.

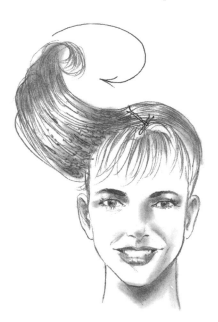

#9 The twist in the back should be
going toward the bride's right side.
The twist on the top should be
going toward her left.

#10 Place a pouf of netting in-between
the two twists. Decorate the seam
in back and the roll on top with
pearls and crystals hot glued to
hairpins.

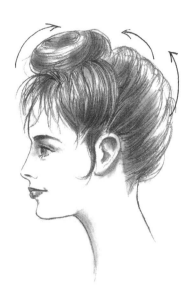

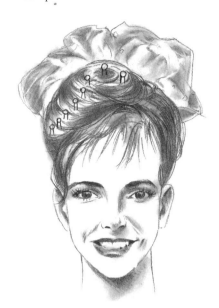

Karen

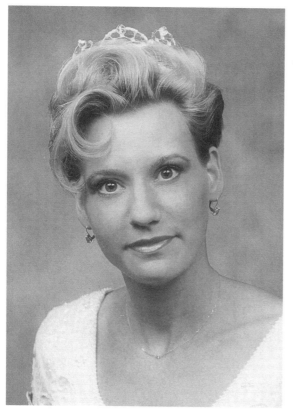
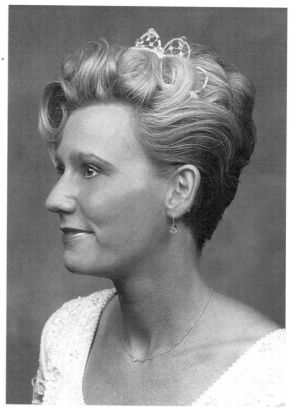

This bridal style lends a dressier look for the bride with short hair. Wash and towel dry the hair. Do not use a conditioner. Put in a light gel and comb through to evenly distribute the product. While combing, look for a natural part or cowlick and how the hair moves.

#1 Comb the sides back, pushing in any natural wave. Extra length will be tucked behind the ear.

#2 Start in the front and place in stand-up pin curls. Take a small square section of hair and hold it upward.

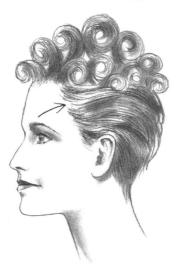
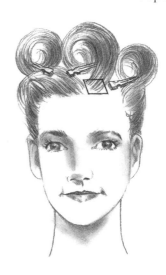

Bend it in the direction you want it to go making a circle. The ends will rest on top of the base of the hair. Put in a clip. The bottom of the clip must slide along the scalp; the top of the clip holds the ends down on the base of the curl.

#3 Do a bricklay pattern with the curls; this prevents holes on the style. On top, keep the curls open and larger side. This provides height. These curls are not intended to create a lot of curl, but fullness and body. Place client under a hood dryer.

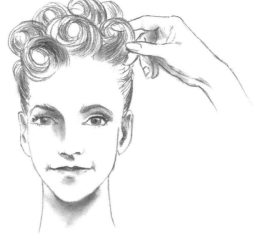

#5 Slightly backcomb the base of the hair depending on desired height. (Do not tease the body of the curl, this will make it frizzy.) Shape curls into desired style and spray.

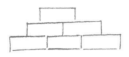

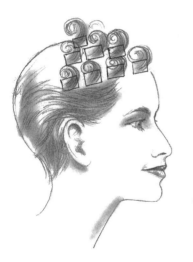

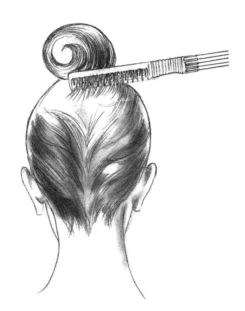

#4 When completely dry and cooled remove the clips and *finger* brush. Do not use a bristle brush because you do not want to remove all of the separation in the body of the curl. Your goal is to get rid of any scalp separation and parts. Spray with a dry aerosol spray as you finger work it.

Headpieces suggested for this style:

Backpiece

Crown

Headband

Tiara

Heather

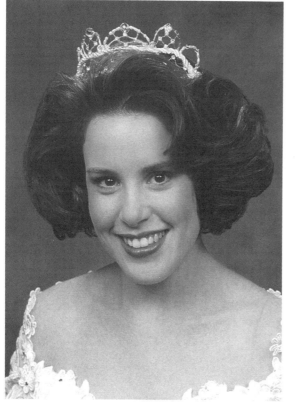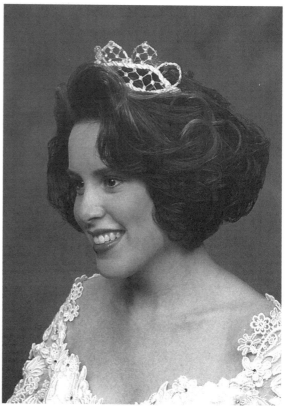

Heather has a layered bob with some great highlights.

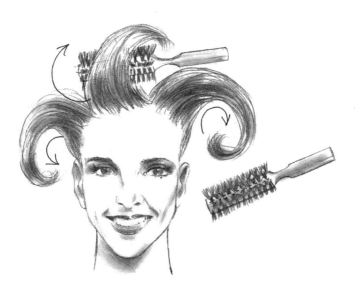

#1 For maximum body, wash and blow dry this style. Using your favorite liquid tool and a large round brush, lift the root area for maximum height.

#2 Set on small to medium Velcro rollers. Overdirect the front for maximum height. Set everything under using tension.

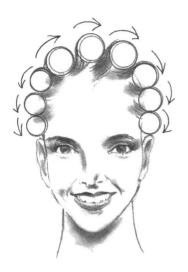

Headpieces suggested for this style:

Crown

Half **headband** with veil

Headband with veil

Picture hat

Pillbox

Tiara

Wreath

#3 Spray gel the set, lightly mist with water and put on a plastic bag. Put under a pre-heated dryer for 5–10 minutes until the bag steams up. Remove the bag and finish drying. Let the set cool before removing the rollers. Brush, shape, and backcomb the base area if necessary. Finish spray well.

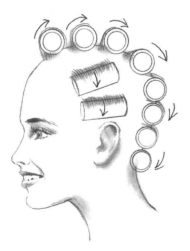

Mary

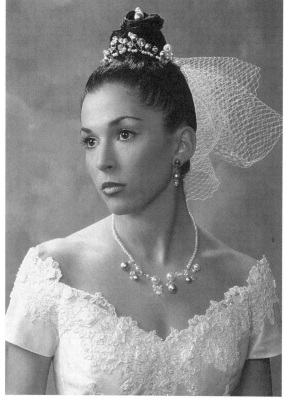 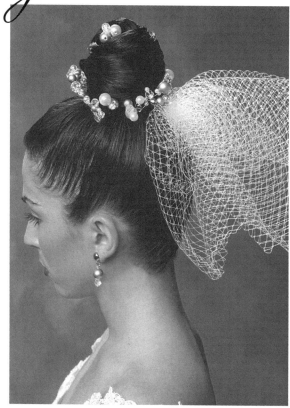

This model has silky fine hair that is not too dense. When a bride has fine hair it is best to put more emphasis on ornamentation rather than the hair itself. Veiling or something dramatic and different takes the focus off the lack of hair.

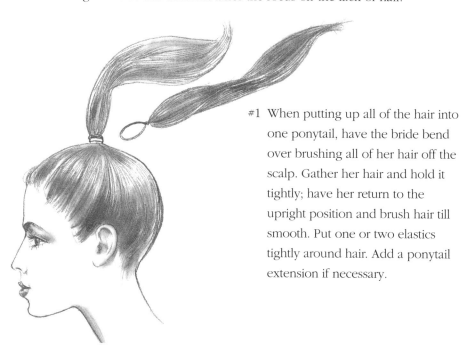

#1 When putting up all of the hair into one ponytail, have the bride bend over brushing all of her hair off the scalp. Gather her hair and hold it tightly; have her return to the upright position and brush hair till smooth. Put one or two elastics tightly around hair. Add a ponytail extension if necessary.

#2 Brush and smooth the ponytail using a gel if necessary. Make sure it is very smooth and free of flyaways. Slightly twist the hair and wrap one large curl around the base of the ponytail. Tuck the ends under and bobby pin all around. It may help to have the longer bobby pins for this hairstyle.

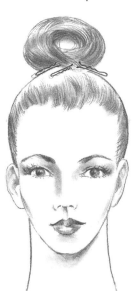

Ornamentation for this design:

You will need:

☙ Russian netting 12 inches by 24 inches

☙ silver colored wire

☙ various sizes of pearls in white and silver

☙ various sizes of crystals

☙ hot glue gun

☙ hairpins

☙ one large clear plastic comb

☙ needle

☙ white thread

☙ needle nose pliers

Lay out the Russian netting flat. Sew by hand a large straight stitch across the edge of one of the long sides. Pull to gather and tie a knot to secure.

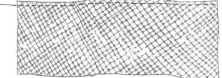

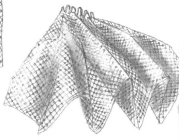

Break the plastic comb into three pieces. Sew one piece onto the Russian netting.

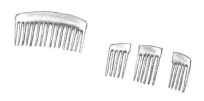

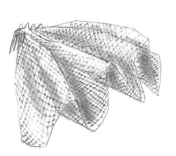

The headpiece is in two sections. There is a tiara section at the front of the head. There is a second section in the back that is attached to the netting. There are pearls and crystals glued onto hairpins that are placed throughout the updo. You can also make a necklace to pull the look together.

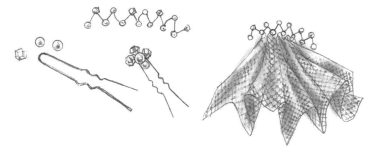

Please experiment with this headpiece design and learn by trial and error. This is a free form look and no two should look the same.

1. Cut about two feet of wire. The wire should be flexible enough to bend easily but not too flimsy so that it looses its shape. It should be thin enough to thread the pearls you want to use.

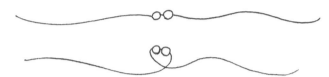

2. Thread a couple of beads into the middle. Hold the two beads and twist a loop, twisting twice. Now thread beads onto each end of the wire and twist and make loops as you go. Sometimes thread only one bead, sometimes thread two or three. Interchange colors and sizes. Make two beaded sections about the same in size. Sew one onto the Russian netting near the comb.

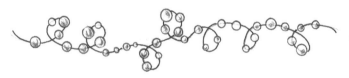

3. Take the two other pieces of comb and glue a piece onto each end of the front section of beaded wire.

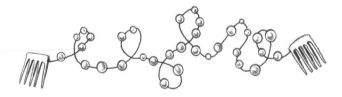

4. Glue pearls and crystals onto a few hairpins. Attach the pieces to the hairstyle where shown. Experiment with different color beads and different color wire to make a variety of looks.

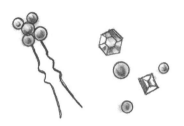

Headpieces suggested for this style:

Backpiece

Crown

Flowers all around the base of the top knot

Half headband with wire

Small **wreath**

Tiara

Nim

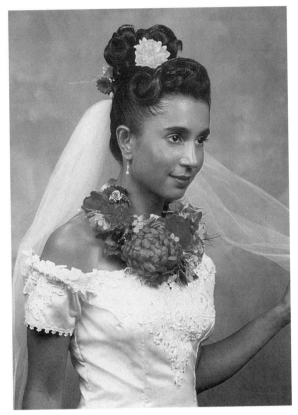

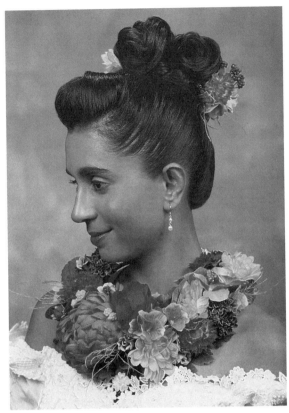

Nim has fine hair, which is great for detail work. Fine hair flows like fabric and looks as smooth as ribbon. I used a ponytail hair addition with this style.

#1 Section the hair behind the ears and

place a ponytail on top of the head. Make sure the ponytail is wrapped as tight as it can go; you don't want it to slip later under the weight of the finished updo.

#2 Draw up the rest of the hair and

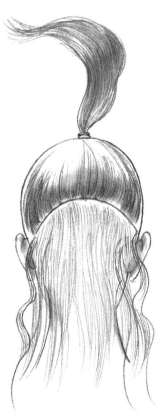

place another ponytail close to the first one. Leave out a section of the bang area and roll it in a hot roller. Overdirect the roller for maximum height in the front.

#3 Use a ponytail hair addition that is

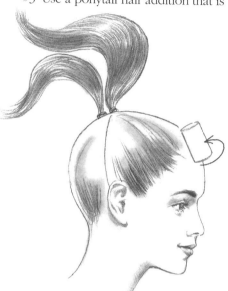

attached to a large elastic. You can choose one close to the bride's own natural hair color. Wrap the elastic tightly around both of the other two elastics. Now you have three sections; the two ponytails of natural hair and one hair addition.

#4 Take out a section of natural hair from underneath the second ponytail. This will be added to the addition to help blend the colors. Take out as much hair as you feel you need or can afford to take away from the rest of the style.

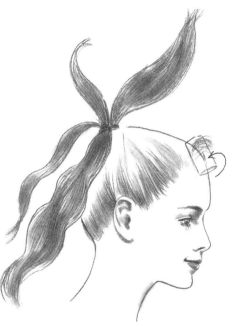

#5 Braid the natural hair into the extension, braiding all of the extension. Use a small rubber elastic on the end.

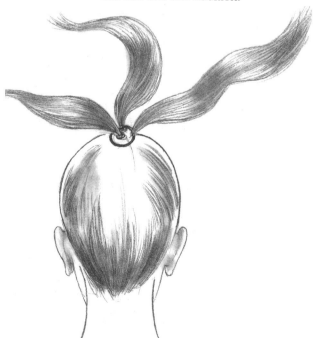

#6 Wrap the braid around the ponytails creating a crown that the curls will sit in. Do not wrap it too tightly. Put the remaining hair into hot rollers.

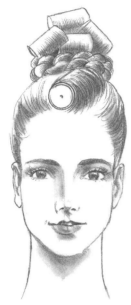

#7 When the curls are cooled separate the hair into three sections. For a nice detailed, clean look, separate the hair all the way down to the elastics. Spray and smooth the sections.

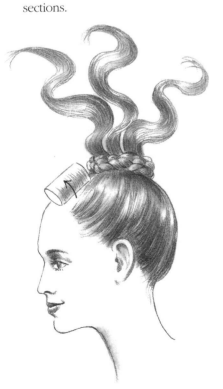

#8 Start in the front. Pick up one section at a time. Allow the hair to coil and fall naturally. Do not force it to take a direction. Wherever the bulk of hair rests on the braid and scalp, pin it there. Use your last section to balance the look where needed. Bobby pin the bulk weight. Use hairpins to finish. Spray well.

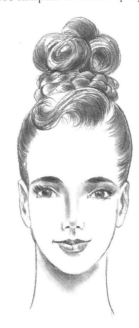

#9 Take out the roller in the front and shape it to please the bride. You may need to bobby pin a soft pin curl to the scalp.

Headpieces suggested for this style:

Crown

Wreath

Headband placed between front curl and updo

Barrette **backpiece** in the back as shown with removable veil

Jill

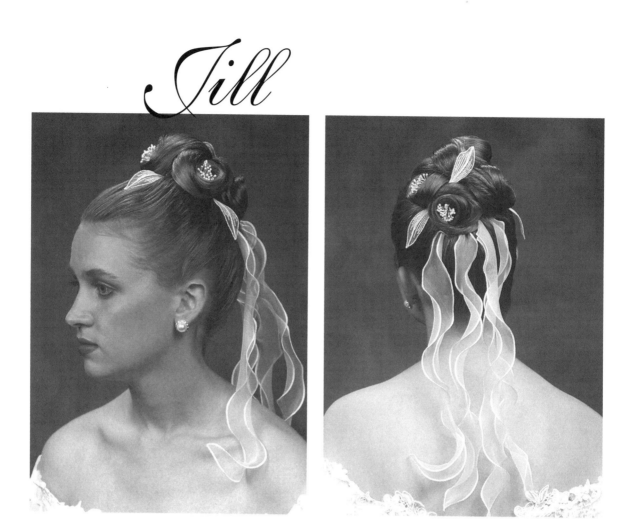

Jill has long one length fine hair. This style is great for thick hair as well.

#1 Set the hair on large and medium hot rollers for body. When cool, brush out the set with a bristle brush.

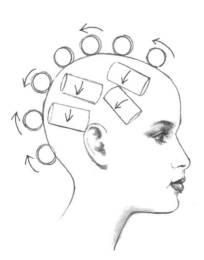

#2 Draw the hair up into four or five ponytails all close to each other on top of the head.

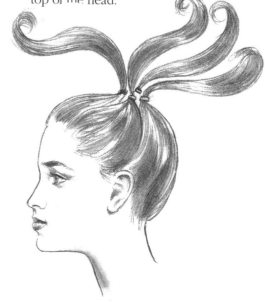

#3 Make the front into two ponytails. This helps keep the sides tighter and the hair from shifting.

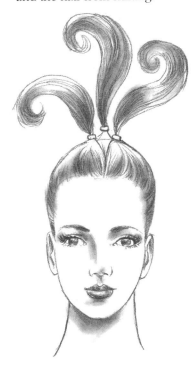

#4 Bobby pin the elastics to the scalp so the ponytails do not shift around. Begin making the ends of the

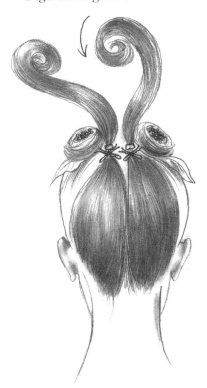

ponytails into large pin curls. Spray with a dry working spray or a spray gel for control. Bobby pin the pin curls, trying to get the pins to grab near the ponytails.

#5 Secure the pin curls with hairpins. Spray well. Decorate the pin curl "flowers" with artificial flower centers. Add white wedding leaves along the edges of the curls. Add veil ribbons or any style veil to the back.

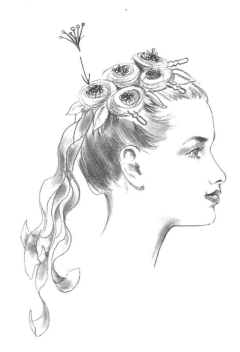

Stacia

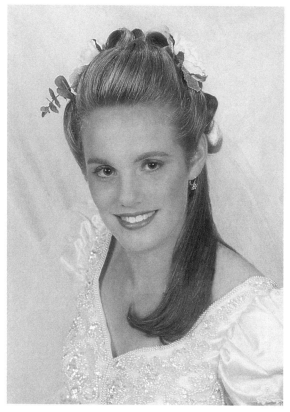
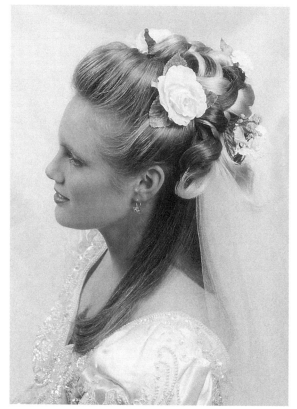

This model has coarse, straight hair. Hair like this would not hold a soft, loose, springy curl without a body wave first. Hair of this texture and weight looses its curl rapidly. This is why most of the curls are pinned up onto the crown. The bottom is left straight because it creates a nice contrast to the crown. If the back was curled it would get stringy and flyaway and visually take away from the crown design. This style also has the addition of a contrasting synthetic hair extension.

#1 Section out a circular area in the crown for the ponytail. Leave out the sides (section 3) and leave out the front area between the temples (section 2). Let the back part hang loose and let its thickness guide you. If the bottom looks thin and wispy put less into the crown ponytail. If there is too much hair hanging down put more into the crown ponytail.

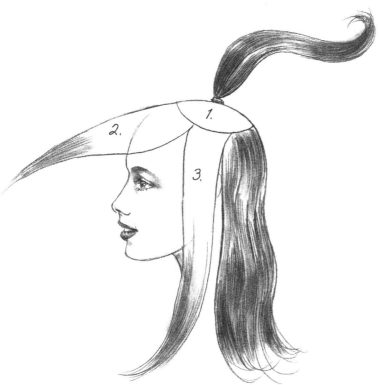

#2 Spray the three sections with a spray gel. Set the crown in small to medium size hot rollers. Spray again. Set the sides (section 3) in one large hot roller vertically going back. Set the front section in one or two large hot rollers going back. Spray again. While the rollers are heating up you can smooth out the back section with products and a blow dryer, or set in large Velcro rollers or leave alone.

#3 Remove the rollers from the hair when cooled. Add the contrasting colored ponytail hair piece onto the crown ponytail.

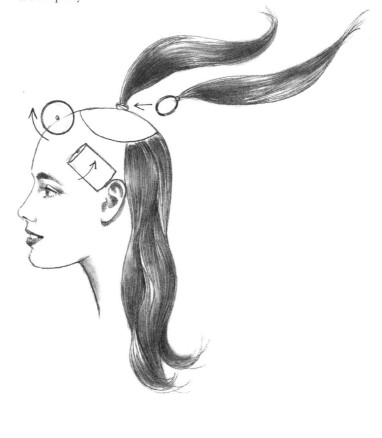

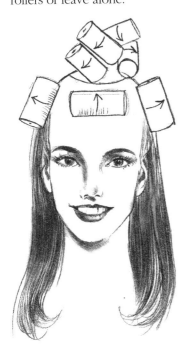

#4 Clip the ponytail section out of the way for now. While standing behind the bride brush the front section up and away from the face. With your hands above the top of the head, twist this section while placing it down to rest just in front of the ponytail. This trick will produce a pouf in the front for the bride without bangs. This step may need a few tries until the bride is comfortable with how the pouf looks. Try twisting to the right or to the left and work with her natural hairline. Once it is in place bobby pin it securely as shown in the drawing.

Some brides may want this section drawn back smooth and tight while some will like a side pouf as shown in the photo. Do not move to the next step until the front and sides are the way the bride likes them.

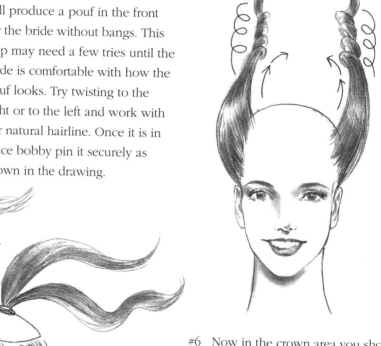

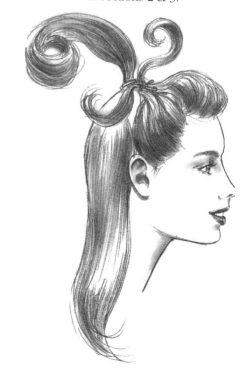

#5 Repeat the same trick for the two sides. This time draw the hair back along the sides of the head. Twist the sides up toward the crown: on the left side twist clockwise, on the right side twist counter-clockwise.

#6 Now in the crown area you should have the hair from the ponytail and the extension plus the ends left over from sections 2 & 3.

#7 Use the ends from section 2 and add a piece of blonde from the extension and make a pin curl. Pin it just behind the front pouf. Do the same for both side sections 3.

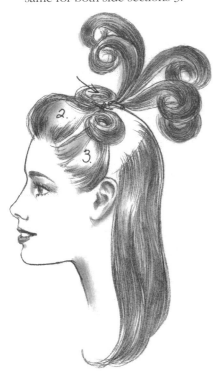

#8 With the rest of the hair be creative. Take a section of the natural hair for a curl and add a piece of the synthetic hair to it. Work the design by making and pinning the curls. Keep the loops tight and compact. This style does not have a lot of volume or height. Create by working the head from side to side to keep the hairstyle even and balanced.

#9 Add silk flowers that have been glued to bits of combs and hairpins.

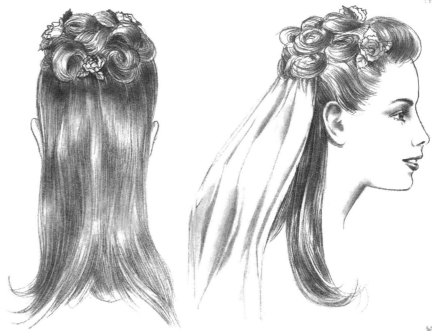

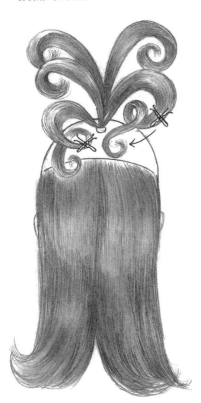

#10 Attach a veil just under the curls and arrange the hair to fall over it.

Headpieces suggested for this style:

Backpiece	**Profile**
Half **headband** with wire	**Tiara**
Headband	**Wreath**

Dana

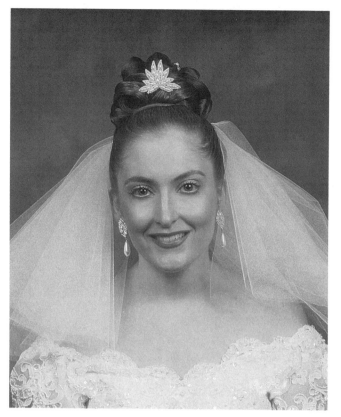

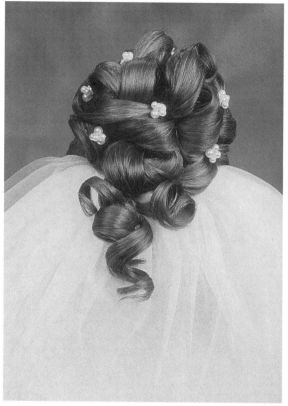

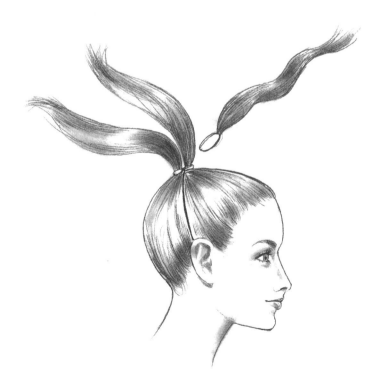

#1 Separate the hair ear to ear at the top of the crown. Make one ponytail on top. Then make a second ponytail just behind the first one. Use a third elastic to combine the two together. In this case the third elastic has a ponytail addition for added volume. It matches the model's hair perfectly or it can be slightly off for subtle contrast.

#2 Take a section of hair about 1 inch thick away from all the rest of the hair. Tease it and spray this piece well with a dry spray until it is thick and matted.

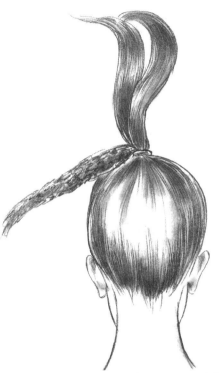

#3 Wrap this matted piece very tightly at the base of the ponytails. DO

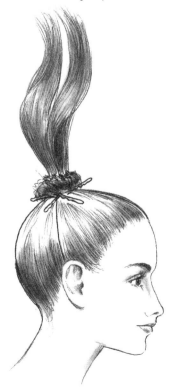

NOT wrap up the ponytail but make sure you wrap going around the lower base ending close to the scalp. The ponytail should not flop over but stand firm and away from the head. The matted piece provides a base where much of the pinning will take place. If your ponytail is flopping over use more hair, tease more, and wrap tighter.

#4 Set the ponytail on medium hot rollers. Setting should be neat, clean, and with tension. Spray gel each piece as you set it. There should be no flyaways. Spray again and let cool.

#5 When removing the rollers DO NOT brush or disturb the curls. To make the curls, take a curl from the front and pinch it 1/3 of the way down the strand, letting the end hang loose.

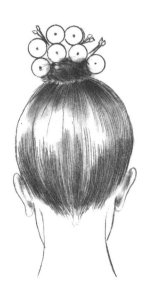

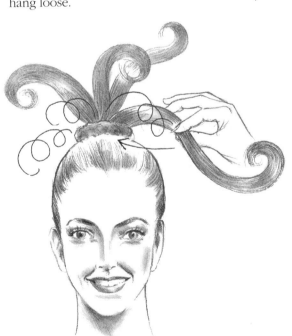

#6 Holding the strand bring it to the base of the ponytail and double pin it at the base in the matted part. Let the end hang free for now. Working the head from side to side pin all of the curls this way. Pin some on top of the elastics. Keep the curls clean and avoid brushing. Spray with a dry spray and smooth with your fingers.

#7 Attach the headpiece just under the hair in the back with bobby pins. The width of this veil prevents it from being put on a comb.

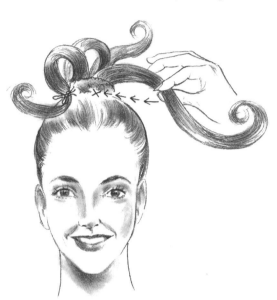

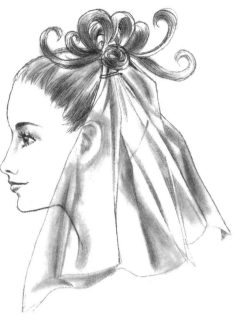

#8 Now work the loose ends into the style. Pinch close to the ends leaving the very end free and pin in more loops. Just hide the ends in the style and leave some free to hang down the back of the veil.

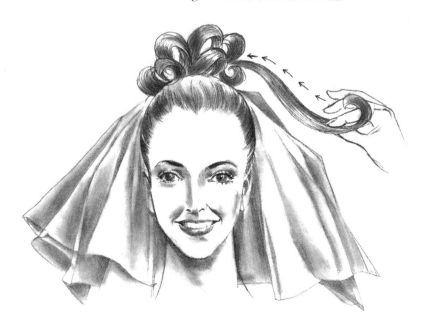

Ornamentation for this design:

You will need:

- hot glue gun

- hairpins

- flat bridal appliqués

- medium size pearls

Bend the tips of two hairpins up to form a right angle.

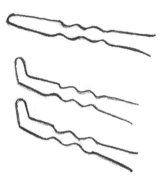

Glue these to the bottom back side of a bridal appliqué. Push the hairpins into the hairstyle. If necessary bobby pin over the hairpins to secure it.

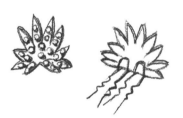

Hot glue four or five pearls onto a hairpin. Make five or six of these picks and place throughout the hairstyle.

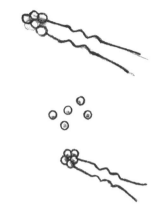

Headpieces suggested for this style:

Backpiece

Flowers

Half **headband** with wire and pouf

Profile

Tiara

Wreath

Carrie

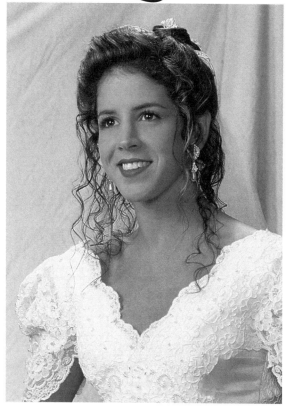

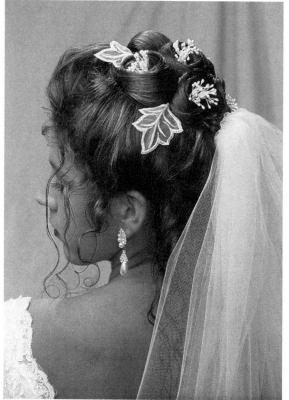

Whenever working on a bride with naturally curly hair who wishes to utilize her curl, ask her to wash her hair at home in the morning. Have her use her regular styling aid and let it dry naturally. When working, try not to disturb the curls and if the entire look is to be curls do not use any tools but your fingers and pins. This design combines smoothness with natural curl.

#1 Remember to leave out curly tendrils all along the hairline as you are working. Make a small circle section at the crown. It needs to be thick enough to make one hair flower. Take a parting from the left front to behind the right ear and draw up to the top of the head (a). Put in an elastic as shown. The ponytail will be loose from the head so bobby pin it into the circle parting from the first section.

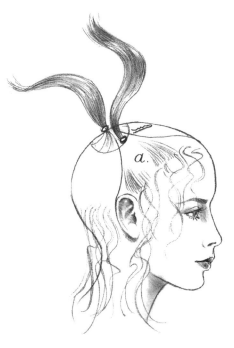

#2 Take a section from the opposite side to behind the left ear (b), put an elastic on it and pin it into the circle.

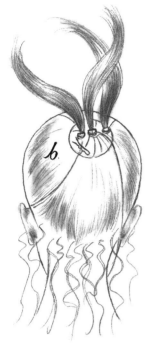

#3 Take the remaining hair and place it into three loose ponytails (1, 2, 3). Do not brush the hair smooth. Bobby pin the ponytails to the

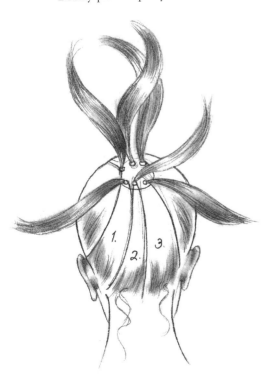

scalp. If the bride's hair is thicker, use more ponytails.

#4 Starting at the top, wrap the first ponytail around two fingers loosely; smooth with a brush if desired. Keeping a center area open lay this

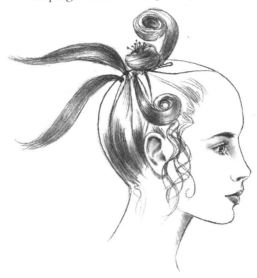

hair flower on the scalp and bobby pin around the edges.

#5 Make hair flowers in this same way all around the head. Check for

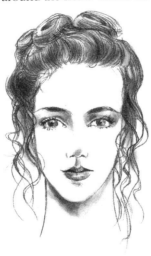

balance. Use hairpins around the edges for control.

off the excess. Slide the end at the base of a hair flower and bobby pin in place.

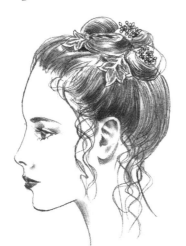

#6 Add flower centers, leaves, and veil on a comb.

Headpieces suggested for this style:

Backpiece made of flowers

Hair flowers inside a **wreath** made of flowers

Ornamentation for this design:

You will need:

🖉 flower center picks

🖉 fabric leaves

Separate two or more flowers centers and wrap together with one of the wires. Cut off the excess stem length.

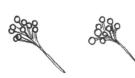

Bend, insert into hair flower center, and bobby pin.

The leaves are also attached to wire. Cut

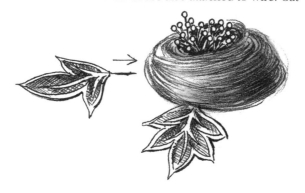

Leslie

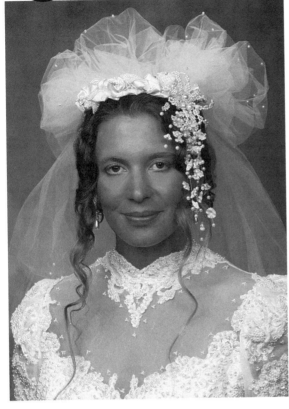
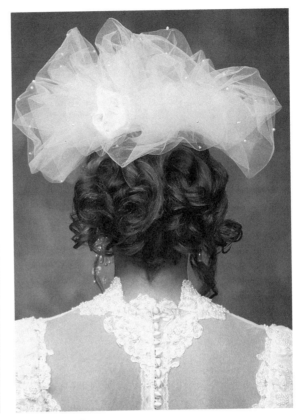

Leslie has very long hair that is naturally wavy. This is a soft loose look done without brushing or backcombing. I had Leslie wash her hair in the morning and put a light gel product in her hair. I asked her to air dry it so the curls were undisturbed. Any bride with natural curls knows her hair and how it behaves. If she wants a natural look, I have the bride help me out in this manner.

#1 If needed, go over the ends with a marcel iron to give them a fresh curl. Then, take a section from temple to temple and put in two loose ponytails in the back, level with her ears. Don't let a part be obvious. The ponytails should be loose and hang down. Leave out the hair at the sides and in the back, plus any tendrils from the front.

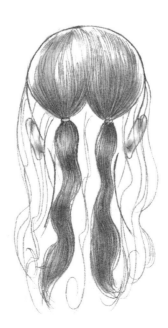

#2 Split the left ponytail in half. Take up all the hair from the left front and behind the left ear and add it to the left half of the ponytail.

long the hair is.) Secure this knot to the scalp by pinning from underneath. Wherever your fingers are holding the hair to the head is where a bobby pin should go.

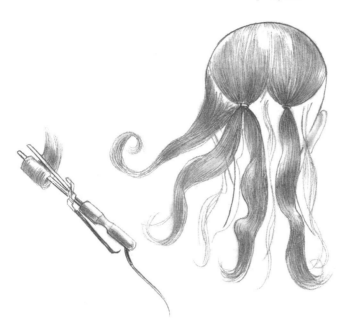

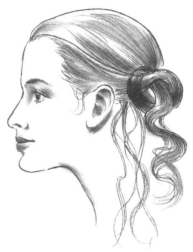

#5 Do the same for the right ponytail.

#3 Take this section and tie a loose knot. The curly ends should be hanging out of the center of the loose knot.

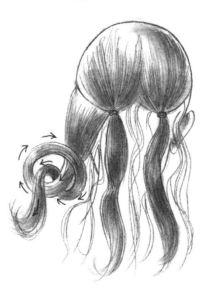

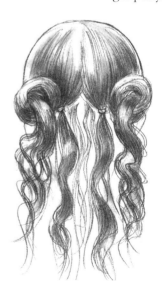

#6 Take the remaining loose hair that is hanging down and split it in half. Add each half to the half of the two remaining ponytails.

#4 Bring the knot up the section until it is close to the scalp. (How long the ends hang out depends on how

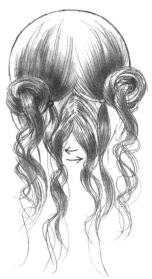

Headpieces suggested for this style:

A **wreath**

Flowers along the knots

Garden hat

Headband

Juliet cap

Pillbox hat

#7 Make two more knots to fill in the middle. Bobby pin to the scalp. To prevent the knots from slipping loose make sure you bobby pin the section that is coming out of the knot securely. Secure the edges of the knots with hairpins. Arrange the curls that are hanging and spray.

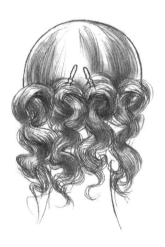

Daniele

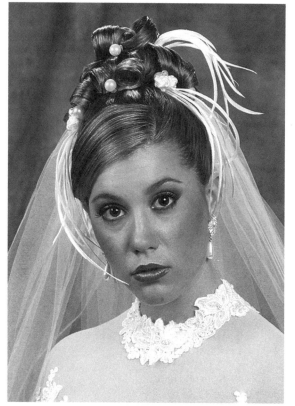
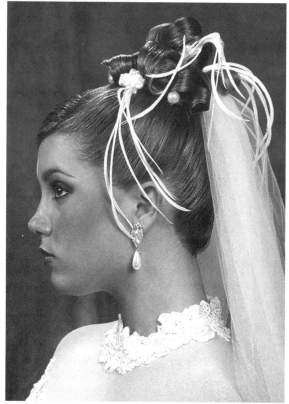

This model's hair length is just past her collarbone with long layers around the face.

#1 Section out the front two sides. This style can have a middle part or a side parting.

#2 Section the remaining top from ear to ear and put in a tight clean ponytail. Draw up all the back hair

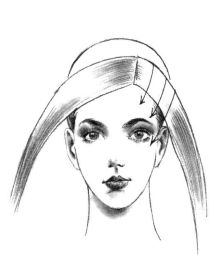
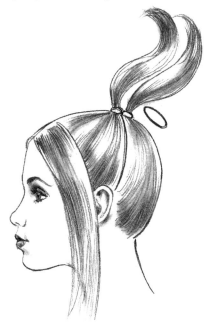

into another ponytail close to the first one. Use a third elastic to secure these two together.

#3 Holding the left side in your hand smooth upward. *Do not brush this hair against the head but in your hand.* When it is smooth lay it against the head and pin it up near the top elastic.

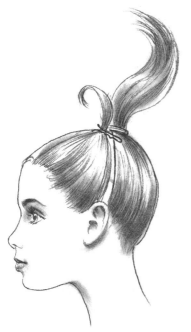

#4 Draw the right side across the forehead draping it along the side and pin near the top ponytail.

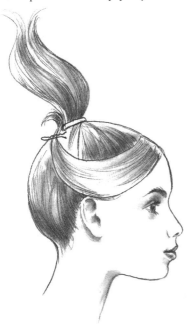

#5 Spray well all the loose hair in preparation to be curled. Use a very hot 3/4 curling iron and very neatly make small tight curls of all the hair. Use spray gel on each section to be curled. The curls should almost sizzle and be crispy when done. Pin the curls to the head at the base of the ponytail. Spritz when done. Attach the veil just under the curls in the back.

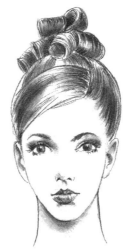

Ornamentation for this design:

You will need:

🪶 firm narrow feathers that come in a flat plastic package

🪶 hot glue gun

🪶 six round braided satin buttons

🪶 large pearls and crystals

🪶 a clear plastic comb and hairpins

Cut or break the clear plastic comb into one-prong pieces.

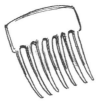 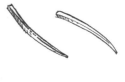

Pick out four or five feathers and hold them together at one end. Glue these ends at the top of the comb piece. Have the feathers follow the curve of the comb so when it is inserted into the hairstyle it will follow the curve of the head shape.

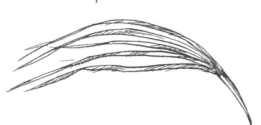

Glue two buttons over the ends of the feathers that are glued to the top of the comb.

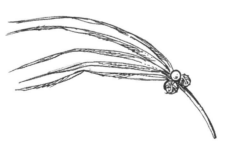

Glue a pearl or crystal between the buttons. This can also be done with all black accessories for bridesmaids.

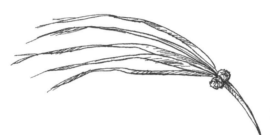

Glue large pearls or crystals onto hairpins to put into the hair.

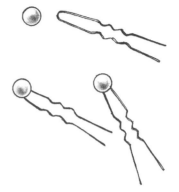

The veil can be purchased premade and hand sewn onto a French clip or comb. Or follow a veil pattern and make your own.

Headpieces suggested for this style:

Backpiece

Crown

Flowers

Half **headband** with wire

Profile

Tiara

Wreath

$\mathcal{J}ill$

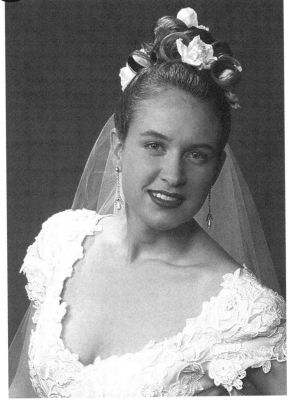

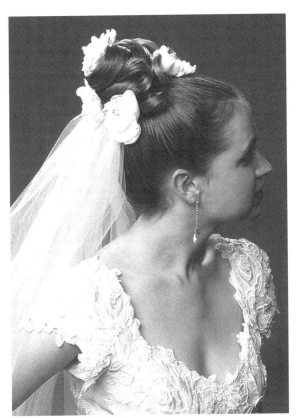

This hairstyle is done much the same as Dana's with different ornamentation and veil.

#1 Separate the hair ear to ear at the top of the crown. Make one ponytail on top. Then make a second ponytail just behind the first one. Use a third elastic to combine the two together. In this case the third elastic has a ponytail addition for added volume. It matches the model's hair perfectly or it can be slightly off for subtle contrast.

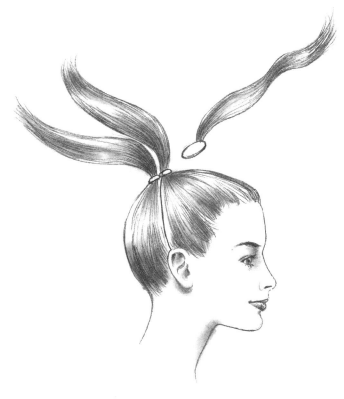

#2 Take a section of hair about 1 inch thick away from all the rest of the hair. Tease it and spray this piece well with a dry spray until it is thick and matted.

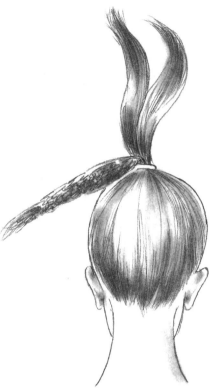

#3 Wrap this matted piece very tightly at the base of the ponytails. DO

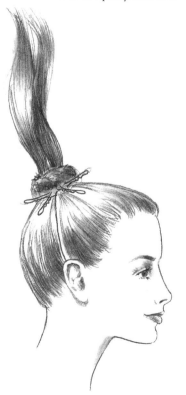

NOT wrap up the ponytail but make sure you wrap going around the lower base ending close to the scalp. The ponytail should not flop over but stand firm and away from the head. The matted piece provides a base where much of the pinning will take place. If your ponytail is flopping over use more hair, tease more, and wrap tighter.

#4 Set the ponytail on medium hot rollers. Setting should be neat, clean, and with tension. Spray gel each piece as you set it. There should be no flyaways. Spray again and let cool.

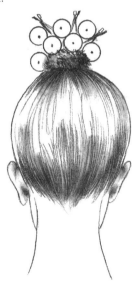

#5 When removing the rollers DO NOT brush or disturb the curls. To make the curls take a curl from the front and pinch it 1/3 of the way down the strand letting the end hang loose.

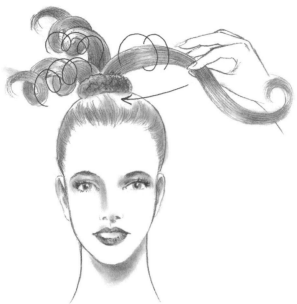

#6 Holding the strand, just bring it to the base of the ponytail and double pin it at the base in the matted part. Let the end hang free for now. Working the head from side to side pin all of the curls this way. Pin some on top of the elastics. Keep the curls clean and avoid brushing. Spray with a dry spray and smooth with your fingers.

#7 Attach the headpiece just under the hair in the back.

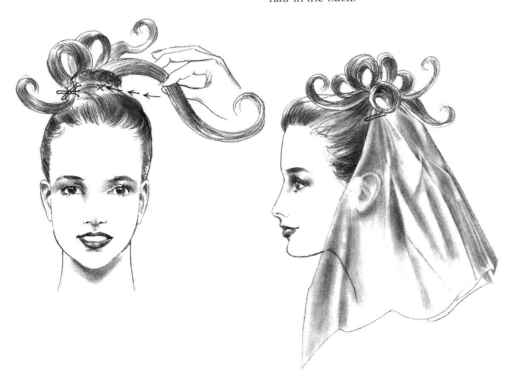

Turn the flower right side up. At the very center place a large drop of glue and attach one large pearl.

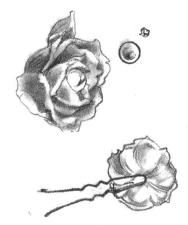

Now glue a small rhinestone on top of the pearl. Place three of these flowers across the back of the style so they look like they are attached to the veil. Use the rest in the updo. Bobby pin over the hairpins if necessary.

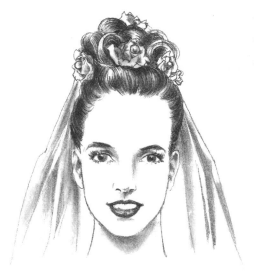

#8 Now working near the ends of the curls pin them into the style leaving some of the loose ends free. Adorn with silk flowers.

Ornamentation for this design:

You will need:

🌿 seven silk flowers

🌿 hot glue gun

🌿 hairpins

🌿 seven large pearls

🌿 seven rhinestones

Pull the stems off the flower. Turn the flower upside down. Put a bit of glue near the base and stick on a hairpin.

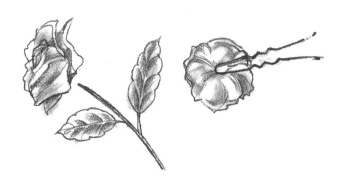

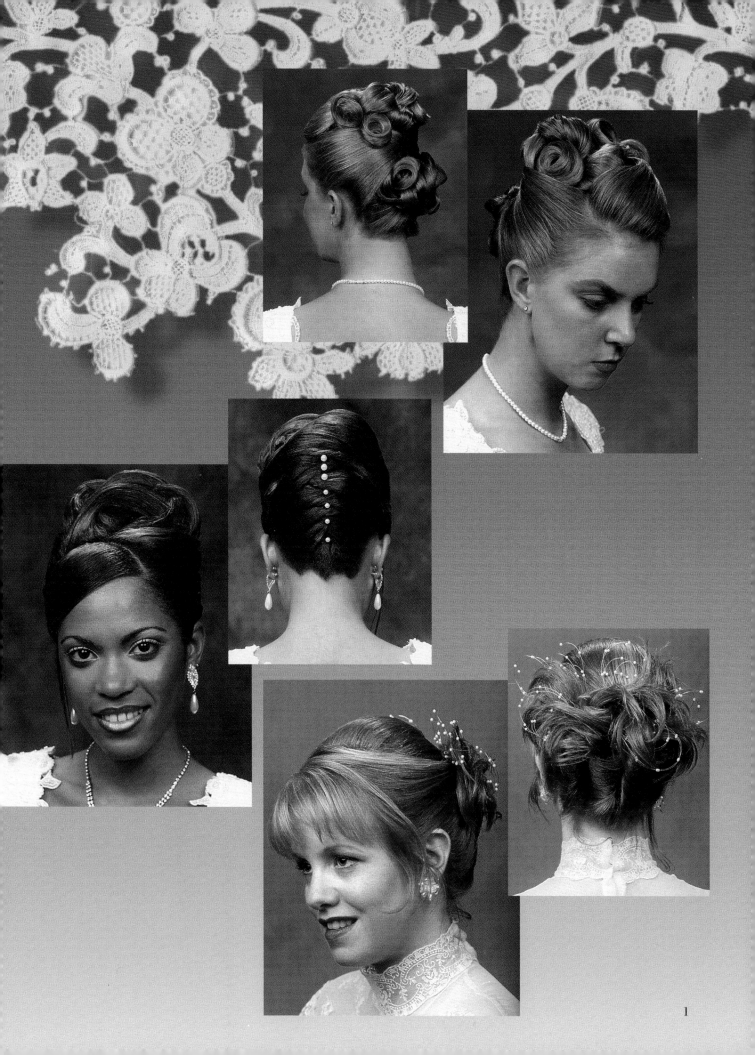

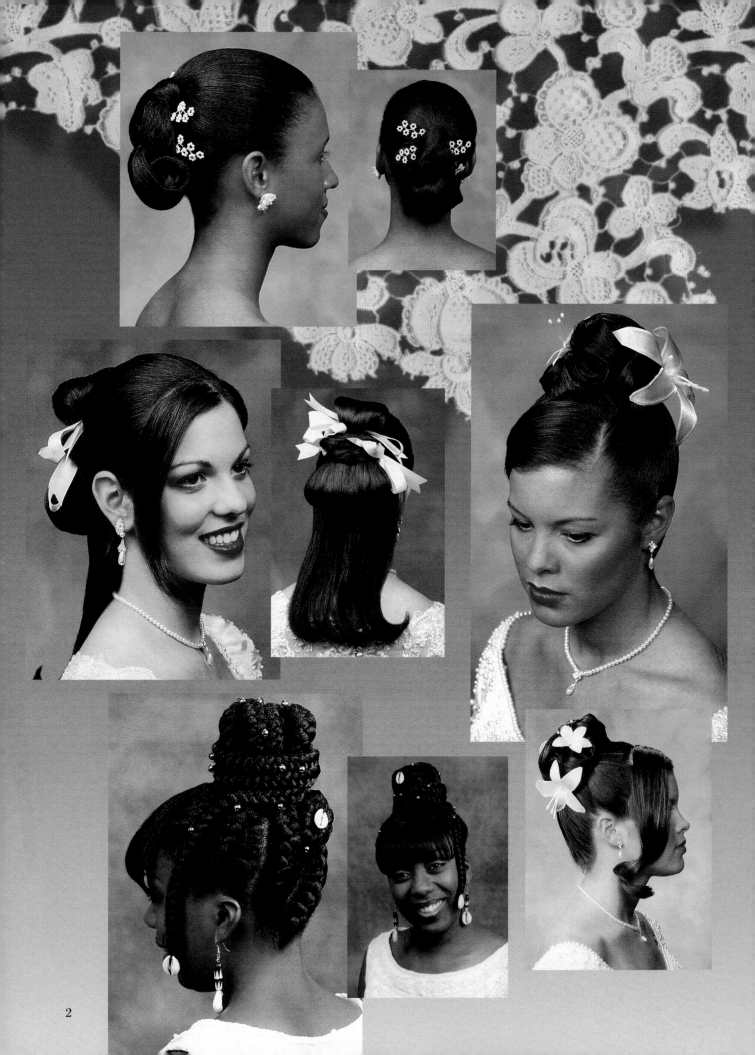

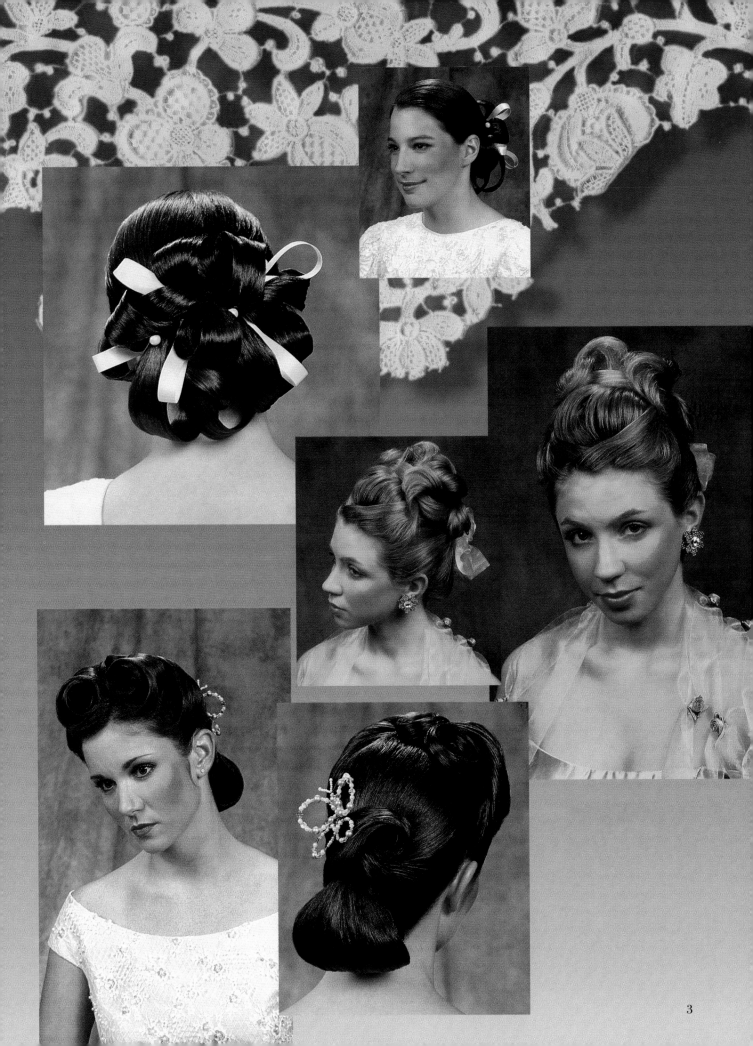

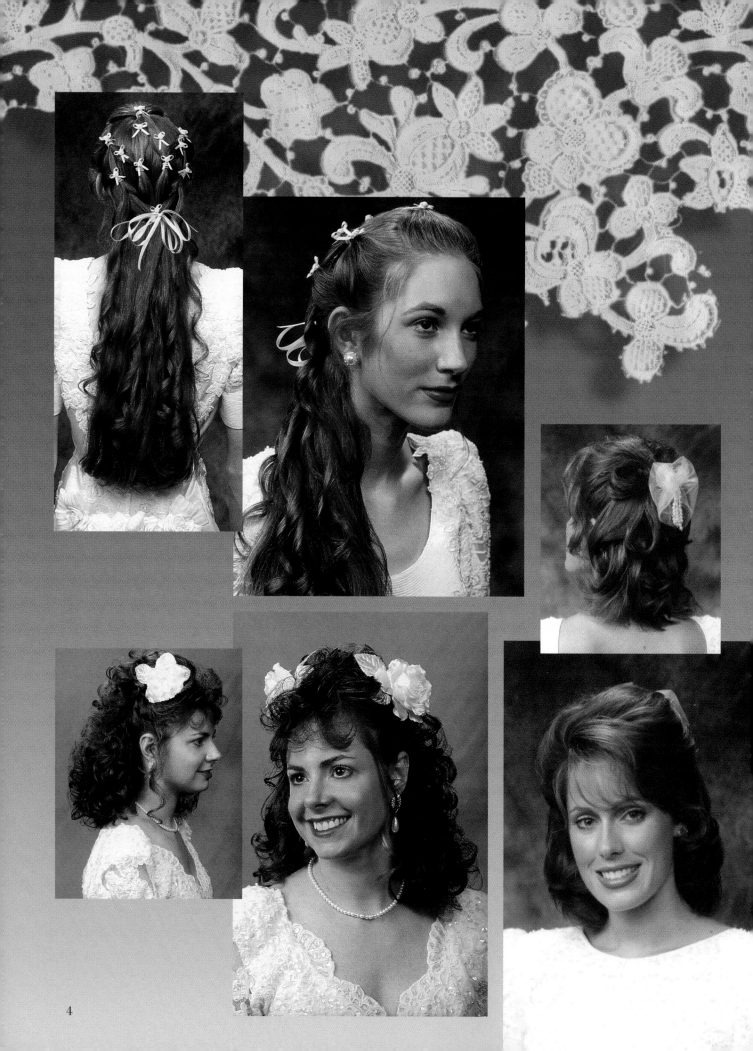

4

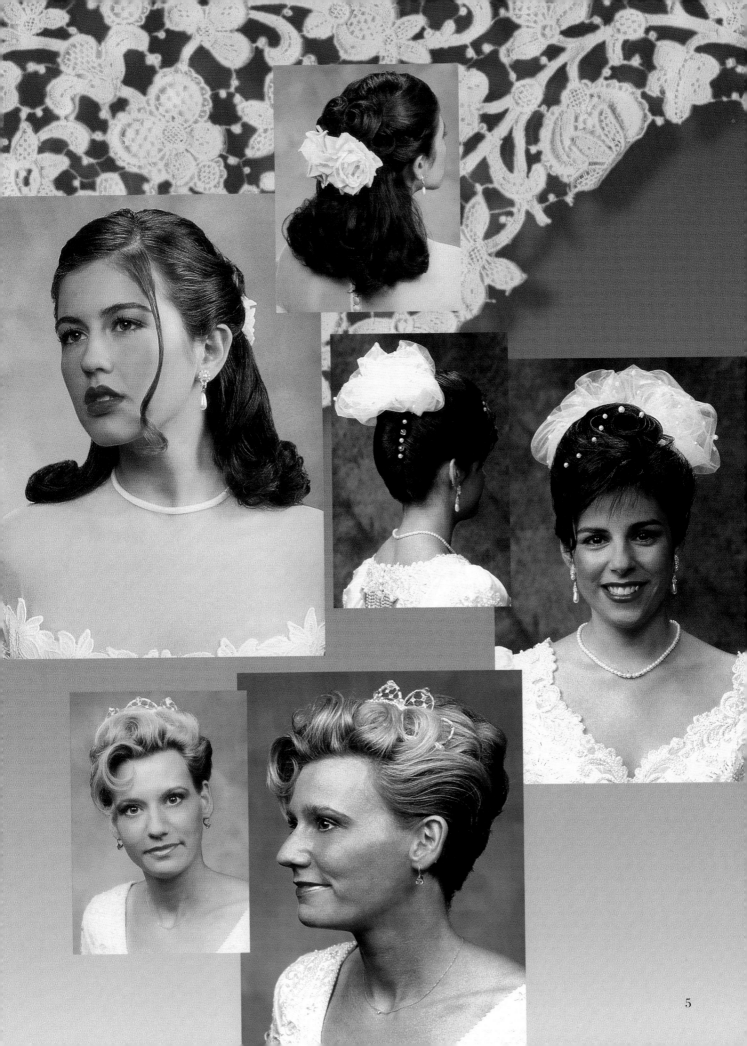

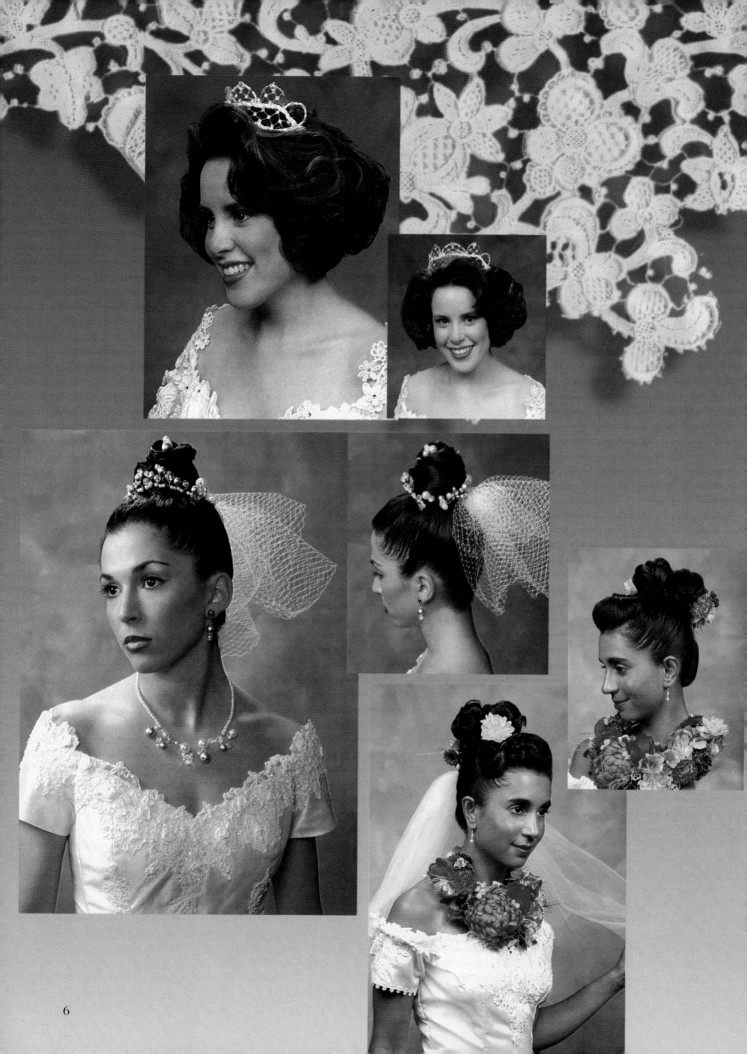

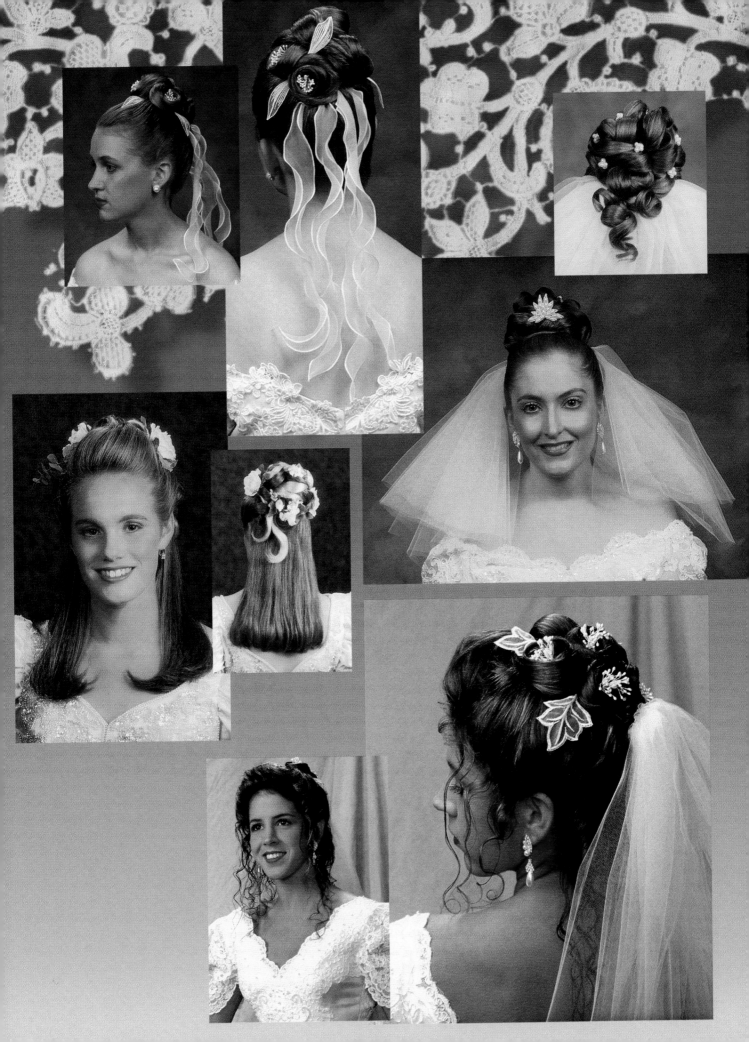

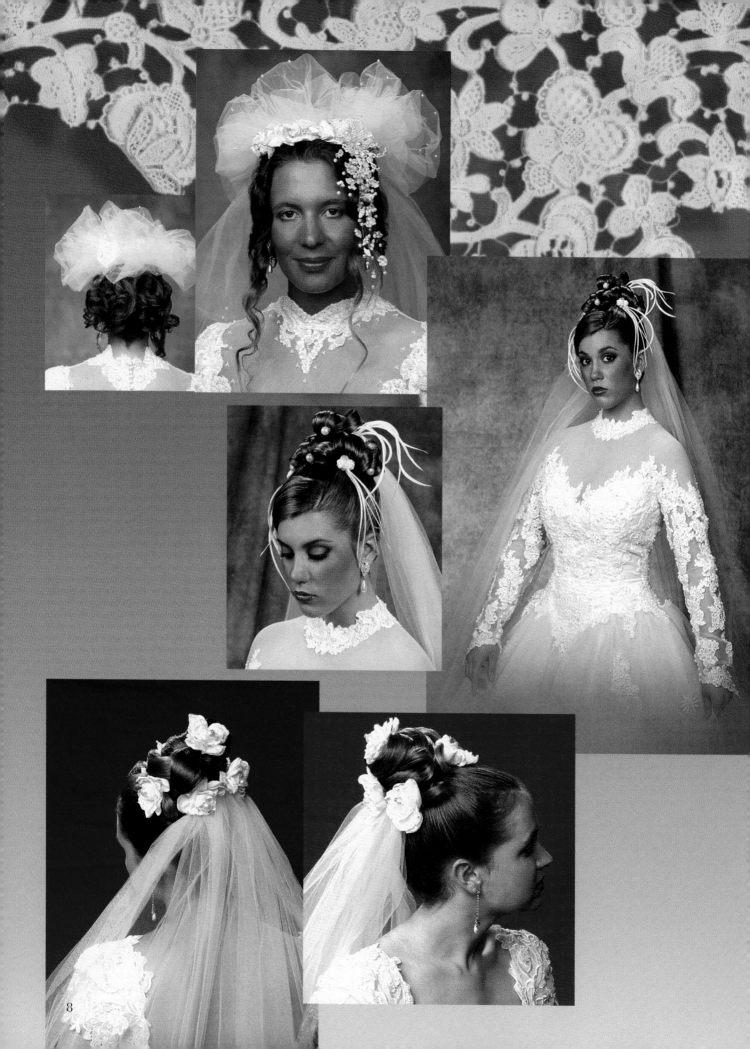

APPENDICES

These following 6 appendices contain reference material pertaining to the bridal industry. They will serve to educate you in some basic bridal terminology and styles. They will prove helpful during the consultation process as well as direct you in determining the best hairstyle for the bride's total bridal look.

APPENDIX A: Headpiece styles

APPENDIX B: Veils—their names, styles, and lengths

APPENDIX C: Fabrics and nettings—their names, descriptions, and textures

APPENDIX D: Bodice styles, waistlines, and gown designs, with names

APPENDIX E: Gown and train lengths

APPENDIX F: Sleeve styles and necklines

APPENDIX A:
HEADPIECE STYLES AND THEIR DESCRIPTIONS

As a bridal specialist it is important to know the variety of headpiece styles and their terminology to assist the bride in choosing a hairstyle.

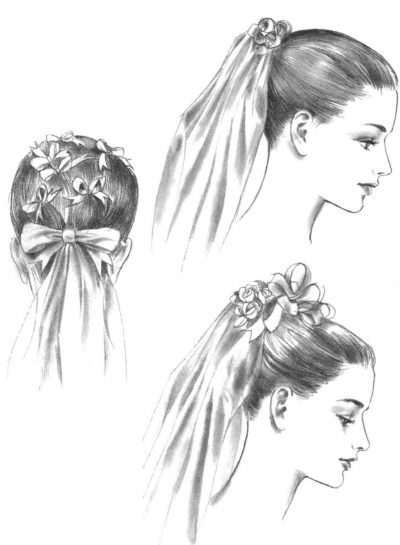

Crown. A small, round headpiece worn on top of the head. It is smaller than a wreath. Some brides think they should have their hair coming out of the center of it but it may be too small. If the bride is petite and has a small, compact updo she may be able to get away with it. It is best to wear a crown directly on top of the head. A bob hairstyle or a style that is tightly drawn to the nape of the neck is perfect. A crown can be made of jewels and wire, fabric and lace, or pearls and crystals. The veil can be attached or placed separately in the updo or not present at all.

Backpiece. This is a small collection of flowers or fabric or a bow that is attached to a French clip or comb. It is worn at the back of the head. It can be worn higher so it can be seen from the front or in the middle of the hairstyle or at the nape of the neck.

If there is a blusher attached to the veil make sure the placement of the back piece is not too low.

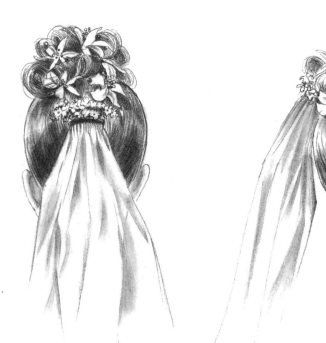

Decorated Updo. This is a hairdresser's dream style. If the bride wants a beautiful updo offer to decorate the hairstyle. You may use a variety of flowers, fresh or silk, pearls and crystals on hairpins, or ribbon on wire woven through the curls. Use the gown style, texture, and pattern for inspiration. The hair itself can even become the flowers. If the veil is long and heavy it can be attached to a French clip or on a comb and attached to the back of the updo.

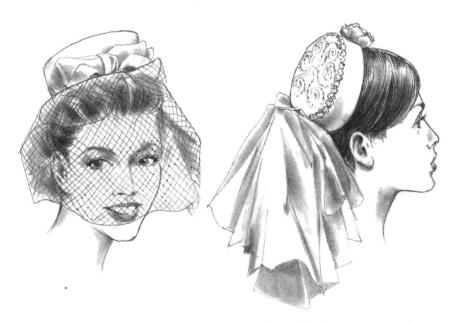

Hats. Hats can be any size, floppy or firm. They can be made of lace, fabric, or netting, and trimmed with beads, pearls, or flowers. Larger, looser hats should match looser gowns and be worn during the daytime or morning wedding. Smaller, firmer, compact hats like a pillbox can be worn any time of day and are better suited to a fitted bodice or suit. They can be placed

centered on the top of the head or
tilted. Place the hat where the bride is
comfortable with it before designing the
hairstyle. The veil can be attached to
the back of a hat that is worn centered.
If it is worn tilted, a Russian netting
covering the face in the front or no veil
at all is best.

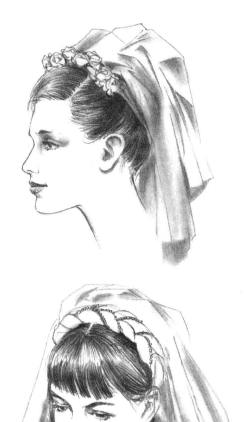

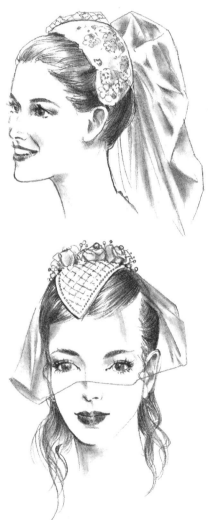

Juliet Cap. A small cap that usually
sits on the head over the parietal bone.
It may also be worn forward and tilted
with netting covering the face. This
style has to have a lower horizontal
updo or roll or chignon at the nape. A
short haircut or bob is also good for
this headpiece style.

Headband. Headbands can be a full
ear-to-ear headband or a half headband reaching temple to temple. If the
bride has long hair and she wants to
wear it down, a full headband is best
for keeping it off her face. If she has a
wide shorter bob I explain to her that a
full headband makes the hairstyle too
tight to the ears and that she may
consider a half headband style. The veil
is usually attached to the headband and
will cover the entire head. The hair may
be designed high to fluff up the veil.
The veil may also be detachable.

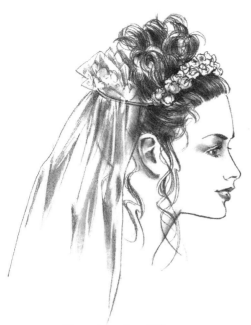

usually no veil attached. The profile can be made from clusters of pearls, flowers, sprays, crystals, and/or ribbons that is worn on one side of the head. It can be large and full, profiling the entire side of the head, or smaller in design. Usually a bob or layered style worn with the opposite side up is best for this headpiece. Larger profile styles can be balanced with an updo to one side.

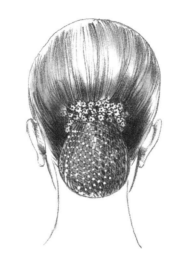

Headband with a Wire. This is a headband style but it has a wire that goes around the back of the head. This allows for a beautiful updo to be designed just behind the headband. Many also come with a pouf at the wire. The entire veil is attached to the wire and falls from the back of the head.

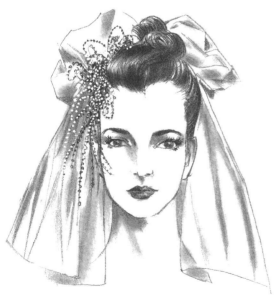

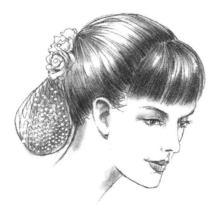

Snood. This is a small bag that is attached to a back piece. It can be made out of lace or Russian netting and holds a chignon in place at the nape of the neck.

Profile. This style is mostly seen with second-time brides because there is

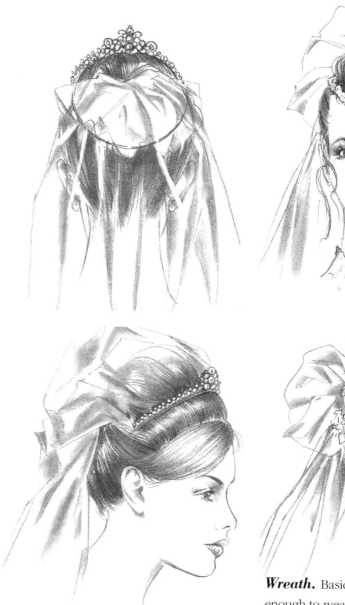

Tiara. This is a small half-circle crown worn on the top of the head. This style can be any variety of wire with pearls and crystals. Rhinestones, gems, and beaded flowers can also make up a tiara. A tiara can be separate or also have a wire attached that goes around the back of the head to hold the veil. They can be small and chic or large and ornate.

Wreath. Basically a wreath is large enough to wear a hairstyle coming up out of the center of it. It can be worn forward on top of the head or worn leaning back over the crown of the head. It can be very country looking, made out of small flowers, soft and wispy. It can also be made out of larger flowers, sprays of pearls, or heavily beaded. Porcelain flowers are also being seen on many designs. A wreath can also be worn down on the forehead coming to a point. Many wreath styles also have a pouf attached to the back with the veil coming down from under the pouf. Fresh flowers make lovely wreaths. Many flower girls wear wreaths.

APPENDIX B:
VEILS—THEIR NAMES, STYLES, AND LENGTHS

Some brides want layers and layers and length flowing behind them; some wear a veil no bigger than a handkerchief; others do not want any at all. Today it is popular to have a removable veil for the reception. If I am making a headpiece with a removable veil I use Velcro or, if it is long and heavy, it is best to use hooks and eyes. Judy Rockwell, who provided all the gowns for this book, also gave me the measurements of the various veil lengths.

Blusher. This is a one-layer piece of veil that is worn over the bride's face as she walks down the aisle. Traditionally it is lifted up by her father as he gives the bride to her husband-to-be.

Pouf. This is the piece that is full and gathered and attached to the back of the head. It can be attached to the headpiece or can be made separate from the veil.

Russian Netting. This is the large, woven netting seen slightly covering the face usually attached to a hat of some sort. It is also lovely by itself pinned into an updo.

Shoulder 18". Also called Flyaway. Just as fashion has no rules anymore, wedding wear is bending a few as well. This style is supposed to be worn with an informal dress but I have made some multiple-layered shoulder styles that have a very chic European feel. When worn with an off-the-shoulder gown it balances beautifully with a full tulle skirt.

Elbow 27". This length comes to rest at the elbows. It is less formal and draws attention to the area of the waist. It is usually seen with a backpiece headpiece, or pillbox hat.

Fingertip 36"– 42". This is a very popular length for most premade veils. The veil comes to the fingertips and usually has a blusher creating a second, shorter top layer. This veil can come decorated with pearls or ribbon along the edges.

Walking 58"– 62". This length falls near the ankles and may have a couple of layers. It can also be called Ballet or Waltz length.

Floor 68"–72". This length would need to be custom trimmed while on the bride. She would have to have her hair done just like it is to be on the wedding day and wear it to the fitting. It just should graze the floor.

Chapel 90". This length flows on the floor behind the bride but is designed to be worn at a chapel, which is a smaller, less-formal church with a shorter aisle. Of course, it can be worn at any size church today. Many brides also like to have a floor or Ballet length veil *over* the chapel length.

Cathedral 108". This veil is designed to be worn at a cathedral or a very large, formal church with a long aisle. This length is definitely for the princess bride.

APPENDIX C:
FABRICS AND NETTINGS – THEIR NAMES, DESCRIPTIONS, AND TEXTURES

Satin. A smooth, shiny, heavy, opaque fabric. It can be made out of silk, nylon, rayon, or the like. Silk is the most expensive and is called Silk Duchess Satin. Satin shows every ripple because its shine bounces light.

Taffeta. A fine, rather stiff fabric made out of silk, nylon, or acetate, with either a matte or satin finish.

Silk Shantung. One of the most popular fabrics, this is a lightweight silk taffeta that has an irregular soft lump in the yarn called a slub. This gives the gown some texture. It is also not pure white.

Silk Organza. A thin, stiff fabric that is transparent with a crystallike surface. May also be used as an underlining for sheer materials.

Silk Chiffon. This is a sheer, soft lightweight fabric.

Voile. A thin, sheer, lightweight cotton fabric.

Lamé. A metallic, lightweight fabric.

Jacquard. Usually used for a gown of period design. This fabric is lightweight with a satin background having a woven floral pattern.

Bengaline. This fabric gets its name from where it was imported, Bengal, near India and Bangladesh. This heavy, woven ribbed fabric is often embossed with a floral pattern.

English Net. This is a soft, flowing net made of cotton.

Tulle. Named for the city in France where it was first made, this is the most popular and inexpensive netting, usually made of nylon. Tulle made from rayon and silk is more expensive.

Stretch Illusion. This is a fine net made with Lycra.

Point d'Esprit. This is a diamond-pattern netting.

APPENDIX D:
BODICE STYLES, WAISTLINES, AND GOWN DESIGNS, WITH NAMES

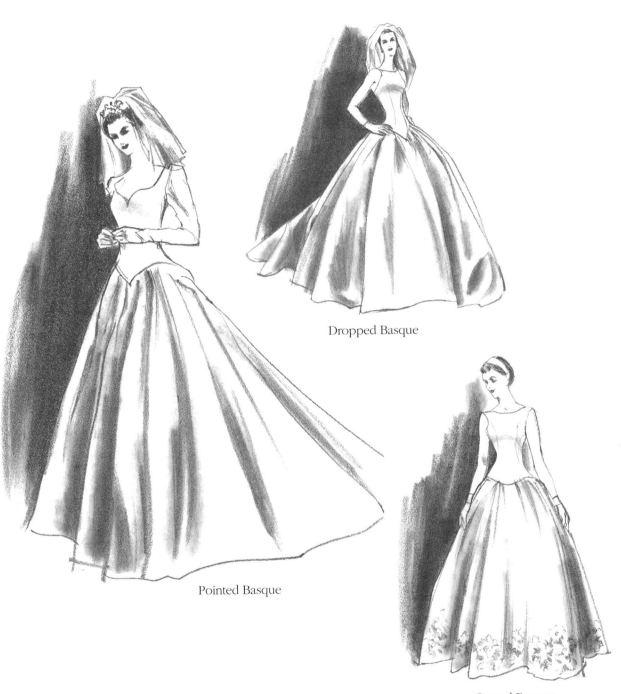

Dropped Basque

Pointed Basque

Curved Basque

Basque. A very popular waistline because it is flattering to most figures. It can be curved, come to a point, or dropped to the hips.

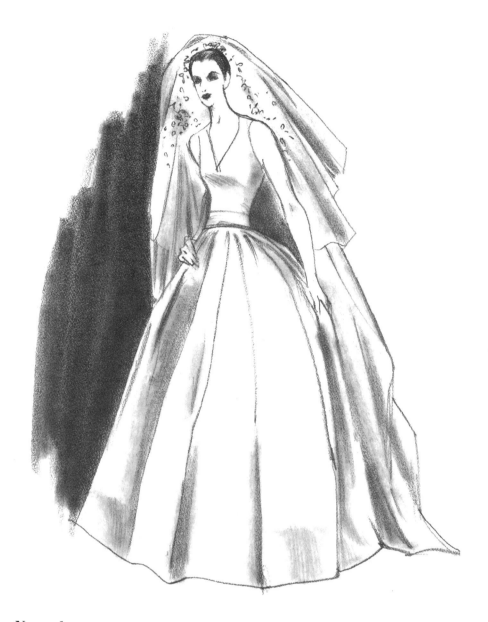

Natural. Perfect for someone with a tiny waist. The gown is gathered and flows from the natural waistline.

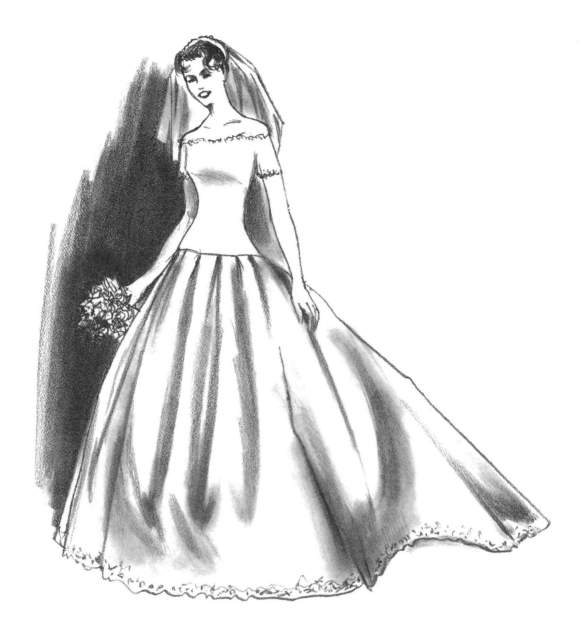

Dropped-waist. The skirt of the gown is gathered and flows out several inches below the natural waistline.

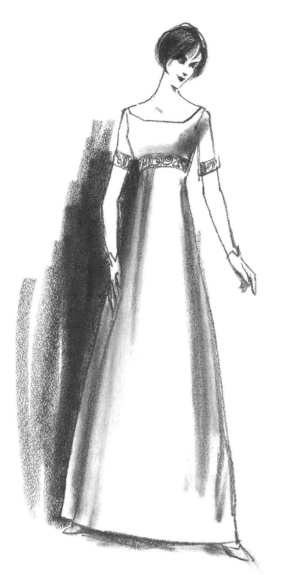

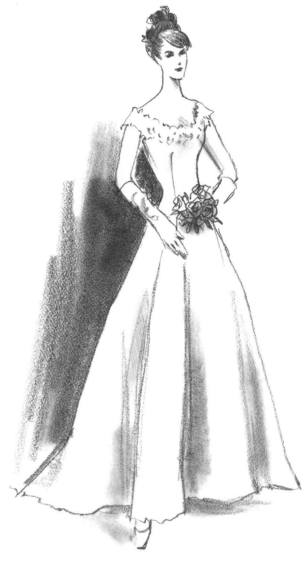

Empire. This is a period-style gown where the high waistline starts just below the bustline.

Princess. A very flattering gown design for everyone. Vertical seams fall from shoulder to hem with no specific waistline.

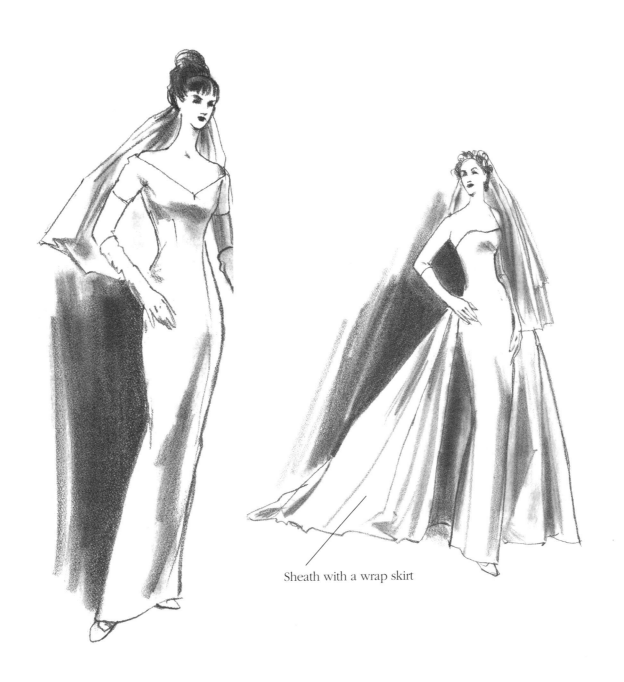

Sheath with a wrap skirt

Sheath. A very flattering slim waistline that is form-fitting to the floor. Many times this gown is accompanied with a wrap skirt.

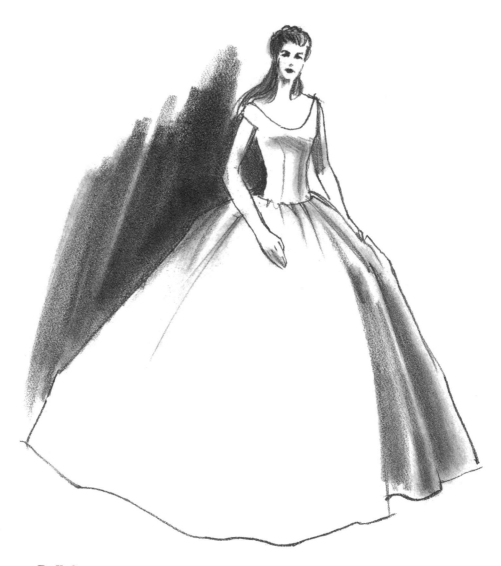

Ball Gown. A very full gown giving a horizontal line to the bride's total look. The skirt can fall from a Basque or natural waistline.

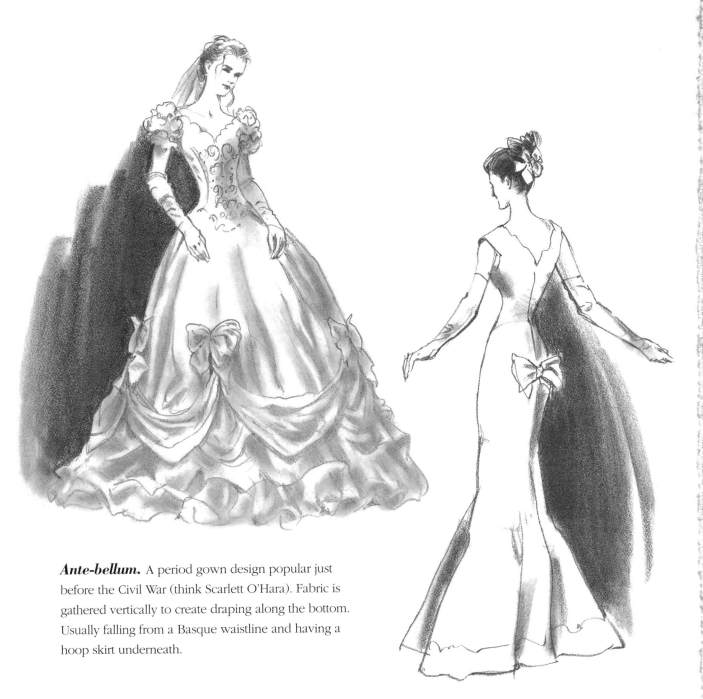

Ante-bellum. A period gown design popular just before the Civil War (think Scarlett O'Hara). Fabric is gathered vertically to create draping along the bottom. Usually falling from a Basque waistline and having a hoop skirt underneath.

Mermaid. Minus the fish scales, this *is* what the gown looks like. A perfect figure and an outgoing personality can carry off this dress style.

APPENDIX E:
GOWN AND TRAIN LENGTHS

Tea Length. 8 to 10 inches from the floor, this hemline is several inches above the ankles.

Ballet. 4 to 6 inches from the floor, this hemline falls to just above the ankles.

Sweep. 8 to 10 inches on the floor, this gown has a short train.

Chapel. This train extends approximately $1\frac{1}{2}$ yards from the waistline onto the floor.

Semi-cathedral. This train extends approximately 2 yards from the waistline onto the floor.

Cathedral. A very formal gown train that extends $2\frac{1}{2}$ or more yards from the waistline.

APPENDIX F:
SLEEVE STYLES AND NECKLINES

Sleeve styles and necklines play an important part in choosing which hairstyle will be given to the bride to best balance her total look.

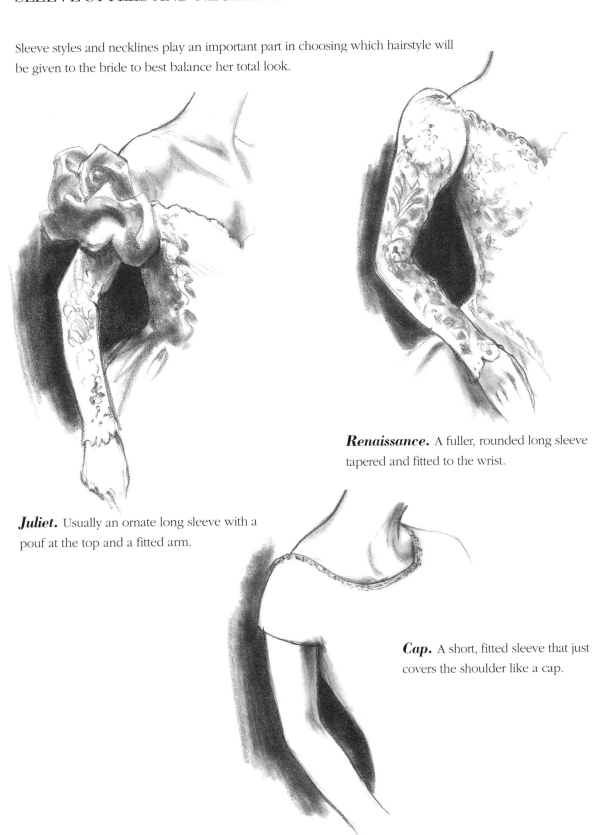

Renaissance. A fuller, rounded long sleeve tapered and fitted to the wrist.

Juliet. Usually an ornate long sleeve with a pouf at the top and a fitted arm.

Cap. A short, fitted sleeve that just covers the shoulder like a cap.

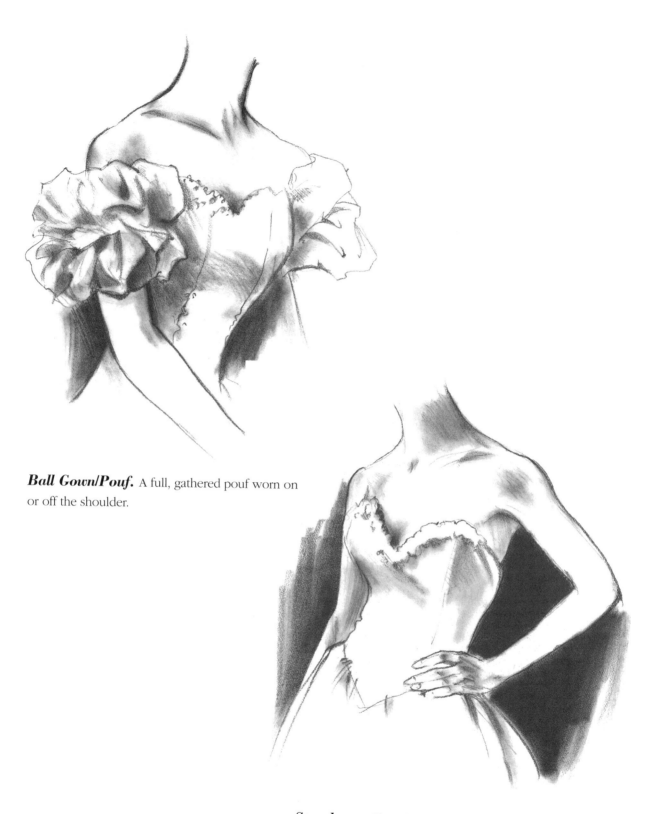

Ball Gown/Pouf. A full, gathered pouf worn on or off the shoulder.

Strapless. Self-explanatory. Many times this style is accompanied by a removable jacket that has a sleeve design that needs to be taken into consideration.

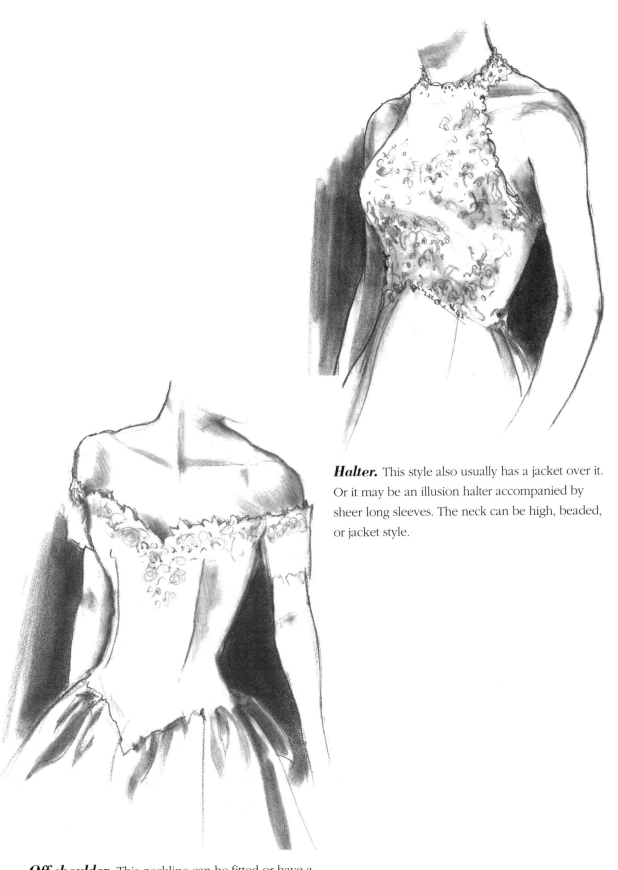

Halter. This style also usually has a jacket over it.
Or it may be an illusion halter accompanied by
sheer long sleeves. The neck can be high, beaded,
or jacket style.

Off-shoulder. This neckline can be fitted or have a
very wide, full pouf.

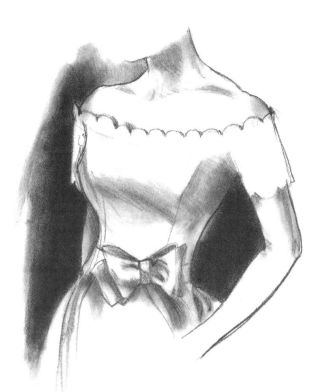

Hug-the-Shoulder. This gown is not quite off the shoulder but falls at the apex of the shoulder.

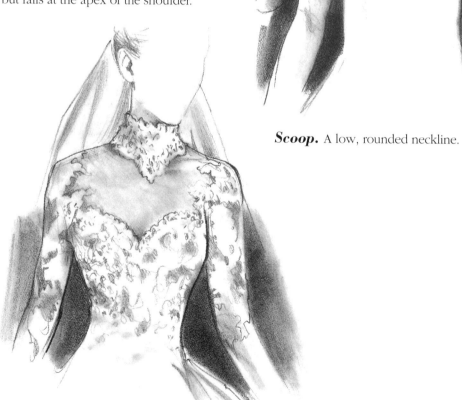

Scoop. A low, rounded neckline.

High Collar. This gown can have a variety of styles at the bustline, but it fits closely around the neck. This is best for a bride with a long, slim neck.

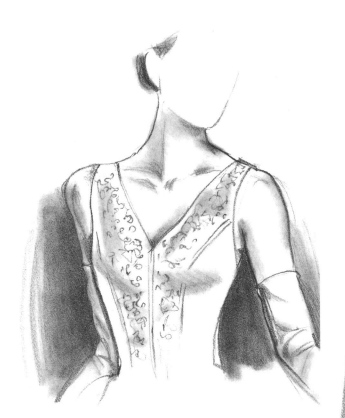

V-Neckline. When the bride says her gown has a V-neckline make sure to ask what the sleeve looks like.

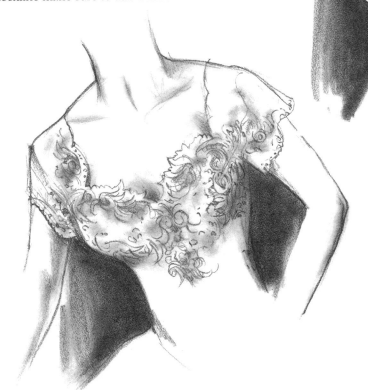

Sweetheart or Keyhole. This neckline resembles a heart shape that dips at the bustline. Some gowns also have this shape in the back as well. Keyhole resembles the outline of an old-fashioned keyhole at the neckline.

Sabrina. This neckline is straight across and usually scalloped or made of lace. It is slightly higher than the collarbone.

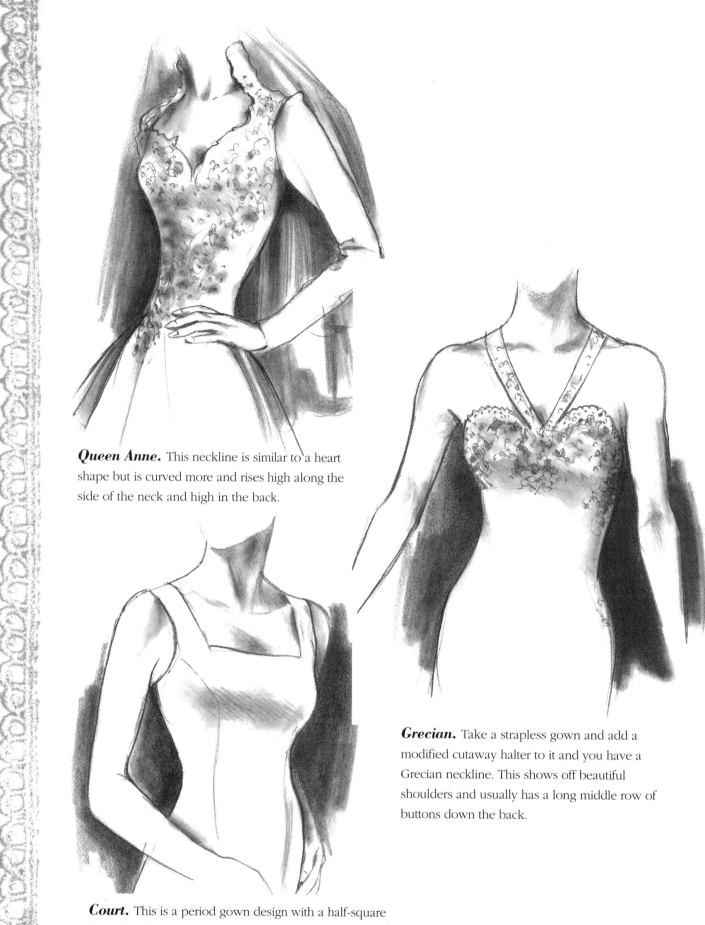

Queen Anne. This neckline is similar to a heart shape but is curved more and rises high along the side of the neck and high in the back.

Grecian. Take a strapless gown and add a modified cutaway halter to it and you have a Grecian neckline. This shows off beautiful shoulders and usually has a long middle row of buttons down the back.

Court. This is a period gown design with a half-square shaped neckline.

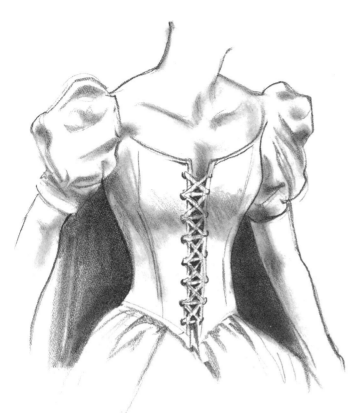

Bateau. This period neckline sometimes has a laced-up bodice. The neckline curves slightly downward below the collarbone and may have a full sleeve that can rest at or fall off the shoulder.

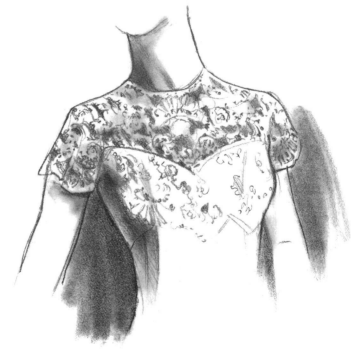

Jewel. A jewel neckline circles the base of the neck.

END NOTES

INTRODUCTION

1. *Modern Bride* Health and Beauty Survey 1996. Conducted by *Modern Bride* Research.

CHAPTER 1

1. *Webster's New World Dictionary,* 2nd ed., s.v. "Image."

2. Paul Hawken, *Growing a Business.* New York: Simon & Schuster, 1988.

3. Vincent Farricielli completed my questionnaire on bridal clients.

4. Paul Hawken, *Growing a Business.*

5. Ruth Roche, *SalonOvations Magazine,* September 1996, 35.

6. Alison Davis, "15 Ways to Get More Confident." *McCall's,* September 1996, 52.

7. Ginger Boyle, *SalonOvations Magazine,* September 1996, 36.

8. Brook Wainwright, "15 Ways to Get More Confident." *McCall's,* September 1996, 52.

9. Cynthia Hanson, "Professional Image Might Need a Boost," *Chicago Tribune,* 1995.

10. Ibid.

11. Gerrieann Murray, "Tricks of the Trade," *ABC Dialogue,* March/April 1995, 6.

12. Ruth Roche, *SalonOvations Magazine,* 36.

13. Ruth Roche, *SalonOvations Magazine,* 35.

14. Denise Pereau, *SalonOvations Magazine,* 35.

15. Career Track Seminars, Produced by Career Track, Inc. (Career Track Publications, Boulder CO). Seminar inquiries 1-800-334-6780.

16. Paul DiGrigoli interviewed with me by telephone.

17. Denise Pereau, *SalonOvations Magazine,* 35.

CHAPTER 2

1. Modern Bride Health and Beauty Survey 1996. Conducted by *Modern Bride* Research.

2. Ibid.

3. David A. Walker, Jr., "Seasonal Strategies," *American Salon,* March 1989, 107.

4. Reader to Reader, *NAILS* Magazine, May 1996, 338.

5. Ibid

6. Denise Pereau interviewed with me by telephone.

7. Victoria Wurdinger, "Professional Salon Management, Target Markets," *American Salon,* May 1989, 86.

8. Vincent Farricielli completed my questionnaire on bridal clients.

9. Joy Gray-Miott, "Personality," *ABC Dialogue,* March/April 1995, 5.

CHAPTER 3

1. *Webster's New World Dictionary,* 2nd ed., s.v. "System."

2. Rocco and Dianne Altobelli, "Super Heroes," *American Salon,* October 1996, 32.

3. DeniseLor Cerullo interviewed with me by telephone.

4. Maggie Mulhern, "Oh Happy Day! The Bride & Grooming," *Modern Salon,* September 1996, 82.

5. Lisé Pradon, "Tricks of the Trade," *ABC Dialogue,* March/April 1996, 6.

6. Pilo Arts salon brochure.

7. G. Gregory Geiger interviewed with me by telephone.

8. Ibid.

CHAPTER 4

1. Jim Smith, "10 Ways to Keep Clients Coming," *American Salon,* July 1992, 32.

2. Susie Fields, "Super Confidence and How to Get It," *SalonOvations Magazine,* September 1996.

3. Karen Sauer, "Letters," *ABC Dialogue,* January 1995, 17.

4. Henry Ford, *My Life and Work,* 1922, quoted in Paul Hawken, *Growing a Business,* Simon & Schuster, 1987.

5. Denies Pereau, "Women's Work," *SalonOvations Magazine,* September 1996, 35-36.

6. Dan Licitra, The Bridal Line Network, A Division of Innovative Telecommunications Services, Inc., *Ten Common Reasons for Insufficient Bridal Sales,* "Recommendations and Commentary on Successful Marketing and Selling in the Bridal Profession."

7. Noel Direnzo interviewed in person.

CHAPTER 5

1. Dwight Miller interviewed with me by telephone.

2. Tatiana of Boston quote taken from advertisement in *Bride's* magazine.

3. Mary Trasko. *Daring Dos: A History of Extraordinary Hair.* Flammarion, Paris–NY 1994.

CHAPTER 6

1. Dan Licitra, The Bridal Line Network, A Division of Innovative Telecommunications Services, Inc., *Ten Common Reasons for Insufficient Bridal Sales,* "Recommendations and Commentary on Successful Marketing and Selling in the Bridal Profession."

2. DeAnne Rosenberg interviewed with me by telephone.

3. Robbin McClain "Steps to Success," *American Salon,* April 1996 (interview of Arnold Zeqarelli).

4. Connie Glaser. *Swim with the Dolphins: How Women Can Succeed in Corporate American on Their Own Terms.*

5. Marcy Blum, ABC Newsletter, "Personality," July/August 1995, 5.

CHAPTER 7

1. Lori Neapolitan, educator for Your Name Cosmetics and consultant to salon makeup departments, interviewed with me by telephone.

2. "Counter Moves," *American Salon,* February 1996, 38.

3. *Modern Bride* Health & Beauty Survey 1996. Conducted by *Modern Bride* Research.

4. Ibid.

5. Ibid.

6. Ibid.

7. Dan Licitra, The Bridal Line Network, A Division of Innovative Telecommunications Services, Inc., *Ten Common Reasons for Insufficient Bridal Sales,* "Recommendations and Commentary on Successful Marketing and Selling in the Bridal Profession."

8. Susan Bergeron McKenna interviewed with me in person.

9. Kathleen T. Hayes, *Today's Black Bride,* Spring/Summer 1995, 15.

10. Laura Geller of Laura Geller Makeup Studios New York interviewed with me over the phone.

11. Kathleen T. Hayes, *Today's Black Bride,* Spring/Summer 1995, p. 15.

12. Susan Bergeron McKenna interviewed with me in person.

13. Victoria Wurdinger, "Target Markets," *American Salon,* May 1989, 87.

14. Louis Salvati, Artistic Director of Education for Graham Webb International, interviewed with me in person.

15. Laura Geller of Laura Geller Makeup Studios New York interviewed with me over the phone.

16. Victoria Wurdinger, "Target Markets," *American Salon,* May 1989, 87.

17. Dee Alicia, makeup artist with Noelle Spa for Beauty & Wellness, in Stamford, Connecticut, interviewed with me in person.

18. Susan Bergeron McKenna interviewed with me in person.

19. Dee Alicia.

20. Diane Young interviewed with me by telephone.

21. Susan Bergeron McKenna interviewed with me in person.

22. Laura Geller interviewed with me over the phone.

23. Dee Alicia.

24. Ibid.

CHAPTER 8

1. Terri Schmidt completed my questionnaire on bridal beauty.

2. Suzi Weiss-Fischmann, executive vice president of OPI Products, North Hollywood, CA, quoted from *American Salon* magazine, Cents and Sensibility (by Kelly Donahue), October 1996, 34.

3. Terri Schmidt.

4. Sue Trischitti interviewed with me in person.

5. Terri Schmidt.

6. Sue Trischitti.

7. Diane Young.

8. Gene Juarez Salon & Spa interviewed with me by phone.

9. Diane Young.

10. *Standard Textbook for Cosmetology,* Albany, NY: Milady Publishing, 1995.

11. Kristin Wall, spa director of the Adam Broderick Image Group in Ridgefield, CT, interviewed with me by telephone.

12. Diane Young.

13. Paula Fierson, a consultant for Noelle Spa for Beauty & Wellness, in Stamford, Connecticut, interviewed with me by telephone.

14. *Modern Bride* Health and Beauty Survey 1996. Conducted by *Modern Bride* Research.

15. Kristin Wall.

16. Diane Young.

17. Ibid.

CHAPTER 9

1. Paul DiGrigoli is the owner of Paul DiGrogoli's Advanced Training Center in Easthampton, Massachusetts, where I have been an updo educator since 1991. He has motivational and educational tapes and teaches haircutting as well.

2. Brooke Wainwright, "15 Ways to Get More Confident," *McCall's,* September, 1996, 51.

3. Victoria Wurdinger, "Fame: How Small Salons Get Big City Coverage," *Modern Salon,* August 1996, 68.

4. Sherry Chiger, "Write Makes Might," *American Salon,* December 1995, 32.

5. Kim Lord of Kim Lord Public Relations, New York City, interviewed with me by telephone.

6. Jayne Morehouse.

7. Information was taken from worksheets produced by Ginger Boyle, Elantis Productions Visual Marketing, 220 South Doheny Drive, Beverly Hills, CA, 90211.

8. John Hickox, as quoted in *Modern Salon* Magazine, August 1996, 72.

9. Andrew DiSimone, of Andrew DiSimone Studio located in IL Makiage, 107 E 60th Street, New York, NY, 10022. Andrew interviewed with me by telephone.

10. Ibid.

11. Paul DiGrigoli interviewed with me in person.

12. Ginger Boyle.

13. Heather Landaw, "Calling Card," *American Salon,* December 1995, 26.

14. Paul DiGrigoli.

ACKNOWLEDGMENTS

Thank you to my husband Fritz, my biggest fan! You have heard the computer keys going until all hours of the day and night without a complaint. Also a big thanks to my two precious future brides, my daughters.

To my parents, your sacrifice throughout the years for me is truly appreciated. I love you both very much.

Paul DiGrigoli, you believed in me from the beginning and have been a great coach, mentor and colleague. God placed you in my life to bring out the potential I had stored inside. Thanks, Paul!

Also thanks to my employers Noel Direnzo and Alan DiMonte who have given me the freedom to travel, teach and pursue my own personal career goals.

To all the salon professionals who contributed to this project, thank you for taking my calls and responding with great information. I am happy to be a part of such a great profession.

To the Association of Bridal Consultants and it's members, thank you for all of your helpful information.

A huge thank you to Judy Rockwell owner of the Bridal Loft in Hamden, CT. and Josie's Bridal in Westport, CT. You were so kind in letting me use your beautiful gowns so many times.

A special thank you to Steven M. Cooper of SM. Cooper Photography in Milford, CT. Your time, talent and patience with me and the models was greatly appreciated. We did it ! Great Job!

To Stephane Colbert of Stephane Colbert Photography, your artistic talent shines through in your work.

A special thanks to makeup artist, Susan Bergeron McKenna who worked with me for a year on many, many photo sessions and also to Dee Alicia.

Thank you to Susan Tricetti for your work on the nail model. You keep me laughing.

To Kathy Villafane, who worked on some of the models. Thank you for your time and talent.

To all my beautiful models. Thank you for your time and smiles and enthusiasm. You make this book a pleasure to look at.

To my brother, John Lott, your time and talent in helping with the photos saved the day! Many, Many thanks! We make a great team.

I also wish to thank those at Milady Publishing who have been supportive and consistently wonderful throughout this endeavor.

Lastly, I am prayerfully thankful to my Heavenly Father.